THE
CULTIVATION
OF WHITENESS

THE

CULTIVATION
OF WHITENESS

Science, Health, and
Racial Destiny in Australia

WARWICK ANDERSON

DUKE UNIVERSITY PRESS
DURHAM   2006

Warwick Anderson is Robert Turell Professor of Medical History, Population Health, and History of Science, University of Wisconsin, Madison. He is the author of *Colonial Pathologies* (Duke, 2006).

©2003 by Warwick Anderson

First North American paperback printing by Duke University Press, 2006

Printed in the United States on acid-free paper

Published by arrangement with Basic Books, a member of the Perseus Books Group.

Library of Congress Cataloging-in-Publication Data
Anderson, Warwick
The cultivation of whiteness : science, health, and racial destiny in Australia / Warwick Anderson.
p. ; cm.
Originally published: 1st ed. New York : Basic Books, ©2003.
Includes bibliographical references and index.
ISBN-13: 978-0-8223-3840-6 (pbk. : alk. paper)
ISBN-10: 0-8223-3840-8 (pbk. : alk. paper)
1. Social medicine—Australia—History. 2. Medical care—Australia—History.
3. Public health—Australia—History. 4. Race relations—Government policy—Australia—History. 5. Science—Australia—History. I. Title.
[DNLM: 1. European Continental Ancestry Group—history—Australia.
2. European Continental Ancestry Group—history—Great Britain. 3. Eugenics—history—Australia. 4. Eugenics—history—Great Britain. 5. History, 19th Century—Australia. 6. History, 19th Century—Great Britain. 7. History, 20th Century—Australia. 8. History, 20th Century—Great Britain. 9. Oceanic Ancestry Group—history—Australia. 10. Oceanic Ancestry Group—history—Great Britain.
11. Prejudice—Australia. 12. Prejudice—Great Britain. 13. Race Relations—history—Australia. 14. Race Relations—history—Great Britain. WZ 70 KA8 A552c
2003a]
RA418.3.A8A546 2006
362.10994—dc22   2006011040

Contents

Acknowledgments

I FIRST REALIZED THAT I needed to write this book when I was lecturing in Melbourne in 1997 and someone in the audience stood up and declared that I was a traitor to my race. The public lecture—on the general history of race science—was a response to the recent rise of racialist and ultra-nationalist groups in Australia. "Race traitor" is the sort of phrase one does not expect to hear any more: As a historian I imagined myself transported back to the 1930s. But unfortunately I hadn't actually been transported anywhere. So how could people still be talking about race in this way in the 1990s? What was the "race" I was betraying, and did it deserve my loyalty after all? What was the "whiteness" that still seemed so valuable to many? Evidently, it was time for me to think again, and more deeply, about the tough fabric woven from ideas of race and nation.

Back in 1987, when I was a medical doctor taking courses offered in the History and Philosophy of Science Department at the University of Melbourne, Rod Home had suggested to me that the development of tropical medicine in Australia might make a worthy essay topic. In later years my interests would drift away from the history (and practice) of medicine in Australia, toward the study of American colonial medicine in the Philippines and American public health more generally. But now I looked again at my Australian research notes and decided to make something more of them, this time focusing on race and medical science in the emerging nation. I am grateful to Rod Home, Richard Gillespie, and Jan Sapp for guiding my initial foray into the subject at Melbourne; and to colleagues in the History and Philosophy of Science Department who also supported my later efforts to write this book, in particular Janet McCalman, Ian Anderson, John Cash, Henry Krips, Monica Macallum, Rosemary Robins, and Geoff Sharp. Janet read the whole of the first draft, providing just the right mixture of skepticism and encouragement;

and Ian commented extensively on the last two chapters. Their engagement with the book has improved it immensely.

I became a historian of science and medicine through graduate study at the University of Pennsylvania, and my teachers there, especially Charles Rosenberg, Rosemary Stevens, Mark Adams, and Riki Kuklick, continue to influence my work. My first academic position, in the early 1990s, was in the History of Science Department at Harvard University, where Allan Brandt and Peter Galison were generating an innovative and exciting program in the history of science and medicine. My understanding of the entwined histories of race and science benefited from discussions with a floating intellectual community in Cambridge, Massachusetts, including Mary Steedly, Barbara Gutmann Rosenkrantz, Jim Moore, Lisbet Rausing, Arthur Kleinman, Evelynn Hammonds, Mike Fischer, and Mario Biagioli. Among the graduate students in History of Science, Conevery Bolton Valencius, Nick King, and Michelle Murphy were the most closely engaged with my research interests, and they kept me intellectually alert. Conevery's work on the medical geography of nineteenth-century Arkansas and Missouri made me rethink my own analysis of the material presented in Chapter 1.

In Melbourne I benefited enormously from the advice of Phillip Darby, Jane M. Jacobs, Marcia Langton, Patrick Wolfe, and others associated with the Institute of Postcolonial Studies. Participants in the history of medicine working group in the Johnstone-Need Medical History Unit at the University of Melbourne, urged on by Cecily Hunter, read and commented helpfully on the first two chapters. Ross Jones shared his unrivaled knowledge of eugenics and social policy in Victoria and stimulated me to reflect further on interwar biology in Melbourne. I spent many evenings chatting with Steve Alomes, a neighbor on Bellair Street, about racial thought in Australia. Jill Kleiner, Charlie Holmes, Ed Newbigin, and Rosemary Robins guided me through central Australia and shared their knowledge of the region. The last two chapters were revised at Krongart, near Penola, where I enjoyed the hospitality of Loane and Graham Skene. I am also grateful for the advice I received over many years from Alison Bashford, Alison Caddick, Michael Cathcart, Jim Gillespie, Lori Harloe, Geoff Kenny, Milton Lewis, Roy MacLeod, and Sioban Nelson, among others.

In San Francisco I have relied on new colleagues and friends to sustain me in the final stages of this project: In particular I would like to thank Philippe Bourgois, Adele Clarke, Lawrence Cohen, Tom Laqueur, Lisa O'Sullivan, James Vernon, and Ros Wyatt. James read the final version of the manuscript and provided timely reassurance. Thanks to Lara Freidenfelds we were able to discuss Chapter 4 at a lively meeting of the Bay Area "Medheads" group.

I am grateful to Jono Wearne, Chris Shepherd, Matthew Klugman, and Martin Gibbs for research assistance in Melbourne. Renae Stoneham and Asmira

Korajkic helped to make sure that administrative duties at the Centre for the Study of Health and Society did not fully take over my life. A small Australian Research Council grant supported part of this research, and grants from the Faculty of Arts of the University of Melbourne and from the Harry S. Symons Bequest aided publication. Ken Wissoker and Anitra Grisales at Duke University Press and Teresa Pitt at Melbourne University Press smoothed the paths to publication. I have revised the book for the American edition, explaining some arcane Australian references and changing the emphasis of the introduction and conclusion.

In conducting research for this book I have incurred a debt to countless librarians and archivists. I would like to thank the staff of the following institutions: the Baillieu Library and Special Collections, University of Melbourne; the State Library of Victoria; the Mitchell Library and Dixson Library, New South Wales; the National Library of Australia; the Australian Archives in Sydney and Canberra; the Barr-Smith Library, University of Adelaide; the Strehlow Research Centre, Alice Springs; the Rockefeller Archive Center, Tarrytown, New York; and the Peabody Museum Archives, Harvard University. Philip Jones at the South Australian Museum archives was especially helpful, as was Ann Brothers at the Medical History Museum, University of Melbourne.

A small part of Chapter 3 appeared in "Immunities of empire: Race, disease and the new tropical medicine," *Bulletin of the History of Medicine* 70 (1996): 94–118, and "Race, geography and nation: Remapping 'tropical' Australia," *Historical Records of Australian Science* 11 (1997): 457–68. Portions of Chapter 4 were first published in "'Where every prospect pleases and only man is vile': Laboratory medicine as colonial discourse," *Critical Inquiry* 18 (1992): 506–29, and "'The trespass speaks': white masculinity and colonial breakdown," *American Historical Review* 102 (1997): 1433–70. I thank the editors and reviewers of the journals for their suggestions. Thanks to Linda Nash, Chapter 4 was circulated at the colloquium on "Nature and its publics in the tropical world" at the University of Washington–Seattle. A shortened version of Chapter 8 was presented at the Institute of Postcolonial Studies, Melbourne, the History and Philosophy of Science Department, University of Melbourne, and the Science Studies Program at the University of California–San Diego; it also constituted the basis of the 2000 Culpeper Lecture at the University of California at San Francisco and Berkeley.

This book would not have been finished without the friendship and support of Susan Sawyer, Mark Veitch, and Fiona Wilson. And as always, my family has helped me in countless ways, direct and indirect. In particular I thank my parents, Hugh and Dawn Anderson, for reading the whole manuscript and providing me with encouragement and guidance, drawing on a half-century of their own research in Australian history. I dedicate this book to them.

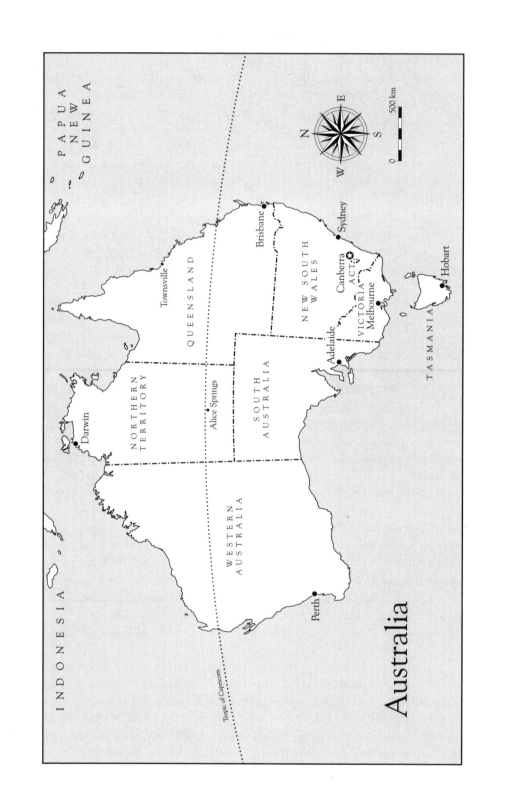

INTRODUCTION

THIS IS A BOOK ABOUT medical and scientific visions of what it meant to be white in Australia during the nineteenth and early twentieth centuries, when the colonial settler society came to refashion itself as a nation.[1] It is a history of medical ideas and practices during that period—all of it filtered through the lens of "whiteness." For hundreds of years now, doctors and scientists have sought to chart the destiny of their bodies and to understand the environment in which they found themselves, but these efforts are rarely subject to historical scrutiny. In this book, I would like first to recapture the sense of estrangement experienced in the nineteenth century by many European newcomers to Australia, and then to explain how biomedical science and public health made their discomforted "whiteness" seem normal—necessary even—in their new world. How did science and medicine more generally give expression to concerns about racial displacement and territorial possession? In explaining health and disease in a new land, how did doctors frame ideas of race and country? Science and medicine are often left out of conventional histories of Australia—or of any other country for that matter. Here I would like to show how they once helped to set a nation's racial agenda.

Perhaps this will seem an unusual perspective in which to view medicine and public health. After all, the history of medicine has largely been a history of institution-building, great doctors, and scientific and technical progress. More recently, we have learned about the historical framing of disease and the experience of illness.[2] What I plan to do is find out what medical science and public health had to say about identity, environment, and nation. I will seek to recover the civic vision of medicine, to trace its pervasive, yet sometimes occult, contributions to the understanding of race and climate, degeneration and progress, nature and nurture, gender and industry, in an emerging nation.[3] Science and medicine produced a civic subjectivity as surely as did literature, art, film, and other cultural enterprises. Doctors were doing more than dealing

1

with disease: They were allowing people to think of their bodies and their surroundings in different ways; they helped citizens imagine a future for their
families and country; and they changed individual behavior, giving new meaning to mundane interactions with others and the environment. Therefore, I
am suggesting that the clinic and the laboratory should be added to those sites
where the nation—any nation—may be imagined.[4]

Until the middle of the twentieth century, medical scientists and public
health officials in Australia regarded the white body as their principal research
interest. They were fascinated by whiteness; the term itself crops up everywhere in biomedical science and public health. But this scientific touchstone
generally stood for more than mere color or hue—indeed, sometimes it seems
to have stood for any corporeal feature *except* color. The "white race" and the
"white organism" were figures of speech that implied a wide range of physical
and cultural signs of European difference. During much of the nineteenth
century, being "white" in the Australian colonies usually meant claiming
British ancestry; in fin-de-siècle Australia, whiteness was re-created as a national type on the tropical frontier; later, it sometimes became diffused into
the general, and more obscure, category of Caucasian, or else it was narrowed
down to subtypes such as Nordic.[5] Until the 1880s, then, being British implied a lineage; after that, whiteness became a type, mobile and standardized;
later still, in the 1930s, whiteness dissolved into variations across a population.
Whiteness might suggest a typical bodily constitution or temperament; a cultural legacy and thought style; a virility or femininity; a head circumference
and brain capacity; a predisposition or resistance to certain diseases; a blood
group; a lamentable inability to sweat off tropical moisture—and so on.
Whites were alternately vulnerable to changed circumstances or impervious to
setting; the racial type was either degenerating or it was triumphant in the antipodean environment. Color was the least of this racial calculus: Most experts
thought skin tone was far too dependent on circumstance to gauge accurately
the deeper meaning of whiteness or to provide a reliable index of its fate.
Whiteness was merely a signpost pointing to a true racial type—the essence of
whiteness—which continued to resist efforts to decipher it. Even so, investigators were reluctant to abandon the search: Indeed, the illegibility of the racial
Ur-script seemed to enhance its value. The scientific definition of whiteness remained as tantalizing as it was evanescent. Until the 1930s, few biomedical
scientists in Australia, or elsewhere, doubted that they would eventually resolve manifold human difference into a few physical and mental types, called
races, one of them white.[6] But none of them ever managed to do so to anyone
else's satisfaction—not for long, at least.

In biomedical science and public health, "white" remained a vulgar and imprecise term—but still a useful one. It provided a simple, if somewhat ambigu-

ous, label for a stubbornly variegated collection of human physiological and pathological features; and it served as an entry point into the major political debates of the day. For most doctors, biologists, and anthropologists, whiteness was not an empty category, defined only in opposition to other races; rather, it was filled with flexible physical, cultural, and political significance. But we have become so accustomed to this assemblage of whiteness—the repertoire has become so commonplace—that we may fail to recognize the work it took to put it together, to make it look normal. What would it take to repopulate the history of settler societies such as Australia with specifically white bodies, to make these bodies visible again, and ultimately to make them as strange as any other body?

I believe that this calls for an unusual history of racial thought. I do not want to provide another analysis of the development, largely in Europe and North America, of flawed yet occasionally sophisticated scientific and social theories of human difference.[7] Rather, I have chosen to study the midlevel, mundane theorizing that commonly occurs when one does science or practices medicine in a society a long way from Europe. Sometimes local scientists and doctors do refer to allegedly "key" figures and concepts in racial thought; mostly they do not. Accordingly, I have tried not to use terms like "monogenism," "polygenism," "social Darwinism," or "eugenics," unless they were used at the time—and mostly they were not. I spent some time trying to separate monogenists, who argued for the single origin of humanity, from polygenists, who postulated many origins, and got nowhere.[8] Neither have I ever been able to get a fix on the colonial forms of social Darwinism. It seems to me that in the Australian context these may be malapropisms that distract us from working out how racial theory—with whiteness as its central figure—was produced and transacted among colonial scientists and ordinary doctors. In my experience, terms of this sort are at best blunt tools that tend to mutilate the racial thought of out-of-the-way intellectuals. But others are perhaps more skilled in their use.

A community expects those who explain and treat its illnesses to be able to account more generally for perceived differences in physical and mental status, to assign responsibility and blame, and to describe continuities of biological type and potential for change. In a colonial (and protonational) society, where so much is still uncertain, the constructive function of medicine is further magnified. To interpret their new world—and to change it—colonial scientists and doctors drew, in part, on contemporary theories of race and environment, as well as on local scientific training, clinical observation, political interests, and their own experiences of well-being and peril. Their understanding of human difference was thus a situated knowledge (the point may seem obvious, but it is frequently forgotten).[9] Therefore, I have tried to convey the complexity and idiosyncrasy of the various local biomedical worldviews, without endorsing them or sneering at them, and to locate those scientists and doctors who sought to explain human and environmental difference in their own communities, institutions, and career structures. What did it mean to investigate and write about race in the disparate academic and medical cultures of Melbourne, Sydney, Townsville, and, later, Adelaide? How was it possible to have a career as an expert on whiteness in the emerging institutions of medicine and science in Australia? Why did notions of whiteness circulate so easily in these local contexts? The scale of intellectual life in Australia in the nineteenth and early twentieth centuries provides us with a rare opportunity to reveal the social patterning of ordinary racial thought and to illustrate more generally how local circumstances can prompt and shape intellectual work.

It is important to realize that medicine, until the early twentieth century, was as much a discourse of settlement as it was a means of knowing and mastering disease. In seeking to promote health, doctors drew on a fundamentally moral understanding of how to inhabit a place with propriety.[10] They advised their communities on how to avoid sources of pathology; they offered guides to hygienic behavior and civilized conduct. Race and environment jostled together in this civic vision. In Australia, most doctors assumed that only whites would ever reach the necessary standard of hygiene and decorum; some of them wondered if there were places—the tropics, for example—that were inimical to a cleanly, self-possessed, white civilization, places that could never be successfully colonized and remain purely white. How might one live in such places in order to remain white? How could whites avoid pigmentation and degeneration? How must citizens behave in Australia if it was to become truly white, even in the tropical north? Medical science and public health came to provide a rich vocabulary for social citizenship in an anxious nation. Scientists and doctors counseled politicians and the public on how to implant and cultivate a working white race across the continent, giving forceful expression to concerns about heredity, masculinity, and industry even while they promised to dissolve the doubts that their theories were crystallizing. Intellectuals sought to unsettle whiteness and then offered to resettle it; they constructed shaky identities that only they might eventually make secure. Medical science was a means of mobilizing people across the globe, of bounding a territory, and of filling it in. How, and where, should valuable—and vulnerable—whites live in a new country? Ask the doctor. Ask the scientist.

The history of the medical construction of white Australia necessarily draws as much from histories of immigration, population policy, eugenics, geography, and physical anthropology as it does from standard histories of science and medicine. It thus allows us to connect histories that previously have appeared surprisingly separate. Why, for example, is the history of ideas about nature so rarely combined with the history of racial thought given that for most nineteenth-century intellectuals race and circumstance, blood and soil, were so frequently compounded? How is it that the development of the white Australia policy, intimately connected with labor history, is rarely associated with the history of the scientists who sought to justify it? What makes a critique of eugenics in Australia so difficult to synchronize with the history of Aboriginal anthropology? Historians generally have focused separately on the presumed antitheses of whiteness—antipodean environment, alien races, Aboriginal Australians—not on the sovereign, yet often invisible, category whose boundary these contrapositions mark in such an excitingly assailable manner. But the medical construction of white Australia provides another lens through which we may view two hundred years of European settlement, a more encompassing way of studying explanations of what this strange project in human displacement might mean, how it might possibly make sense.

In the first part of the book, I describe fears of white degeneration in the antipodes, whether from an exhausting, depleting environment, from contact with other races, or from urban life. Chapter 1 attempts to rediscover the geographical viewpoint of nineteenth-century colonial medical practice, to find again that potentially tragic vision, a vision now lost to us. In Chapter 2, I trace the importation and inflecting of germ theories in Melbourne in the 1880s, describing the gradual exoneration of the southern environment, as well as the increasing apprehension about the social, and in particular the urban, causes of disease. With the emergence of germ theories, a shared repertoire of belief about health and disease begins to segment into lay and expert spheres, and the emphasis here is increasingly on medical debates rather than on ordinary experience. After this, the scene shifts to the north, with Chapter 3 examining white anxieties about the Australian tropics, the last bastion of geographical pathology and an alleged impediment to the whitening of the whole continent. In Chapter 4, I relate how medical scientists in Townsville conducted research to prove that the white Australia policy—a tenet upon which the nation was founded—not only would prove feasible in the northern tropics but also was in fact a medical necessity, especially in the tropics. Chapter 5 explores the efforts of national hygienists in the 1920s to register and regulate tropical white bodies, even as the category of whiteness was disaggregated by some scientists into subtypes and broadened by others into Caucasian. In Chapter 6, I follow medical scientists as they slowly head south again in the 1930s to study the degeneracy of the urban white child, by then the principal threat to white Australia, and I describe the complex mixture of hereditarian and environmentalist policies designed to resolve this national predicament. Although some geographers in the 1930s continued to challenge claims of white triumph in the tropics, and some tried to set environmental limits on European settlement, only a few aging tropical scientists and bureaucrats were left defending the project; most researchers had moved on. My general argument to this point is that virile, energetic whiteness was defined in nineteenth-century Australia largely in relation to an exhausting, weird environment, later in terms of urban social pathologies, and then, in the early twentieth century, it was more often figured in opposition to supposedly disease-dealing non-white races. By the 1930s a medically informed binational self-assertion allegedly had circumvented or dissolved these, and other, inflated threats, thereby producing a normative white citizenry that worked even in the tropical north.

And yet just as the white race was represented as achieving a triumphant form in Australia—as having become imperviously self-possessed, virile and denatured—its character and claims were being hollowed out from within. Aboriginality has always occupied a surprisingly ambiguous and unsettling position in relation to the figure of whiteness. Medical scientists had etched more deeply the demarcation between whites and the land, and between whites and other races, but recognition of persistent Aboriginality, especially in the 1920s and 1930s, caused them instead to attempt to reframe the boundaries of whiteness, incorporating Aboriginal Australians into the category as distant relatives and object lessons. Aboriginal Australians were scientifically reconfigured as archaic, or simply dark, Caucasians.[11] Medical scientists and physical anthropologists were thus able to discern a number of alternative indigenous Caucasian destinies, each of which retraced the imagined features of their own white development. Chapter 7 discusses the scientific significance of these Caucasian theories, the fascination with notions of Aboriginal purity or heterogeneity, and the consequent physiological and hematological investigation of the people of the central deserts in the 1930s. For some scientists, especially those in Adelaide, the entry of the "full-blood" into the biomedical present allowed them to express their own ambivalent estimate of white modernity. Other scientists, again mostly from Adelaide, chose to focus on the destiny of the "half-caste" and to urge the absorption of hybrid Aboriginals into whiteness as probationary or second-class citizens, a group that might constitute a proletariat particularly well adapted to work in central and northern Australia. But even as medically supervised assimilation commenced, the proliferation of hybridities among the previously unitary white Caucasians and the previously homogeneous dark Caucasians, and between these racial subgroups, began to destabilize the whole edifice of racial classification. As I argue in Chapter 8, the final chapter, race science in Australia was undermined in the 1940s as much by its own proliferating contradictions and sophistry as by celebrated British and North American critiques of the concept of race.

The popular appeal of the concept of race has apparently withstood its postwar decline in scientific validity. If only the scientists who had put so much effort into constructing, and popularizing, racial classification had taken more time to dismantle the conceptual framework—but they had mostly shifted their attention to other problems. In any case, it is evident that facile, ever-flexible typologies of human difference still help to organize and channel public self-satisfaction and prejudice.[12] Perhaps this account of how such simplistic categories were invented by earlier generations of doctors and scientists will make some contribution to their eventual dissolution.

PART ONE

THE TEMPERATE SOUTH

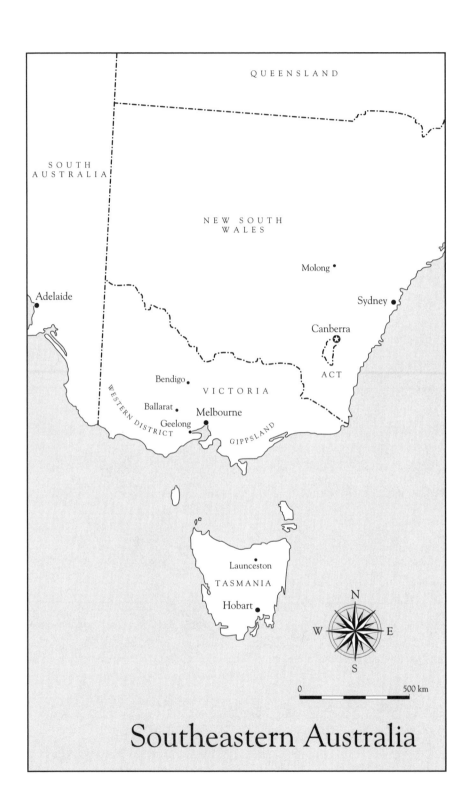

QUEENSLAND

SOUTH
AUSTRALIA

NEW SOUTH
WALES

Molong •

Adelaide •

Sydney •

Canberra ✪

ACT

Bendigo •

VICTORIA

Ballarat •

Melbourne •

Geelong •

GIPPSLAND

WESTERN DISTRICT

Launceston •

TASMANIA

Hobart •

N

W   E

S

0   500 km

Southeastern Australia

CHAPTER 1

ANTIPODEAN BRITONS

THE EARLY AUSTRALIAN COLONISTS found themselves drawn deep into the cross-currents of their new environment. They felt their bodies move along with the strange elasticity of the air; their spirits shifted with the direction of the winds; at certain times of day the clear light irritated their eyes; thought, muscle power, vital energy—all could become unreliable and fickle in circumstances so unlike those of home. Many immigrant Europeans seemed out of balance with the new climate, while some of those whites born locally, developing in ill-matched circumstances, appeared gradually to diverge from the ancestral type. New fevers and fluxes were challenging the basic economy of alien bodies, overstimulating and then depleting racial reserves of energy. The climate was foreign, social life appeared disordered, the diseases varied, and it sometimes seemed that a new biological type might emerge from the colonial turmoil.

Whether as convict, officer, or free settler, coming to Australia was no simple transposition. Those who first stepped ashore at Port Jackson (later Sydney) in 1788 had entered a new territory, unsure of the character of the seasons, the prevailing winds, the fertility of the soil, the quality of the water. As later colonists moved inland from Sydney or established other outposts along the coast, they too were assaying the land and climate as they went, using their own bodily sensations, their feelings of comfort or unease, to judge whether the land they coveted was a properly British territory. Until late in the nineteenth century, newcomers would attempt to match their personal sense of bodily terrain with their novel environment, adjusting their diet, clothing, housing, and physical activity in order to establish a harmony of individuality and circumstance. Some, such as Dr. George Wakefield, called this unavoidable process "acclimatisation" or "seasoning." From his tent at Emerald Hill, near Melbourne, in 1853, the young doctor wrote home to let his father know that "this certainly is the most extraordinary place ever beheld, everything being reversed to what it is in England."[1] For many years his body was not in harmony with this environment, and he suffered terribly, like most of his patients, from rheumatism, dysentery, and intermittent fever. But his constitution eventually seemed to adjust, and in 1861 he wrote that "I am afraid that I should not be able to stand the cold after having become acclimatised to the heat of this country . . . besides there is a certain charm to colonial life, a kind of independence."[2] Wakefield, like so many other Britons in the southeast of the continent, had become inured to the hot summer winds, the damp winters, the sudden variations in weather, the droughts, the floods, the poor soils, multitudes of insects, and monotonous eucalyptus forests. He found that he was drinking and eating more, smoking more, and washing more often, his clothes were looser and more casual, he wore a wide-brimmed hat, and he went out riding as often as possible. He still felt British—very much a white man—and he increasingly yearned for "home" as he aged, but his body and habits had changed perceptibly in the foreign environment. Like most—but perhaps not all—of his fellow colonists, he had acclimatized.

In seeking to explain the excessively high death rate of white children in the new country, Dr. J. William McKenna observed in 1858 that "nature presents herself under aspects most remarkably distinct from what she does in our native land." Without physical and behavioral adjustment, without acclimatization, white families were in peril. It had to be recognized that immigrants, "being placed under new conditions of life . . . have also a new class of knowledge to acquire." If they failed to do so, then the harsh Australian summer would remain a season of "grief, mourning and desolation" for the poorly adapted transplanted Britons.[3]

McKenna, like many local physicians, put his faith in cold baths and ice water, but the medical experts who had stayed behind in Britain could afford to show more detachment, and thus be less optimistic, when pronouncing on the fate of the race in foreign climes. Frequently they warned of racial limits to acclimatization. In his influential survey of medical climatology, R. E. Scoresby-Jackson, an Edinburgh physician, treated Australia as a vast experiment in racial transplantation, just one part of "the inquiry which is at this moment being carried on in every quarter of the globe relative to the effects of migration from one portion of the earth's surface to another upon every variety of organised creatures." Evidently, the death of a few infant organized creatures in Melbourne would cause him little grief: They must simply have "abrogated the laws of climate." Scoresby-Jackson believed that it was highly probable that

> *all* who leave their native soil to reside in foreign climates would ultimately *die out* were this not prevented by the return of their offspring to spend a portion of their lives in the mother country, or through the transfusion of

new blood into the veins of their descendants by intermarriage with immigrants fresh from the parent stock.[4]

The individual Briton might visit the antipodes with impunity, but it was quite likely that an isolated white race permanently resident there would eventually degenerate and die out. A medical responsibility thus supervened on British colonialism: How might doctors transform Britons from sojourners into settlers, how might they make them feel at home in such a strange place—how, indeed, would they ever acclimatize such alien whites?

Looking into the past from an age of mundane global traffic, it may be difficult to comprehend the nineteenth-century medical vision of British settlement in Australia: It is perhaps hard today to imagine that bodies once appeared so vulnerable, so sensitive to circumstance, that tragedy might await those who had merely wandered from their ancestral environment. But if location seems to us medically trivial, it was not so for most of the nineteenth century. To explain the basis of health, and the causes and expressions of disease, medical doctors and lay people alike drew on a language of place and circumstance. An individual's constitution, the sum of heredity and education, was always responding dynamically to fluctuations in local conditions—to the prevailing temperature, the direction of the winds, the shift in seasons, the character of the soil, the presence of filth or rotting vegetation.[5] The body functioned as an amazingly sensitive system of intake and excretion, of give and take with its changing environment. When that system was in balance, a state of health was achieved; but when the exchange went awry, disease was the result.

In this conceptual framework there was little room for reductionist notions of extraneous disease entities; rather, ill health was seen as an imbalance, or disease, of the whole bodily system, a disorder whose character might shade subtly from one diagnosis to another during the course of an illness. On one day the symptoms and signs would suggest typhoid, but on another the manifestations might assume more an aspect of typhus. It was the doctor's duty to attempt to restore the balance of assimilation and excretion, to stimulate a lowered (asthenic) systemic tone with a strengthening diet and tonics, or to deplete an overstimulated (sthenic) constitution with purging and bleeding. Diagnosis and treatment were titrated against the patient's experience of illness and the doctor's local knowledge. The patient could affirm the systemic imbalance implied in any diagnosis and feel the effects of restorative treatment; and the doctor generally was well aware of the family history and circumstances and would modify his intervention accordingly. Both doctor and patient shared a cognitive framework that related bodily experience to predisposition and environment.[6]

"The body was always in a state of becoming," writes Charles E. Rosenberg, "and thus always in jeopardy."[7] In a person's homeland, the crises generally were seasonal or developmental or behavioral; but these challenges to constitutional stability would dwindle into insignificance when compared to the effects of migration from one climatic zone to another. It was commonly believed that each race had a distinctive constitutional character or temperament that was best suited, whether through providential or evolutionary mechanisms, to its ancestral environment. Any disruption to this nexus through emigration would threaten bodily integrity.[8] The constitutional balance of British bodies, finely attuned to circumstances of Britain, might thus destabilize in the antipodes. Colonial physicians watched vigilantly for any signs of imbalance in the bodily systems of themselves and their alien charges. They described modifications of white bodies, alterations in their ailments, and the necessary innovations in treatment. Prospects for permanent European settlement remained unclear, a cause of considerable anxiety among medical experts. Would the old race become increasingly diseased and disordered in Australia and eventually die out? Would British bodies and minds prove basically resilient, demonstrating an unanticipated stability of type? Or would an altogether new biological form emerge, finely attuned to its weird circumstances?[9]

STRANGERS IN A STRANGE LAND

During the first thirty years of British occupation, doctors began with some trepidation to take stock of the healthfulness, or salubrity, of New South Wales. On the whole it did not seem, at first glance, especially hostile to the British bodily economy, but medical men qualified their praise with the reservation that there had been insufficient time to observe its long-term effects. The country was still too unsettled; people came and went and rarely stayed long enough to put down any roots. In the first few years at Sydney, malnutrition—even starvation—and not the foreign climate seemed the chief cause of illness and death among the thousand or so convicts and their warders. During the next thirty years of settlement, the preponderance of convicts would draw medical attention more to immorality and intemperance, and less to displacement, as the likely causes of any constitutional derangement. Not surprisingly, doctors expected that the convict version of the British bodily system would more often be buffeted by excess and indulgence, whether in drink or sex or other vice, than reflect the changes in atmosphere and soil. Hippocratic medicine—the concern with airs, waters, and places as causes of disease—was essentially a discourse of settlement, requiring some familiarity with the lie of the land and knowledge of weather patterns, and presupposing a people of previously sound constitution, most of them conducting themselves responsibly, behaving in a settled and temperate manner.[10] Not until after the 1820s did colonial doctors believe these conditions had been achieved in Australia.[11]

The lack of long experience of settled conditions did not, of course, stop the first British colonists in New South Wales from making occasional efforts to understand the territory and the climate, whenever more pressing duties permitted them the leisure to speculate on their displaced destiny. John White, the surgeon-general of the First Fleet and then of the settlement at Port Jackson until 1794, had kept a diary of the winds and temperatures as the ships sailed from Britain to New South Wales, but on arrival in 1788 he was compelled to set this aside and concentrate on improving the nutrition of the convicts, in an effort to abate an epidemic of scurvy.[12] It was not until a few years later—after nutritional worries had diminished and death rates had declined—that Governor Arthur Phillip felt confident enough to write to Lord Sydney and assure him that "a finer and more healthy climate is not to be found in any part of the world."[13] Many others in the infant colony, including David Collins, the judge-advocate, shared Phillip's good opinion of the "salubrity" of New South Wales.[14] Watkin Tench, a young captain of the Marines, found the climate "undoubtedly very desirable to live in. In summer the heats are usually moderated by a sea breeze, which sets in early." Everyone was relieved that it was not an Indian climate. "Those dreadful putrid fevers by which new countries are so often ravaged, are unknown to us," wrote Tench within a few years of arrival. "And excepting a slight diarrhoea, which prevailed soon after we had landed, and was fatal in very few instances, we are strangers to epidemic disease."[15] The cautious John Hunter, governor of the colony from 1795 until 1800, admitted that the "sudden vicissitudes" of heat and cold might make the English "too apt to pronounce this colony very unhealthy," but his experience had convinced him that this was not the case. Indeed, he had never seen "the constitutions either of the human race or any other animal more prolific in any part of the world": Multiple births were common, and women at an advanced age had produced children.[16]

Even so, most of the early colonists still feared the hot winds that frequently blew from the inland. In March 1789, for example, Collins reported that "those persons whose business compelled them to go into the heated air declared that it was impossible to turn the face for five minutes to the quarter from whence the wind blew."[17] Watkin Tench, otherwise so breezily optimistic, also deplored the "intolerable heat" that was, he thought, "occasioned by the wind blowing over immense desarts [sic]." During the great heat of 27 December 1790, Tench found that "our dogs, pigs, and fowls, lay panting in the shade, or were rushing into the water." But "no lasting ill-effects, however, arose to the human constitution; a temporary sickness at the stomach, accompanied with lassitude and headache, attacked many, but they were removed generally in twenty-four hours by an emetic, followed by an anodyne."[18] Still, it seemed that the new country, often surprisingly pleasant, could suddenly turn into a most un-British cauldron. In November 1791, Collins observed:

The extreme heat of the weather during the month had not only increased the sick list, but had added to the number of deaths. On the 4th, a convict attending on Mr White, in passing from his house to the kitchen, without any covering upon his head, received a stroke from a ray of the sun, which at the time deprived him of speech and motion, and in less than four-and-twenty hours, of his life.

And yet such environmental catastrophes continued to appear insignificant in comparison to the ill effects of convict vice. Collins and others especially deplored the common overindulgence in rum. When "dysentery" broke out in 1793, the severe judge determined that many "were affected after drinking, through want of a sufficient stamina to overcome the effect of the spirit."[19] With such poor stock it would remain difficult to assay with confidence the quality of a foreign soil and atmosphere.

Free settlers, arriving in greater numbers during the 1820s, attracted by the developing pastoral industry, seemed generally more robust in constitution and more restrained and resolute than the convicts. Almost 10,000 free settlers arrived in the penal colony in the 1820s, but immigrant numbers began to dwindle at the end of the decade as the result of a decline in wool prices. Many of the newcomers, concerned that they might yet become the innocent victims of migration, wondered if their displacement from home gave any legitimate cause for apprehension. What sort of effect might the airs, waters, and places of New South Wales exert on their alien British bodies? How should they adjust to changed circumstances? Might not a hot wind cancel out even the most fastidious conduct?

Peter Cunningham, a navy surgeon who had spent two years in New South Wales in the 1820s, tried to encourage prospective emigrants, proclaiming the "extraordinary healthfulness of the climate." It was a happy place where many European fevers and diseases, including "intermittents, remittents, typhus, scarlet fever, small-pox, measles, hooping cough, and croup," were unknown.[20] Cunningham admitted that the hot northern winds often left influenza and eye blight in their wake, and dyspepsia frequently was "aggravated in the low, warm, portions of our country." He also conceded that "on reaching the age of puberty, phthisis [tuberculosis] is liable to supervene from the rapid sprouting out in stature of our youths at this period; but the European phthisis is uniformly cured or at least relieved by a removal hither, if early resorted to."[21] And as for dysentery, the major expression of British discomfort in the antipodes, Cunningham assured his readers that "deaths even from this cause are exceedingly rare among the sober-living portion of the community, and far from common even among the debauched"—dysentery was "seldom productive of danger to any but the imprudent and intemperate."[22] So long as one behaved prudently it would be safe to tend one's flocks on the pastures of Australia Felix.

Guides for British emigrants repeatedly trumpeted the health advantages of Australian residence. The Reverend John Dunmore Lang, whose promotional energies never fluctuated, saw Britain "vomiting forth" its convicts and sinners onto a land that "yields to none other on the whole face of the globe for the salubrity of its climate and the serenity of its sky."[23] Although Europeans arriving in the northern parts of the country might "find their system somewhat relaxed at first, and be tempted to give way to lassitude," Lang thought that they would soon overcome the challenge.[24] In the 1830s, another popular emigration booster, Samuel Butler, extolled the Australian summer, a season when "the atmosphere, however heated, only displays its power in spreading luxuriance over the face of nature, without producing any debilitating effects upon the human frame." It was a land where "the atmosphere is pure, dry and elastic"; even when the hot winds blew, "the lungs play freely, and no difficulty is felt in breathing."[25] The new British colonists were liable to few diseases—principally ophthalmia (or eye blight), influenza, and dysentery—and those who succumbed usually were tainted with immorality. Admittedly ophthalmia could occasionally arise unbidden within the innocent, the result of hot winds, the glare of light from white surfaces, or working in the open air with the head uncovered. Similarly, influenza might be explained as a reaction to "the miasmata issued by the marshes of the interior combined with the extreme aridness of the atmosphere inducing inflammation of the throat." But in cases of dysentery, so prevalent among the convicts and lower-class settlers, "dissipation is found to be the master cause."[26] In New South Wales, in contrast to home, excessive indulgence appeared to "undermine the constitution, and to blast the prospects with more fearful and fatal rapidity." "Here the lamp of life burns brightly and strongly in its own pure air," warned Butler, "and is extinguished without the long feeble flickering which characterises the protracted duration of helpless senility."[27]

Dr. George Bennett, in describing his wanderings in New South Wales during the early 1830s, was somewhat more ambivalent toward British prospects. A great supporter of acclimatization projects, whether plant or animal, Bennett nonetheless admitted that:

> To an emigrant, one who has left behind the land of his fathers, to rear his family and lay his bones in a distant soil, the first view of this, his adopted country, cannot excite in his bosom any emotions of pleasurable gratification; despondency succeeds the bright rays of hope, and he compares with heartfelt regret the arid land before him with the fertile country he has forsaken.

But all was not lost, for "as industry gives him wealth and independence, and he finds his family easily maintained, he becomes reconciled to his choice, and remains comparatively if not entirely happy."[28] As a medical man, Bennett could reassure his readers that few diseases arose from the climate of Australia. Predictably, "dissipation and numerous vices introduced from home" had caused some ailments "to prevail extensively in the populous town of Sydney, but in the interior they are comparatively few." Moreover, even in the 1830s, Australian ladies "may compete for personal beauty and elegance with any European, although satirised as 'corn-stalks' from the slenderness of their form."[29]

When Sir James Clark, Queen Victoria's personal physician, came to write his remarkably influential book, *The Sanative Influence of Climate*, he relied on promotional literature in assessing the wholesomeness of the antipodean atmosphere. He had heard that in Van Diemen's Land, soon renamed Tasmania, "all diseases, both acute and chronic, are generally mild, and of comparatively short duration, and yield easily to the usual remedies." The climate of southern Australia was generally pleasant, except in summer, "when the heat is disagreeably great." Even so, Clark reported that "Europeans enervated by a residence in India become very much invigorated and improved in health by a short stay in this country."[30] But other doctors, such as Thomas Bartlett, an army surgeon who visited the colony during the depression of the 1840s, were prepared to challenge Clark's anodyne authority. It was clear to Bartlett that the climate of Australasia did not "approach that exemption from grievous diseases of which so much has been noised abroad." White people would find the heat exhausting; the soils were poor; flies and mosquitoes abounded in summer. Bartlett lamented the "sufferings of the settlers under a withering, scorching sun"—as they struggled with their flocks and crops, "the rays of its powerful, burning, summer sun shoot down" on their vulnerable British heads.[31] "In consequence of the extreme heat during the summer, and the rapid changes of temperature, the wear and tear of the constitution is considerable." The prospects for the transplanted race were poor: "As it is with vegetable, so it is with animal, life— the quickness of growth can only be equalled by the rapidity of decay. Children shoot up into men and women with singular rapidity, but their constitutions cannot long withstand the inroads of the climate."[32] While emigration agents continued to describe Australia as an antipodean paradise for Britons, many doctors, after 1840, were suggesting that it might prove instead a colonial purgatory, no place for a white man or woman.

Certainly the experiences of some unfortunate doctors gave testimony to the power of the Australian environment to exhaust even the most fastidious of British bodily systems. In becoming unwell, doctors would naturally tend to exonerate themselves and condemn their noxious circumstances. When Dr. David Wilsone left Adelaide in 1839, heading for the new settlement of

Melbourne, he was departing from "one of the most straggling, dusty, uninteresting places I ever was in." For months he had endured "*three* very great annoyances, myriads of sandflies (*a biting one*) by day, fleas in dozens *literally* at night, and the unhealthy roasting, hot Northerly wind . . . so oppressive and hot, obliging us to go to the sea shore to enjoy the cool air."[33] But the Port Phillip District (later Victoria) was little better, and he soon was suffering from "feverish attacks with bowel complaint." In March 1840, on his run near Werribee, the ailing doctor expected to die, but within a few weeks he announced that "it has pleased Almighty God to give a check to the Dysentery." "It took all my manhood to bear up under it," Wilsone, the son of a Glasgow surgeon, wrote to his brother in England.[34] He decided to move into Melbourne itself—a new town of 4,000, crowded with fourteen medical men already—"to try the effect of a change of air to aid in re-establishing my health." Initially he felt "a decided amendment in health and strength" and hoped "as the weather gets warmer I will get rid of these troublesome symptoms."[35] But his weakness and ill health continued, and within a year he was dead—the innocent victim, so he had thought, of a climate horribly unsuitable for his race.

FEVERED COLONIALS

Patrick Divorty, an Edinburgh-trained surgeon who visited Sydney in the 1850s, encountered a treacherous and influential environment. Soon after his arrival, the barometric pressures and temperatures were "reeling in endless confusion"; the winds were "variable and capricious in their direction." Periodic gales, blowing up red dust and called "brickfielders," beset the inhabitants, and in summer hot winds would blow for days from the northwest, only to be followed by a southerly buster carrying rain. Divorty wondered if the Omnipotent had placed the constitution of the western European into a "ruthless clime."[36] The sun and heat were so severe that "the cutaneous glands, as well as other sebaceous follicles, are called into more active operation, as is frequently evinced by the unctuous feel of the skin." But then the climate would suddenly change, with "the oleaginous substances secreted by the follicles becoming congealed," and as a result "the surface of the body, especially the parts exposed, becomes, as it were, hermetically sealed."[37] According to contemporary medical theory, any such impediment to intake or excretion would throw the bodily economy out of balance and thus into disease and distemper.

To Divorty's trained eye the new climate seemed generally to lower the tone of the European bodily system. On arrival, the immigrant had rosy cheeks, a fresh complexion, and a "plump-elastic appearance"; but after a few years the complexion became harsh, the face turned gray, and skin seemed "shrivelled and unctuous." Most colonists lost weight and experienced a "languour and depression of spirits." Divorty had noticed "the slight anaemic appearance of the female," her "relaxed fibre," decaying teeth, and poor mammary development. White men as well as white women seemed to age prematurely. The prevailing diseases, in keeping with these altered constitutions, were generally "adynamic" and subacute in character. And the recent finding of gold had caused the Australian mind to take on an even more morbid cast.[38]

There can be no doubt that with gold discoveries in the 1850s the colonies of New South Wales and Victoria were changing rapidly, almost beyond recognition. In 1820, the population of New South Wales had amounted to 25,000 or so, most of them convicts—rough in conduct, heavy-drinking, badly fed, and poorly housed. But convict transportation was in decline, and the development of the wool industry had attracted increasing numbers of free settlers: In 1840, almost half the population, by then 130,000, either was born locally or had emigrated in search of land. Squatters soon occupied all the good grazing country in New South Wales and Victoria.[39] In the 1850s, as soon as news spread of vast fields of gold, especially in central Victoria, men deserted the colonial towns to head for the diggings, and thousands took passage from Europe and California. Within a few years there was a doubling of the population of the new colony of Victoria, which had achieved self-government only in 1851, just one month in advance of the onset of gold fever. At the beginning of that year, the population of Melbourne scarcely amounted to 20,000, yet in 1861, 140,000 resided there; during the early 1850s, 90,000 people were arriving at its port each year. The influx of gold-seekers—mostly fit young men—was absorbed generally without great difficulty, but many of them soon succumbed to the usual colonial problems of dysentery, alcoholism, injury, and eye blight.[40]

Among the gold-seekers were many poor or adventurous young doctors—by 1850, one person in 500 in Victoria was medically qualified, though few of them saw patients.[41] In December 1852 on the Castlemaine diggings, in central Victoria, one of the many dispirited young doctors recently arrived from England noted in his diary that he was "still suffering from diarrhoea—most unpleasant weather—rain and wind nearly all day." After finding little gold, and hearing that he would "make much more by my profession than gold seeking in the earth," Dr. James Selby eventually began a lucrative medical practice back in Melbourne.[42] In May 1856, Dr. George Wakefield wrote from Ballarat to his father in England, reassuring him that "I have been digging and got on famously with it, and was never better in health since leaving home." But Wakefield did not strike rich and, like Selby, gradually drifted back into medical practice: "Really qualified medical men are extremely scarce here," he wrote, and yet he would soon feel the competition keenly.[43] Others, like the earnestly sentimental and religious Dr. Thomas McMillan, had left their local medical practice to try their luck on the diggings, and soon they too rejoined Selby and Wakefield in the doctoring trade. McMillan was more successful than many other refugees from the diggings, later becoming president of the Medical Society of Victoria.

McMillan's response to the disrupted, uncultivated landscape, and to the capricious climate, was typical. Working in Brunswick, a northern suburb of Melbourne, not long after his arrival in the new colony, McMillan had observed:

> Hot winds still more violent today, a perfect typhoon, Melbourne has been darkened with dust all day. Truly this is a disagreeable climate and country to live in and has been very much misrepresented. I feel that I am not to have very firm health in this town of Melbourne if I am to pursue a sedentary occupation.[44]

His diary entries reiterate his sensitivity to harsh surroundings: "a very hot day and felt very feverish and unwell" (23 January 1854); "I believe I have got a cold on account of the rough weather yesterday" (4 February 1854); "the weather much cooler and health still improving" (14 March 1854); "I hope it will be more favourable for health than the late hot winds" (13 April 1854); "a most extraordinary hot day, the heat not only depressing *but sickening*" (13 February 1855); "I have no expectation of good health until the weather clear up and improve" (14 May 1857). McMillan, who had trained in Edinburgh, was carefully attentive to the influence of the strange weather on himself and his patients. The hot winds, as always, presented the greatest shocks to the British system: "A terrible day with hot wind and dust. Everyone appears to feel as if life was a burden. This is certainly a most unwholesome and disagreeable climate." And a few days later: "Felt rather unwell. A very hot day, wind and dust. Felt worse during the forenoon and very unable for my duties. After wind changed and rain fell, felt a little relieved" (16 and 21 February 1855). Even winter in colonial Victoria felt hostile. "The weather still showery and miserably cold," McMillan wrote in Geelong in June 1855. "I never suffered more from it either in Scotland or in America."[45] It was proving a singularly "disagreeable" climate.

Doctors on the goldfields observed puzzling diseases in themselves and among their patients. Changed circumstances had altered the character of old diseases like typhoid and ague and given rise to new ailments such as colonial fever, nostalgia, sunstroke, gold fever, and bush-mania. Dr. James Robertson believed that the fever prevalent around Melbourne until the 1860s was a form of enteric or typhoid fever, yet it was usually known as colonial fever. It was generally supposed "to be a fever *sui generis*, different from those met with elsewhere. In fact, it was regarded as the 'seasoning fever,' incidental to the climate."[46] Robertson was skeptical of such claims of novelty, but Dr. Edward Hunt recalled the appearance in Bendigo in 1854 of a new continued hemorrhagic fever, a condition that began more like typhoid but then assumed an aspect of typhus, ending usually with death. By 1857, this colonial fever had become more mild and seasonal, separating gradually into a number of different forms. Its initial character had reflected the peculiar interaction of the European constitution with the conditions of life on the goldfields, where the system was liable to "overwork and anxiety" and to "exposure and fatigue." This mysterious ailment, which Hunt had not seen since 1862, was "different from any described, and may be considered as truly 'Colonial' or 'Australian.'"[47]

But when the elderly Dr. D. J. Thomas joined the debate at the Medical Society of Victoria, he gruffly discounted Hunt's remarks. Thomas had diagnosed a true colonial fever long before the gold rushes, and it was completely different, more "bilious intermittent, often of an adynamic state."[48] In the 1840s, pioneers had noticed during summer a loss of appetite, general weakness, and dejection of spirits. Within days, fever, shivering, headache, and vomiting set in, and a great "vital depression" lasted for the next few weeks. The crisis occurred late, marked by diarrhea of a violent character, followed by a long convalescence. The fever had occurred because in the early days of the Port Phillip settlement "much rank vegetation abounded throughout the town. . . . Luxuriant grass grew in our streets, and all the leading thoroughfares contained a chain of mud-holes." This led inevitably to "decomposition and the emanation of germs and gases which had the power of producing bilious remittent (colonial) fever." But with increased cultivation and grazing of sheep and cattle, colonial fever and other constitutional disorders had almost disappeared.[49]

White Destinies

From the 1850s, local medical societies in the Australian colonies provided a forum for the discussion of the intimate connections of race, environment, and well-being.[50] In explaining health and disease in the antipodes, physicians such as Hunt and Thomas were also reframing ideas about race and location. Indeed, it could be argued that until the 1870s, and even later, all medicine was inherently local, and the chief task of Australian practitioners was to chart an Australian medical distinctiveness, to explore the peculiar local amalgam of race and place.[51] In so doing, colonial doctors were bringing together their experiences of local practice and their knowledge of heredity and adaptation. Most doctors had learned from clinical practice, and perhaps from personal experience, to accept a dynamic view of the interaction between racialized bodies and the environment. Accordingly, colonial medical theory—at least until the 1870s—was concerned with the prospects for *adaptation*, focusing on the best means of achieving, if possible, an *acclimatization*, or a restoration of systemic balance, which might preserve the essential features of the race.

Many colonial physicians, themselves disturbed by the turmoil of gold-seeking, expressed doubts that an unmodified southern Australian atmosphere and soil would ever prove a natural habitat for healthy Britons. Dr. James Kilgour, of Geelong, reported in 1855 that most immigrants were "conscious of some change in their constitution after a short residence." Soon after their arrival, they typically noticed a "buoyancy of spirits and a desire as well as a capacity for muscular exertion," but soon they lost this "vital energy," their muscles shrank away, and they succumbed to "an asthenic irritability not to be cured by bleeding or any other active depletory means."[52] Indeed, Kilgour had observed that the "vital powers have not the vigour in setting up reactionary processes in the system which they possess in the colder climate of our Fatherland." In the heat of summer delicate whites suffered badly from exhaustion and debility. Often they developed one of the colonial fevers, characterized by their "uncertain duration, the general absence of crises or changes occurring at fixed epochs of the disease; the deficient reaction and early implication of the nervous system; the little tendency to putridity and frequency of local congestions."[53] Evidently the new environment had sapped the white race's reserves of energy. Kilgour's answer was to advise a better diet and to call for more shade trees, the extension of cultivation, and the provision of spaces for public recreation.

Some of Kilgour's colleagues were more optimistic. "This colony," thundered Dr. Mingay Syder, a rival Geelong practitioner, "was not selected by its discoverers and first settlers as the nursery for the idle, dissipated, scrofulous, phthisical, dyspeptic, hypochondriac, neuralgic, worn-out constitutions." Those who arrived as invalids would remain invalids. It was difficult to determine the cause of ill health in the colonies: Syder suspected that intemperate habits and a bad diet did more damage than any number of hot winds. Given the extent of drunkenness, self-pollution, gluttony, uncleanliness, and poor ventilation in Victoria, it was indeed fortunate that the climate was so good. Certainly, immigrants might suffer from the change in circumstances if they were not careful, but during his five years in the colony Syder had observed that most Britons had great "physiologic powers of climatic adaptation."[54]

In spite of Syder's protests, concerns about the loss of vital power and an excessive languor of whites in southern Australia abound in the medical literature between 1850 and 1880. Dr. W. J. Sterland, like so many of his colleagues, had hoped to find better health in the new colonies, but he was sorely disappointed. When he arrived in Sydney in the 1850s a hot wind was blowing. "The effects upon the human frame," he reported, are "extremely depressing; all energy is gone, one feels utterly exhausted, and gasps for breath like a fish out of water."

The glare of the sun and the dust in summer gave most colonists a severe oph-thalmia. Sterland was to suffer much "from the depressing influence of the hot winds," and twice he was laid up with a "low typhoid fever" as a result.[55] At Molong in New South Wales, Dr. Andrew Ross, a local physician and politi-cian, had observed in summer "an indescribable degree of lassitude" among his patients and constituents. This "lowness of spirits, flagging appetite, loss of flesh" rendered "the subject more susceptible of acquiring new and local forms of disease." With prolonged residence the skin of the British immigrant "be-comes tanned; the plump plethoric frame becomes attenuated; the blood loses fibrin and red globules; lines deepen around the eyes through the iron glare of the hot burning sunshine; the adipose tissue soon melts away; the voice be-comes lower and feebler—in fact the man of forty looks fifty years old."[56] In such a trying climate, the colonist had become as exhausted as the land.

Not surprisingly, many physicians feared that the quality of British blood was rapidly deteriorating. According to Kilgour, immigrant blood was becom-ing more diluted and "its properties poorer" than in Britain; when he looked at it through a microscope he could see fewer "coloured corpuscles." It seemed to him that congestive forms of inflammation were lamentably common be-cause "the tide of blood in the capillary or small blood vessels is checked more by a want of power to move on."[57] Such pathological detail is rare, but Kil-gour's general concerns were becoming a commonplace of colonial medical theory. Many physicians were inclined to attribute their patients' perceived de-ficiencies in energy to a dilution or thinning of the blood—the "loss of fibrin and red globules," as Ross put it. This common anemia was a consequence of enduring a hot, draining climate. And yet there were a few practitioners, like Dr. James B. Clutterbuck, who held onto old habits and were still free with the lancet. Clutterbuck's colleagues in Victoria had warned him that "the blood in fever in this climate is very loose in texture," but he had never seen it so. In any case, he thought that the understandable reluctance to spill precious colonial blood had been overdone.[58]

The nervous system also could become unbalanced and exhausted in foreign circumstances. Under Australian skies, the most sober and reliable British im-migrants frequently developed a nervousness and irritability that might even shade into an evanescent mania. For Divorty, the morbidity of the Australian mind shifted uneasily between depression and melancholia to the extreme moral and mental disturbance of gold fever.[59] "Persons who passed at home for good tempered," wrote Kilgour, "here become remarkable for irascibility." The Victorian physician and pastoralist was convinced that "the increased action of the nervous system is more easily excited here than at home as a consequence of greater irritability and less power."[60] It was a truism of colonial practice that the antipodean climate could both deplete and overexcite the otherwise phleg-matic British constitution. Dr. S. J. Magarey, in Adelaide, proposed that the "hot dry air of our long South Australian summer" caused a "fluxionary hyper-aemia of the brain," which led to a deterioration of the child's nervous system and, sometimes, even to death.[61] In New South Wales, Ross felt that "strong solar light" was capable of altering "the structure of the body" and that it frequently acted through the eyes and on the brain to produce "nervous prostration" in Europeans. The discovery of gold merely compounded the mental and physical havoc wrought by climate. Fantasies of finding gold caused an overexcitation of an already weak and unprepared nervous system, putting it into "a kind of perpetual motion of feverish anxiety."[62] This "gold fever" could be as serious a disease as any other manifestation of systemic imbalance. It was just one of a number of disorders of colonial mentality brought on by a hostile physical environment and stressful social life. In 1869, for example, the *Australian Medical Journal* reported the development in remote districts of a "harmless lunacy," or "bush-mania," presumably the result of "the blank mental activity and the dreary solitude of life in those parts." At Wagga Wagga, a man had been seen "running about in a state of nudity, at times on his knees praying, and at other times dancing wildly."[63] The effects of the climate, alcohol, and social isolation, whether operating singly or in combination, could make any white man mad—or worse.

Some colonial doctors, especially in the 1850s, believed that the sun was the chief cause of the mental and physical derangement they witnessed among their patients. Dr. C. Travers Mackin had no doubt that the irritation of the sun's rays was conveyed through thin white skulls to the brain beneath, causing a range of symptoms from confusion, loss of vision, vertigo, and nausea through to "congestive apoplexy."[64] He recalled the case of a man, thirty-five years old and of "sanguino-nervous temperament, moderately full habit, and a rather free liver," who went out to bathe on an excessively hot day in February 1855. After an hour or so in the water, mostly floating on his back, he noticed an unusual sensation on the front of his head. When he got out he suffered from "dizziness of sight [and] confusion of ideas and giddiness." Despite copious purging, he became "impetuous, contradictory and snappish." Suddenly, he felt a rush to the head, with "numbness of the lower limbs, and an indescribable tingling down both arms, with prostration of muscular energy." Within an hour he was nearly comatose, and to relieve the congestion Mackin had to apply sixteen leeches to his temples and cold wet cloths to the head and to induce more purging. To the doctor's astonishment, the patient was worse the next morning, with delirium, staring eyes, and a "tendency to raving." But after more bleeding and a blister to the nape of his neck (as a counterirritant), the reckless bather made a gradual recovery.[65]

Mackin could supply his colleagues with many more examples of the evil effects of the sun on the British system. The outcome was largely determined by the robustness of the individual constitution and the severity of the insult.

One of Mackin's medical friends, "a young man of spare frame and remarkably temperate habits," lost his hat when out sailing. He felt an odd sensation in the head, his vision dimmed, and he became faint and giddy. The young doctor sank into a coma that lasted for days but from which he recovered with no lasting ill effects. Less fortunate was Mrs. W., thirty-five years old and a schoolteacher of temperate habits, but "her health habitually delicate from dyspepsia." She was returning home from church in April 1855, exposing herself to a hot wind from the north. "She fell down suddenly, exclaiming, 'O my head!'" When Mackin saw her she was comatose, with pupils widely dilated and stertorous breathing. He opened the external jugular vein, "but the patient did not rally, dying comatose six hours after the seizure."[66] It seems as though wherever one looked colonists were falling down in the streets and in the fields. Mackin saw a middle-aged, stout bullock driver who had been struck by the sun and developed a "partial mania" and "incoherent ravings." He was complaining of an intense heat in the scalp. As quickly as cold lotions could be applied to his head they would evaporate into steam.[67] And so it went on: a laborer, forty years old, thin and muscular; a man driving a cart to town; a farmer in the Barrabool Hills; the cases of solar suffering in southeastern Australia could, it seems, be multiplied indefinitely.

Just as the climate disturbed the racial system, so too did it disorder gender roles in the colonies. Most of Mackin's sun-struck male pioneers had been laboring, or recovering from hard work, when they were afflicted; the only woman sufferer was returning from church. The problems of working white males predominate in most colonial accounts of the health effects of climate. Kilgour lamented the lack of muscular and nervous power—the increasing "effeminacy"—in the Australian male; Ross also detected a diminution of strength, "durability," and muscular development. "I submit," wrote Ross, "that under our mean maximum temperature, it is impossible to expect the same amount of manual labour from one man here as it is in England with a cooler atmosphere."[68] Male labor efficiency was a common gauge of racial adaptation, and it would remain so for a hundred years or more. As previously industrious white men weakened, they were also becoming unnerved, sometimes showing signs of melancholy and nostalgia, at other times raving incoherently and dancing naked in the bush. Masculinity, whether it was defined in terms of virility and capacity for manual labor or as self-mastery and moral resolve, was clearly threatened in such trying foreign circumstances. Colonial doctors diagnosed a lack of intrepidity, an aversion to the strenuous life, a failure of nerve force, among many of the British male immigrants.[69] Among the women, they commonly saw a failure to reproduce and care for the home. Divorty, for example, believed that local women had become bloodless, louche, and flat-chested: He had observed that white women reached puberty earlier than in England but deteriorated rapidly after they reached twenty years of age.[70] Kilgour feared that "a deficiency of power frequently exists in the nerves of the womb," with an "increased excitability in the uterine and ovarian systems."[71] Evidently, the colonial racial crisis was also a gender crisis.

Colonial doctors pointed to the local Aboriginal population as an object lesson in adaptation to Australian conditions. Given the prevailing adaptationist assumptions, the pitiful condition of the original inhabitants represented a possible future for the British race in Australia—not until after the acceptance of Darwinism would anyone come to recognize Aborigines as representing its past. Throughout the nineteenth century it was generally assumed that Aboriginal Australians, unlike Europeans, had become well-suited to the harsh antipodean environment; but this only convinced white observers that harmony with such a depleted land would never allow the development of a high level of muscular and nervous energy. The country was difficult and trying; its people in their natural state were enervated. It was true, however, that the Aborigines could withstand many of the hazards of the climate. Mackin thought that their "thick *brain-case*, close woolly hair, and oily skin" protected them against sunstroke. "Does this not supply a farther proof of the adaptive providence of the all-wise Creator?" Mackin asked.[72] But would a previously white population welcome the same anatomical providence? Ross believed that for a European body to be healthy, it "ought to be uniform and well developed, especially furnished with broad shoulders and well-formed chest, characters, however, utterly at variance (except in the Hawkesbury ones, the finest race in the colony), with the generality of the natives." He worried that the "muscular broad frame of the immigrant" was dwindling into the "attenuated slender frame" of the native-born.[73] Like many of his colleagues he detected a frightening degeneration of racial type.

It seemed that the Aboriginal type was not robust enough to withstand the stresses of civilization. A few radical physicians, such as Mingay Syder, deplored the ravages of "man's interest, ignorance, appetite or depravity" on such delicate physiological systems. Syder attributed Aboriginal decline chiefly to "the life-destroying agencies, introduced among, and entailed upon them, by a 'race' calling itself 'Christian.'" He condemned his fellow colonists:

> What, in truth, have we done for the coloured natives? Robbed them of their land and of their food; made them drunkards; debauched, and diseased their women to a state bordering upon barrenness; driven them to murder their offspring to an extent promising a speedy extermination of the "race': and this is our Christian guardianship.

Europeans had "inoculated them with [their] moral and physical poisons" and then did nothing "to arrest the progress of those frightful maladies, consequent upon 'Christian' contamination."[74] If they had been more robust specimens, they might have had a chance; as it was, they did not have the physiological capacity to resist the perils of civilization.

Such concern is rare in the 1850s and seems almost to disappear in later decades. In general, when Aborigines cannot be presented as object lessons, they are ignored completely in colonial medical texts.[75] Most medical geographers seem to have held implicitly to a doctrine of *terra nullius*. Until the 1880s, the Chinese also rarely rate a mention in the *Australian Medical Journal*, even though they were popularly associated with leprosy, venereal disease, and smoking opium.[76] Instead, when colonial doctors wanted to discuss the health of the race, and the constitutional changes arising from its displacement, they resorted to a geographical vocabulary, a language of system and circumstance, of adaptation and alienation, of balance and disorder. Until the 1880s, the health of whites was assessed chiefly in relation to their environment and less often in opposition to another race. But that would change.

CLIMATE AND CONSUMPTION

In view of the common disparagement of Australian climates and circumstances, it may seem paradoxical that many British doctors could still prescribe emigration for some of their ailing patients. But of course such recommendations might equally be consistent with the underlying assumption that disease developed when the bodily constitution was out of harmony with its environment, irritated into imbalance by its surroundings. If a British body was already disordered and unwell in its natural clime, then a change might help to restore order in the system. If it was already healthy, then change might prove detrimental. Although southern Australia was perhaps, for many previously well Europeans, a land of dysentery and low fevers, of nervous irritability and prostration, of sunstroke and exhaustion, it had nonetheless developed a reputation as a potential haven for those who in Europe had already been afflicted by chronic illness.

The southern parts of Australia thus became a refuge for those suffering from phthisis, or consumption of the lungs, a disease later known as tuberculosis.[77] The leading cause of disability and death in Europe during the nineteenth century, phthisis was generally believed to be hereditary and noncontagious. A sufferer had presumably inherited a constitutional predisposition to the disorder, a consumptive tendency that could be irritated into periodic clinical exacerbation. The disease, marked by coughing, hemorrhage, weight loss, and fatigue, was thus the product of the interaction of a constitutional tendency with the individual's environment and habits of life. Life in a mild, dry, and uniform climate—circumstances unlike those in which the disease developed—

seemed likely then to reduce the irritation to the consumptive's physiological system, perhaps to the extent of permitting a remission in the disease. Accordingly, British consumptives were advised to travel to the Mediterranean or to Australia in search of health. Thus we find an alternative medical diagnosis—one clouded with reservations and ambiguities—of the apparent healthfulness of an antipodean climate.

Many colonial doctors had traveled to Australia to improve their health. W. J. Sterland, for example, in England suffered "a delicacy of chest without the presence of actual disease, and an extreme susceptibility to take cold." He found the Australian climate prevented these conditions, although he believed it also produced a profound exhaustion and depression and excited in him a continued, low fever.[78] But other chesty migrants were less disappointed in the southern climate. In 1870, "Medicus" recalled in a letter to the *Australian Medical Journal* that near the end of his medical course at Edinburgh he had discovered tubercle deposited in the apex of his right lung. He was advised to take time off and travel in the highlands of Scotland. While there, a Free Kirk minister gave him a book on the Australian climate. "On reading it, I determined that if on enquiry I found that half of it was true, I should at all hazards go to Australia." His Edinburgh professors suggested that he visit Queensland or New South Wales, as the weather in Victoria would be too cold and variable. But the young doctor disregarded their advice and bought a ticket to Melbourne, where after a few months he felt his chest symptoms begin to resolve. He thought that "the open air, the stimulating and tonic atmosphere, and the cheerful sunlight" counteracted any Victorian climatic variability and the occasional hot wind. "I have gained flesh," he wrote, "am fit for a considerable amount of work, and though not so robust as once, I consider myself in good health."[79]

In the Scottish highlands, "Medicus" had been reading the work of Dr. Samuel Dougan Bird, one of the more celebrated chest physicians in Victoria. Like most of his colleagues, Bird believed that "the modification of disease by climate is a subject which must always claim the special attention of pathologists." Indeed, for the colonists of a land that was "to be the permanent home of a large and powerful section of the Anglo-Saxon race," such observations were not merely a professional inquiry; they were also a "patriotic duty."[80] His own studies had demonstrated that the Australian environment could alter the incidence, character, and course of phthisis among Europeans. The nature of their constitutions had changed, and the new environment produced novel effects on them. Bird's clinical experience led him to believe that chest complaints were rarer in Australia than in Europe, and when they occurred they tended to be milder. It was even possible, he thought, that whites born in Australian possessed a degree of constitutional immunity to phthisis. Some new diagnostic features had also become evident in the antipodean climate: Bird had found that the tubercle was more commonly deposited in the lower lobes of the lungs of residents. Moreover, there was "usually a prominence of dyspeptic symptoms," requiring mineral alkalis, bitters, and digestives. Bird recommended the tonic effects of mercury and antimony in small doses and had found strychnine very useful, "particularly in hot weather, when the nervous system is relaxed and digestion torpid, with cold extremities, poor appetite, and sluggish bowels." Though Bird, like most of his colonial colleagues, thought that stimulants were generally more effective in such a depleting climate, the exact treatment would always depend on the constitutional idiosyncrasies of the patient.[81]

Later, in response to critics of his facile environmental optimism, Bird qualified his praise of the local climate.[82] In the 1870s, he was forced to concede that "there is no standard of excellence in climate for consumption; its merit is entirely relative to the individual case." The greatest benefits came not from a certain type of climate but from a change in climate, a migration to an environment as dissimilar as possible from the one in which the disease had originated. If darkness, damp, and chilliness prevailed, as in Britain, then the sufferer should leave for a place of light, dryness, and warmth. Bird could provide examples of hundreds of migrants whose chest problems had improved in southern Australia. "Freely we have received the bounties of the Almighty," he declared, "in our brilliant skies, our pure light air, our wonderful immunity from miasma and preventable endemic disease." Admittedly, the hot winds of summer were "prejudicial to many invalids," but Bird pointed out that they occurred no more than a few times each year. In summer, he usually recommended "the bracing southerly breezes of the coast, or the highlands of Gipps' Land or Tasmania"; in spring and autumn, the neighborhood of Melbourne; and in winter he sent patients beyond the Dividing Range to the plains of the interior, where the climate was "heavenly."[83]

Many consumptive men had come to Australia dreaming of physical regeneration. They expected that the change in climate and an alteration in their way of life—especially the opportunities for hiking, camping, riding, fishing, outdoor work, and other manly pursuits—would combine to restore their health.[84] Fantasies of Australian frontier life as pure, wholesome, and invigorating tussled in their minds with older theories of the harsh, enervating climate. Promoters of British migration to Australia were still trying to discount medical concerns about the malign effects of the climate on vulnerable alien constitutions, and stories of its curative effect in tuberculosis gave them an opportunity to wax lyrical. Dr. Carl Faber, for example, admitted that the north of the country was too dry and arid, that the "monotony and dreariness of the scenery" was depressing, and that the environment placed a strain on the European nervous system. But he went on to extol the antipodean atmosphere: "It is the serenity of the sky, the transparency of the air, and a certain exciting something in it which perhaps most appropriately might be termed elasticity." Faber promised the prospective immigrant that "the step seems to rebound from the ground; the heart to expand and overflow from joy in everything around, even were it only the most common Australian landscape."[85] After a long, arduous sea journey, how disappointing the arrival in Melbourne—by the 1870s a coarse and malodorous metropolis—must have been for the lonely consumptive in search of good health and a sprightly gait.

Geographical Pathologies and Pleasures

For most of the nineteenth century, colonial medicine was another way of knowing the country; its topographical and climatological theories were filling up the new space, positioning Europeans in a dynamic and reciprocal relation to a foreign landscape. Immigrant doctors in Australia were attempting to diagnose and to stabilize a new and puzzling order of body and environment. In this sense, geographical medicine was, in part, a discourse of racial adaptation and colonial settlement, a means of structuring, and reforming, the intimacies of blood and land.[86] At times, the landscape and climate might appear threatening or cruelly sublime, no place for a previously healthy white man; then again, the country would seem more picturesque and homely, a medical prescription for European strength and vitality. Opinions differed, but until the 1870s few doubted that the language of medicine would necessarily draw on a vocabulary of climate and circumstance. Doctors routinely spoke the Hippocratic diction of airs, waters, and places; they painstakingly accumulated meteorological and topographic detail with a vigor that would have impressed even Alexander von Humboldt, that most celebrated and prolific of scientific explorers.[87]

What sort of milieu emerges from these medical accounts? It is clear that some medical commentators initially found the country unsettling; the climate and the landscape seemed to contest the European presence. On first impression, Dr. W. J. Sterland had found the atmosphere to be brilliant and buoyant, and he praised the "extreme rarity and dryness of the air." But he was concerned that the interior of the continent appeared "to be an interminable waste of sandy and rocky desert," from which blew dangerous hot winds.[88] Everyone seems to have been discomforted by the hot winds. John Dickson Loch, writing in the 1830s, had noticed that a hot wind might blow over Adelaide for days. "A lady, and by no means a languid one," he wrote, "said she felt a wish to do little but lie down and read in the hot weather." Disappointed, Loch felt that this was "clearly not the climate I left India in search of."[89]

When he set up practice in Victoria, George Wakefield soon learned that it was "the hot weather that brings patients, especially children."[90] In Sydney, Divorty had found the hot winds from the northwest almost unendurable. In combination with the surrounding lack of vegetation and the "dry and barren nature of the soil" that gave "that dull, dreary and sadly monotonous appearance to the country," the result was a profound depression of the European spirit.[91] Andrew Ross also viewed Sydney in an unfavorable light, as its geological formation was "composed chiefly of carboniferous sandstone," and its situation in a "naked, sterile neighbourhood" meant that the summer was "more oppressively hot than it otherwise would be." Furthermore, Ross believed that the flat and alluvial character of the rest of New South Wales would favor the production of "deleterious exhalations of mephitic air."[92]

Even the most dedicated promoters of emigration shrank from hot winds. Dr. R. G. Jameson, who had been a medical officer on emigrant ships, claimed that Australia generally possessed a "delicious climate, a fertile soil." But he also recalled a hot wind in Melbourne, where he experienced:

> An overwhelming lassitude, a disposition to pant for breath, and to adapt the recumbent posture. . . . Cattle lay down with lolling-out tongues— poultry sat motionless with open beaks, and there would have reigned a deep unbroken silence but for the dry hiss of the wind as it swept over parched grass and through the straggling branches of trees.[93]

When William Kelly was caught in a dust storm in Melbourne a few years later, he recoiled from "the terrific blasts of roasting granulated atmosphere" that swept over a town by then "chiselled, carved, columned, and corniced in a fashion of ornate but correct finish"—to no avail.[94] "I felt an involuntary pang of horror," he wrote, "thinking that the sharkskin aspect of my legs was the incipient symptom of elephantiasis." And yet Kelly too adhered to the conviction that the climate of Victoria was otherwise "fine and salubrious."[95]

Like many of their medical colleagues, Divorty and Ross contrasted the depressing geographical monotony and the crushing summer heat with a disturbing unpredictability of the climate. For Sterland, "the extreme vicissitudes of the Australian climate, the great and sudden changes in temperature," as much as the dreariness and the hot winds, were likely to injure the European constitution and excite disease.[96] "A storm of dust in the morning and rain in the afternoon," Thomas McMillan ruefully remarked in May 1855. "Australian weather."[97] Ross also deplored the "oscillating colonial seasons," which so strained the constitution in New South Wales.[98] In Melbourne, Dr. James Neild reported that:

A fall of fifty degrees of the thermometer in eighteen hours communicates a shock to the system it is not always prepared to withstand. The body is taken by surprise, by a sudden check to the circulation upon the surface. The internal organs become surcharged with blood, and unless there be extreme elasticity and very considerable tonic force in all the tissues, there can hardly help but be extreme congestion.[99]

Evidently there were great numbers of surprised and congested European bodies in the volatile climate of the southern metropolis. In providing information about the incidence of such constitutional disturbances, medical treatises often came to resemble meteorological analyses of the region. Conversely, many meteorological reports could be read as medical tracts, and they frequently appeared in the local medical journals.[100]

Already at odds with a freakish atmosphere, disconcerted by hot winds and sudden variation, the British bodily system was also responding uncertainly to the defaced and disrupted colonial landscape. It seemed that ambiguous surroundings, encounters with anything in-between, might especially discompose alien constitutions.[101] Thomas had attributed colonial fever to the abundance of rank vegetation and mudholes in the early days of settlement; therefore, both he and Kilgour welcomed further cultivation and stabilization of the soil, convinced that the remaking of the land would aid British adjustment. The most dangerous period seemed to occur when the soil was first opened up, when the country was between a state of nature and a state of culture. It was at this point that powerful emanations, or miasmata, might beset bodily systems more accustomed to settled conditions. Accordingly, the medical prescription was either to avoid the process altogether or, if the lure of gold proved irresistible, to complete it as soon as possible, as well as to establish in the wake of terrestrial turmoil paved roads, lawns, ornamental gardens, and cultivated plots to make the place more English. Just as personal hygiene worked to maintain the bodily system in balance, so might the completion of cultivation eventually make the environment less irritating and disruptive to any such balanced constitution.[102] In this physiological and territorial homology, the cultivation of both body and soil was self-evidently healthful, with a natural order being repeated in a constitutional harmony.

When William Howitt visited his brother, Dr. Godfrey Howitt, in Melbourne in the early 1850s, he observed that the town still had "a straggling, unfinished appearance, with a considerable number of churches and chapels, standing in open waste spaces." The growing suburbs were "a wilderness of wooden huts of Lilliputian dimensions; and everywhere around and amongst them, timber and rubbish, delightfully interspersed with pigs, geese, hens, goats, and dogs innumerable."[103] On the diggings—"no language can describe the scene of chaos"—he camped with his sons at a place where "an unwholesome miasma arises" and was thus attacked by dysentery. "For three days I lay prostrate with the disease, and broiling with the heat, the whole day persecuted by the incessant attacks of the Australian devils—the little black flies, the most intolerable, unabashed, and shameless vermin that ever were created."[104] Englishmen found themselves "labouring under an almost Indian sun at the severe labour of the diggings," and as a result they suffered "the most frightful effects of cramps and rheumatism, of fever and dysentery." In its unfinished state it was "a most terrible crampy country."[105] But Howitt hoped that the completion of cultivation, the march of civilization, might yet improve it:

> Now, I do not believe that any country, under any climate in the world, can be pronounced a thoroughly healthy country, while it is in this state. The immense quantity of vegetable matter rotting on the surface of the earth, and still more of that rotting in the waters, which the visitants must drink, cannot be very healthy. The choked-up valleys, dense with scrub and rank grass and weeds, and the equally rank vegetation of swamps, cannot tend to health. All these evils, the axe and the plough, and the fire of settlers, will gradually and eventually remove.

It might even fix the dreadful fly problem: "In the advance of cultivation and population the diminution of this insect nuisance must be looked for."[106]

An Australian Medical Distinctiveness

As they became familiar with the topography and climate of southern Australia, doctors felt more confident in advising their communities on how to avoid the common local causes of disease. Conventionally, they urged their charges to become more temperate in behavior and to show moderation in diet and alcohol consumption (though they often recommended a little alcohol to stimulate a run-down system). Immigrants should dress more in accordance with the new climate; they must don hats when working outdoors and wear looser, lighter clothing—though always within the bounds of modesty. Housing needed to be much better ventilated and shaded from the sun. After years of practice in the country, doctors could tell which places were especially unhealthy, where bad vapors or noxious emanations were most likely to arise, and they might instruct their communities accordingly. They would warn colonists to stay indoors when hot winds were blowing, counsel settlers to guard against the sudden variations in the weather and to cultivate and cover the soil—to open up new country—with caution and diligence. Some doctors even asked potential emigrants to think carefully about whether they were sufficiently robust to withstand an initial shock to the system on arrival in the antipodes. But despite all their attempts at health education, doctors still found that they had plenty of patients to call on, as well as a large variety of novel expressions of disease that they might treat.

For most of the nineteenth century, the task of the doctor was the regulation of intake and outgo in order to preserve or to reestablish a physiological equilibrium in his patient. Therefore, treatment was necessarily holistic and idiosyncratic, carefully adjusted to the peculiar characteristics of bodily system and local circumstance. What worked for an individual of one race would be futile if imposed on another; what was expedient in one environment would often be unrewarding when tried on the same person in a different place. Until the 1870s, and perhaps later, colonial doctors had sought to devise a uniquely Australian mode of practice, a local distinctiveness in diagnosis and therapy that would reflect the new circumstances. When comparing the active English treatment of dysentery and diarrhea with the French system of strict repose, Dr. J. W. Mackenna concluded that in Australia "the influence of climate had changed the character of the diseases, and, by consequence, the efficacy of the old practice."[107] New methods must be determined through trial and error and close observation at the bedside. In 1857, Christopher Rolleston, the registrar-general of New South Wales, was concerned that "the analysis of diseases is very imperfect in this Colony," and he felt that "the practice taught in the European schools of medicine may require modification, to adapt it to the peculiarities of an Australian climate."[108] In the 1870s, Andrew Ross was still criticizing a fraudulent universalism or routinism in medicine, the local tendency to resort to a remedy discovered in England "as if the climate, constitution, situation and circumstances, were one and the same as in London." According to Ross, local doctors, if they were to practice with sensitivity, had to emancipate themselves "from such quixotic notions of the universal power of medicine" and to develop instead a medical science "from an Australian point of view."[109]

What, then, was distinctive about Australian therapeutics? From the 1850s, most Australian physicians were advocating supportive measures to counteract the depletive and exhausting local conditions, to compensate for the effects of steady heat and hot winds. In part, this reflected the trend in Europe and the United States during this period toward a more stimulating therapeutics, but it also represented an idiomatic adjustment to an especially harsh environment. The climate seemed generally to act on Europeans to produce a more asthenic, or weakened, physical and mental state, but each outcome was singular, a variable function of the individual constitution and the particular environmental circumstances. On the whole, doctors tended to avoid the usual depletive measures, which included cathartics, emetics (such as tartar emetic), counterirritants (blisters), venesection, and a low diet; instead they resorted more often to stimulants such as quinine, strychnine, iron compounds, cod liver oil, alcohol, and a strengthening diet. The doses might still be generous, but they were generally less so than in Britain or the milder parts of the United States.[110] Divorty, for example, believed that the local diseases all were of the "substhenic type," requiring no depletive measures; fevers usually assumed the "typhoid type" and therefore did not require phlebotomy, unlike in England.[111] Ross noted that widespread "constitutional debility" had led to the near universal colonial use of stimulants, especially alcohol, and the avoidance of depletory treatments.[112] But there were always exceptions, as Mackin's aggressively depletory treatment of sunstroke illustrates so vividly. And the eccentric Dr. James Clutterbuck continued to believe that diseases of the cranial and abdominal cavities assumed in Victoria "a violence of form, and a rapidity of termination unknown in England," which led him, perversely, to propose an even more violently depletive therapeutics. "In this colony alone," Clutterbuck reported, "I have bled some hundreds of persons in different forms, and in various stages of disease; and in no instance have I traced those evil consequences said to arise from such practice."[113] All the same, most of his contemporaries regarded such heroic therapeutics as ill considered, if not dangerous, in an already depleting environment.

BRITAIN IN THE ANTIPODES?

Even as some colonial doctors were searching for a distinctively Australian practice of diagnosis, prevention, and treatment, the grounds for such medical exceptionalism were slipping away, undermined by a rising sense of the ordinariness of the climate, landscape, and social life along the southeastern edges of the continent. It took more than fifty years of closer settlement, but by the 1880s most Australian doctors, and most of their patients, felt more or less at home on the mediocre soils and in the tempestuous atmosphere of the coastal regions south of Capricorn. The great influx of newcomers during the gold rushes had for a time disrupted this process of European domestication, but it soon resumed in the 1860s as gold-seekers wearily gave up fossicking on the diggings and returned to a settled life. Many of them converged on Melbourne, which was becoming a major manufacturing center, soon rivaling many of the English provincial cities in size, squalor, and civic pride. The Australian population began to age after the decline of gold fever, and toward the end of the century in the more settled areas there were almost as many women as men—during the 1850s men had outnumbered women almost two-to-one. As cultivation was established and cities grew, as social life became more normal and stable, calls for an Australian medical distinctiveness became ever more muted, at least in what had become known as the "temperate region" of the southeast.

For some, it was as though they had never left England. By the 1860s, George Bennett was remarking that in Sydney "the style is English, and of course agreeable to English feelings." Gone were his earlier reservations about British acclimatization. In places like India, the colonizer must "adopt new customs, learn a foreign language, and form new ideas of society; but in Australia everything is English, and consequently the feeling of separation from home is less keenly felt, if not dissipated altogether."[114] In 1871, the Reverend James Ballantyne, extolling the prospect of *Homes and Homesteads in the Land of Plenty*, declared that "Melbourne is London reproduced; Victoria is another England. Hence many a one on coming to Melbourne has said that he felt as though he had scarcely gone from home."[115] Plants, animals, and social customs introduced from England had all thrived, often far too vigorously.[116] Thus in his travels through western Victoria, the "Vagabond" could imagine himself "in England once more but for the magpies flying about, and the white flock of cockatoos who are devastating the farmers' corn in the valley. The hayfields and cornfields are English, the fruits are English, the home-life is English."[117] Who in such easy familiar circumstances would need special treatment?

With the gradual normalization of the southeastern Australian climate and topography, the expectation of a local distinctiveness in disease causation and expression also declined, though it was never completely eliminated. A gust of hot wind could always unsettle glib assertions of another England down under. But the environmental differences, and hence medical differences, that in the 1850s had been harshly amplified were by the 1870s almost unaccented in the southeast. Mingay Syder wondered if draining the land and removing the forests had meant that "the climate of Victoria has undergone some change, since 'civilised' man first adopted it as his future haven and home."[118] William Kelly was quite convinced that settlement had altered the character of the weather. "Rains are becoming more equably diffused over the seasons," he wrote, "and hot winds are being gradually driven back into the interior by the increased humidity of the climate, which is easily accounted for by the increase of cultivation and agriculture, causing the rains and moisture to percolate through the soil instead of running off the surface."[119] In the 1880s, the ebullient "Garryowen" confirmed that "there were greater extremes of weather in the old than in the modern times—more sudden transitions from heat to cold, and from wet to dry, more baking hot winds, and swamping floods."[120] James Bonwick believed that the colonial hives of sickness were "undrained swamps, impervious scrubs, unrestrained inundations, wastes without surface water, and townships destitute of ordinary sanitary conditions."[121] All of these lamentable nuisances were improving. Most medical authors praised the beneficial long-term effects of planting shade trees and cultivating the land. As time passed, it seemed that the cultivated, temperate parts of Australia would require less adaptation or reformation of Europeans than previously thought. White bodies, as long as they remained clean, pure, and productive, had come to seem natural, even innocent, in the more hygienic and purified environment of southeastern Australia.[122] After the 1880s, the older medical vision of a mismatch between race and region—which for immigrant societies had commonly pointed to a tragic conclusion—was gradually transformed into the celebration of a new territory for the self-possessed white man.

The emerging sense that southeastern Australia was becoming a natural habitat for the British was, of course, as much perceptual as real. There can be little doubt that the landscape was made more picturesque and more deciduous during this period, but these alterations do not wholly account for the changing perceptions of place. As people settled down, they simply adjusted, got used to things as they were, made homes where they could. The increasing "acclimatization" of Dr. George Wakefield provides us with a compelling example of a change in the perceptual environment. Arriving in Victoria during the gold rushes, young Dr. Wakefield had felt his English system become disconcerted—matter out of place—and he frequently complained of disease. But within a few years he was more comfortable. In 1861, he assured his father that "the climate here has much changed since I came, formerly it was so fearfully hot at this time of year, as to be nearly unbearable and caused the deaths of many from sunstroke, disease of the heart, etc. Now the weather has been quite cold, and wet, in fact much like English weather at this time of year."[123] Later the same year, he observed that we "have wonderful cool summers (the last most particularly so) and very few hot winds, formerly it would last a whole week, and continue off and on for 5 or 6 months. . . . I shall give up all thoughts of ever living in England again and will stick to the southern hemisphere."[124] But Wakefield sometimes wondered whether the place was changing or whether it had in fact transformed him: "Whether the climate is changing or I am getting used to it I don't know, certain it is that it does not affect me as formerly: how I shall bear the air of England I don't know, I am afraid I shall be shrivelled up, for even here, I can stand no amount of cold."[125] When Edward M. Curr, a squatter with "a somewhat vagabond turn of mind," recalled the early colonists of the Port Phillip District, he observed that "our cloudless skies, the mirage, the long-sustained high range of the thermometer

. . . troubled them a good deal more than they do us, and helped to make them look on the dark side of things."[126] But as William Howitt had predicted, the Australian climate had "become a natural fact," which "agreed admirably with the native constitution."[127]

By the 1870s, an increasingly cultivated society and a booming economy were prompting climatic rhapsodies, especially from those who wanted to encourage British migration to the new colonies. James Ballantyne assured his readers that the Australian air "is pure, dry and exhilarating"; he understood that "its hot days are tempered by cool sea-breezes, its skies are brightly blue, its evenings soft and serene, and its winters delicious."[128] Of course the British immigrant might notice an occasional hot wind, which "certainly makes one feel rather uncomfortably warm, stirs the bile a little, and disinclines to much exertion; at the same time, it is by no means the terrible thing that some people fancy it to be." Indeed, it could even be "drinking up any miasma that may be floating in the atmosphere."[129] James Bonwick, that other indefatigable booster of Australasian prospects, argued that the rare hot wind was surprisingly healthful, because it "sweeps off pestiferous vapours into the ocean; it dries up foul and stagnant pools; it comes fresh and pure from inland wastes; it proceeds generally from open country, and brings into civilized parts no products of decomposition."[130] Bonwick admitted that Melbourne weather might be capricious, but the local soils seemed eminently favorable to health, and the Victorian hot winds were "so perfectly pure from miasma." The northerlies "may tend to languor, inflammation of the bowels and nervous irritability, but also tend to relieve the system, by perspiration, with no waste of tissue, and by doing so lessen the action of the kidneys."[131] John Hunter Kerr, a long-term resident of Victoria, joined the exoneration of the hot winds: Although they may be "so exhausting while they continue, [they] are pronounced by the learned to be highly beneficial in their effects, purifying the air and removing all pestilential exhalations." Moreover, the winds made residents like Kerr appreciate other days when "nothing more delightful could be imagined, when the air is pure and buoyant, and all nature basks in a glow of life and soft sunshine; when every respiration is fraught with sweetness and enjoyment, and it seems a privilege to live and breathe."[132]

Medical discussions of the natural conditions of southeastern Australia still could be ambivalent in the 1870s, but optimism was beginning to prevail. Even so, a climate that generally was pure, elastic, and effervescent might suddenly turn volatile, harsh, and irritating. The land seemed more pleasant and restorative than ever before, but it could also be dry, barren, and monotonous. The medical perception of place depended largely on where one was, and *who* one was. By the end of the century, one finds an increasingly sophisticated and detailed differentiation of Australian climates and regions in medical and geographical narratives, with the disparity of tropical and temperate habitats becoming especially marked. The more temperate and cultivated places, those more like Britain, were deemed the more salubrious; but those doctors who still attended to geographical factors continued to disparage desert and tropical environments. And yet anyone who had ever cared about the matching of race and region could show mixed feelings even about the effects of the same bounded environment. One particular Australian landscape and microclimate might elicit any number of conflicting sentiments in an immigrant observer.

In geographically sensitive medical narratives, the new land in all its particulars was an object of fear and desire, and to inhabit it was to experience a range of physical and mental states. Trepidation and anxiety drove settlers to seek a dominance of the environment, just as their desire for intimacy with their new home allowed them to imagine a dynamic relation, a physiological flow, between their bodies and the land.[133] In the nineteenth century, colonial doctors were torn between narcissistic identification with the new country and a voyeuristic distance from it. In this medical vision, now lost to us, the race was longing for reunion with environmental plenitude while simultaneously fearing incorporation into a foreign, consuming topography.[134] Whatever emigration agents might proclaim, British bodies were never completely at ease in the new environment, and the shift from incorporation to alienation, from order to disorder, from health to disease, and back again, might be sudden. As Europeans struggled for material possession of the country, it could turn quickly—a hot wind—and dispossess them biologically. The race was not yet at rest—and not yet at home.

CHAPTER 2

A CULTIVATED SOCIETY

ARRIVING IN MELBOURNE IN 1852, young Dr. Walter Lindesay Richardson first ventured to the diggings to fossick for gold. But it proved not the life for an Edinburgh graduate, so instead he set up a medical practice in the central Victorian city of Ballarat, and eventually he prospered. Although Richardson soon married, he never felt properly settled in Australia Felix, and he pined for more familiar surroundings, for "home." In the 1860s, having returned with his family to Britain, he eventually found himself wandering around Edinburgh, yet even there he was a stranger, a ghost revisiting the scenes of his youth. Back in Victoria, facing financial ruin, the increasingly erratic doctor moved from town to town, finally succumbing to general paralysis of the insane in 1879, leaving his family in genteel poverty. As his daughter Ethel—"Henry Handel Richardson"—recorded in her panoramic trilogy, *The Fortunes of Richard Mahony*, this gauche and unguarded immigrant would never truly find his way home.[1] Like so many of his colonial colleagues, Richardson had become disoriented in a new land: At one moment it could make him effervescent and optimistic, and at another, fearful and apprehensive. In Victoria, he wrote in 1869, "the majority are young, strong and active; they live in an atmosphere abounding in ozone, they are employed much out of doors, their hours of work are short, they partake plentifully of animal food and beer, and, as may be supposed, are full-blooded."[2] But even so, he took these apparent blessings to mean that antipodean disease, when it came, would assume more acute and painful forms. "The sky is cloudless," he advised his Scottish readers, "the air dry, the sensible perspiration from the body is rapidly absorbed, while the process of evaporation keeps the surface at a uniform temperature." And yet these dry British bodies were sadly out of place in the new environment—in particular, the combined influences of heat and dentition were often fatal to colonial infants. Richardson reported that everyone feared "death by solar heat, which at present retards the increase of population in one of the most flourishing colonies of the British kingdom."[3] And then again, just as the country seemed to contest British presence, it would repeatedly draw him back.

Even in 1869 many of Richardson's more "advanced" medical readers must have found his environmental preoccupations a little simplistic and old-fashioned. Late in that decade, social and behavioral explanations of disease causation had come largely to displace such environmental and climatic pieties. Of course, the old Hippocratic lexicon of airs, waters, and places had never completely supplanted social and moral concerns, even during the environmentalist enthusiasm of the 1840s and 1850s; and it would be a long time yet before physical and climatic influences were fully discounted. Disease causation was always a complex matter and rarely, if ever, singular. In explaining a fever or a flux, a doctor might adduce physical or geographical influence, or hereditary disposition, or life stage, or social circumstance, or intemperate habit—or any combination of these and other factors. The weighting attributed to each component of the etiological complex depended on the inclinations of the particular doctor, the class of patient, and the fashions of the time. In the middle of the nineteenth century, European and colonial doctors like Richardson had tended to favor environmental explanations, though they still managed to infuse their interpretations of bodily dysfunction with moral commentary and monitory advice. In expounding on the origins of disease, especially epidemic disease, a later generation of physicians would attend more closely to the contribution of social conditions—to poverty and overcrowding, to personal contact, to stress and friction in closely settled populations.[4]

In this chapter I will describe the partial substitution in late-nineteenth-century southeastern Australia of theories of social pathogenesis for older beliefs in the environmental causation of disease. This explanatory shift has generally been attributed to a rising confidence in the multiform doctrine of *contagionism* that gradually eroded the prevailing *anticontagionism*. According to this schema, anticontagionists, who argued that sickness arose from emanations of filth or other environmental influence (often called "miasma"), gradually lost ground to contagionists, who postulated that most diseases derived from some specific poison or seed or germ, which could be passed from person to person, perhaps through a physical or biological intermediary.[5] The fact that smallpox and venereal disease were somehow directly contagious had long been recognized; by the 1870s this route of transmission was looking less like an epidemiological anomaly and more like a model for all ailments. In other words, medical doctors had become less inclined to map the physico-moral disease topography than to trace a socio-moral distribution of pathology; they spoke less of the *nature* of illness and more about the social *norms* of health.[6] That is, disease seemed less likely to arise from a mismatch of bodily constitution and physical circumstance, or from a sundering of the natural bonds between blood and soil, and more commonly to be caught from mundane contact with others. For most doctors, the milieu that mattered by the 1880s was more likely social, less often physical; more commonly interpersonal, and rarely environmental—at least in those places where geographical difference from the race's ancestral region had come to appear specious and insignificant. (Not surprisingly, most Europeans still distrusted the tropics and felt debilitated between Capricorn and Cancer.)[7] Increasingly, doctors were urging each vulnerable human bundle of ancestry and character, of endowment and will, to regulate personal contact, not environmental exposure. It was the social terrain—especially the congested urban terrain—that counted medically.

Of particular concern was the irresponsible conduct of others—especially other classes and other races, as well as those in the crowded, pullulating cities. In southeastern Australia, then, it became ever more difficult to imagine the expanding urban centers as comforting Europeanized refuges for displaced bodies; they were increasingly represented as uncontrolled social aggregates that threatened the health of a well-behaved bourgeoisie. Among medicos, the southeastern Australian countryside would gradually lose its insalubrious reputation, its sense of brooding, its alien threat, and become instead a haven for worn-out city folk seeking recuperation and social distance in the bush. Hot winds, sudden shifts in temperature, bright sunlight—all were dwindling, little by little, into minor nuisances.

With the rise of contagionist doctrines in the 1860s and 1870s, doctors began to speculate on the character of the disease agent that was being transmitted, to investigate what it was that went from body to body and, occasionally, lodged within. In England, John Snow had suggested during the early 1850s that some agent in human feces might contaminate drinking water and cause cholera outbreaks; William Budd later in the same decade argued that typhoid similarly was spread from case to case, probably by something in excrement. By 1867, Jean-Antoine Villemin had demonstrated that there was a factor in the tubercle of consumption—in the chronically inflamed tissue—that could generate the same disease in another.[8] But what was this seed of disease? Each ailment seemed to have its own special cause, each bred true, but would the agent prove to be a specific poison or a specific living organism—that is, a germ? If contagion explained the pattern of most diseases, then what was the causal mechanism? Was it chemical or biological? Was the agent zymotic, a substance derived from a process of fermentation in the body, or microbial, a tiny life form that could pass from person to person?

Microbiological investigation was proliferating alongside the developing interest in contagion.[9] In Paris, Louis Pasteur had determined that minute organisms were responsible for fermentation and spoilage; by the late 1870s, he had identified the germ of anthrax, a disease that occasionally afflicted humans. As early as 1865, Joseph Lister, a Glasgow surgeon, was using Pasteur's notion of microbial pathology to justify the liberal application of carbolic acid, a disinfectant, in the operating room. In Berlin, from 1880, Robert Koch grew the germs, the minute organisms, of human diseases on solid media in his magnificent laboratories. In 1882, he announced the discovery of the tubercle bacillus, the cause of consumption or tuberculosis, and in 1883 the identification of the cholera vibrio.[10] After the etiological disputation of the 1870s, the air was clearing, revealing a profusion of portable germs, some of them coating the conventional environmental landmarks of pathology—filth and drains—and some of them hitching rides on insects and other fauna, but most of them colonizing human bodies. Increasingly, doctors were relying on the bacteriological laboratory to diagnose disease and track down its cause. Previously, the inciting factors of disease had mostly been obvious—they looked dirty or foul, they smelled bad; now they were minute and invisible—they might lurk in unexpected places and even in meretriciously healthy bodies. Only the laboratory could determine the healthfulness of a place, a thing, or a person. Until a clean bill of health was provided, doctors and lay people alike resorted to old assumptions about what sort of people were more likely, even typically, dangerous, what sort of people were most likely to transport these intangible enemies—often the poor and other races. The knowledge that the socially marginal, or outcast, were nasty and uncouth, or lacking in civilization, became compounded with the apprehension that they might also be complicit in the spread of invisible disease organisms. The suspicion of a human carriage of germs, the anthropomorphic mobilization of disease agency, thus could give pathological depth to long-standing social anxieties that previously had focussed on surfaces, manners, and appearances.[11]

Bacteriology was principally a science of disease identification and prevention—the new science did not initially lead to any major therapeutic advance. In the intimacy of the clinic, it provided a fresh understanding of the origins of sickness, and it suggested a causal mechanism that might stimulate a sufferer to reflect on past conduct and possible points of contact. In the broader field of public health, microbiology revealed a need for meticulous registration of bodies and their excretions, as well as for surveillance of food, water, and milk; it proposed new guidelines for behavior in public and in private; it rationalized the self-regulation of personal contact; it reappraised collective customs and habits; and it justified their reform.[12] Germ theories could help to reshape people's understanding of their bodies, places in the world, and ways of life; knowledge of microbes was also a resource for an interventionist state, dedicated to improving national efficiency and disciplining a potentially refractory population. In seeking to prevent disease, the clinic, the laboratory, and the public health office were thus also saying something about what it would mean to be a good, hygienic citizen; they were suggesting the medical forms that national pride might properly assume. Above all, the votaries of the laboratory claimed a technical capability that might safely alienate, or protect, well-behaved citizens from their circumstances, prevent their contamination, and actively transform the biological and social conditions of human existence. This was especially good news for an immigrant society striving to overcome perceived environmental and social defects and to merge six separate colonies into a new nation. Bacteriology suggested a program of social and behavioral reform that might circumvent, or render irrelevant, any apparently fixed environmental or climatic impediments. By the early twentieth century, the older "Hippocratic agenda"—which David Livingstone has called an "ethnic moral topography"—would become a dead letter in Australian medicine and public health, at least in the temperate south.[13] Poor Dr. Richardson, like other environmental pessimists, could do little but retreat to Britain; a later generation would stay and attempt to create safely hermetic microenvironments—social havens—in the new nation.

In this chapter, then, I will try to identify the point at which biomedical science ceased to be an environmental discourse in Australia and became primarily a discourse on hygienic white citizenship. This demands not only an account of the emergence of new theories of mobile, microbiological disease agency; it will also require some attention to the development of more insulated, particulate notions of heredity. During this period, disease and degeneration come to appear increasingly separable; and yet both, as we shall see, were attributed more and more to the proliferation of bad seeds, of different sorts, within the social body, not to bad interactions with the physical environment. With the muting of environmental interests, at least among the medical elite in temperate southern parts, we can watch as white citizens evolve out of British immigrants and become more mobile and autonomous across an innocuous, or uninfluential, national landscape.

FEVER REFORM IN SLEEPY HOLLOW

With the gold rushes, a growing southern upstart rapidly overtook Sydney in population, in geographical spread, and in the establishment of institutions of learning. A complex and sophisticated city was taking shape in the colony of Victoria, developing all the attributes of modern urbanism, including ornate stone buildings, a web of arcades, factories, a railway network, formal parks, museums, libraries, a zoological garden, a university, and a class structure that mirrored the British social order. In Melbourne, one could find grand buildings, broad avenues, and flamboyant displays of wealth but also slums and destitution, crowded tenements, and crushing poverty. By the 1890s, the small provincial town that had struggled into existence before the discovery of gold was sprawling into a vast metropolis with nearly half a million residents.[14] When Nehemiah Bartley, a colonial rover and speculator, visited Melbourne in 1881 after thirty years' absence, he was astonished:

> Heavens! What a metamorphosis was there in those thirty years of gold-fostered development! Long ere I got to Spencer Street, and after I got out into Hobson's Bay also, there loomed the domes of the Supreme Court and Exhibition Building. Heavenward pointed the tall steeples in Collins Street; towering buildings and factory chimneys marked the site of a city, indeed; where all was dull, tame, flat and empty, in 1851.

Wandering through the more prosperous section of the city, Bartley saw "glorious, garden-strewed, flower-decked, tram and train-served suburbs; where, in 1851, a punt and a dusty, desolate road alone marked the site."[15] Until the depression of the 1890s, Melbourne would remain the preeminent city in the Australian colonies.

From the 1870s, foreign visitors rehearsed Bartley's Melbourne odes. Anthony Trollope in 1871 traveled to "the great metropolis of our Australian empire," discovering impressive edifices, wide streets, extensive public gardens, and vigorous civic institutions. There was, he thought, no town in the world where the ordinary working man could do better for himself and his family.[16] On first impression, Richard Twopeny, an itinerant journalist, wondered whether "a slice of Liverpool has been bodily transported to the Antipodes." He admired the adventurous and enterprising spirit of Melbourne, the high level of literacy, and the generous intellectual life.[17] Writing in the late 1880s, Francis Adams, another journalist, assured his readers that "Melbourne has what might be called the *metropolitan tone*. The look on the faces of her inhabitants is the *metropolitan look*." If Sydney still felt very British and provincial, Melbourne resembled more a combination of London, Paris, and New York. Adams contrasted the "illuded progress" of Victoria with the "deluded stagnation" of the rival colony of New South Wales.[18] He praised, somewhat ambiguously, "Melbourne with its fine public buildings and tendency towards banality, with its hideous houses and tendency towards anarchy"; he saluted the southern "leanness and rigidness, the hardness and nakedness."[19]

As Adams's ambivalence suggests, there was a dark side to Melbourne that its other boosters rarely mentioned. In particular, the health of the people, even during the best of times, was not good—indeed, the spirit of speculation that led to the land boom of the 1880s was not the only contagion abroad in the city. From the 1870s, epidemics of typhoid fever, measles, scarlet fever, and diphtheria swept through Melbourne; smallpox struck in the 1880s; and phthisis, or tuberculosis, had become rife, especially among young adults. Between 1870 and 1890, the annual infant mortality in Melbourne was generally more than 150 for every 1,000 live births, a figure that matched London's (whereas rural rates in Australia were considerably lower than those in Britain). Commonly, infants suffered and died from various diarrheal diseases, usually acquired from contaminated food or milk or water. Among those who survived, rickets and other deficiency conditions were widespread. Urban growth in the working man's paradise had outpaced water supply and sewerage; the poor were appallingly overcrowded in badly constructed dwellings; industrial conditions and wages were in fact little better than in Britain; and hygiene generally proved inadequate.[20] By the late 1870s people were talking about a sanitary crisis in the city. Among its inhabitants, Melbourne was gaining an insalubrious reputation at odds with its marvelous appearance.

In the late nineteenth century, Melbourne owed much of its outward civic decorum to a growing middle class, which consisted principally of merchants, civil servants, lawyers, and doctors. In particular, the number of medical practitioners—those who would be called on to resolve the emerging sanitary crisis—was increasing rapidly during the booming 1870s and 1880s.[21] During the early years, the doctors had all been immigrants, and they comprised an unusually well educated cohort of newcomers, most of them having trained at London or the Scottish universities.[22] The majority worked as general practitioners dispersed throughout the colony, whereas the elite of the profession clustered around Collins Street and Lonsdale Street, striving for appointments to the Melbourne, Alfred, or Lying-In Hospitals.[23] The leaders of the intensely competitive Melbourne medical world had wasted little time in establishing the Medical Society of Victoria (1855) for the exchange of clinical information and the discussion of medical theories. They also had founded the most important antipodean medical publication, the *Australian Medical Journal* (1856), and established the first Australian medical school (1862) at the new University of Melbourne.[24] Although their culture was oriented predominantly around clinical concerns, many of these unusually self-confident and assertive physicians had discerned that an inchoate sense of community unease in the new environment might provide them with a topic and an opportunity for creditable theoretical speculation. They wrote copiously, as we have seen, on the relations of man and nature in southeastern Australia, on the likely effect of the foreign environment on an alien race's physiological system, and on the proper medical means to restore balance and integrity to a disordered constitution. Influenced by their constant exposure to disease and their intimate knowledge of the failures of adaptation, most doctors, until the 1870s, were perhaps rather more pessimistic about the future of the race than their fellow citizens. But the rising social status of the profession and its undisputed claim to represent science in the colonies had allowed these medical men to shape the prevailing understanding of the antipodean environment and the place of Europeans within it.

Melbourne had become a buzzing hive of disease and disease theories. As in the gold rush of the 1850s, the major concern was with typhoid and phthisis, and of these two afflictions, both so prevalent in the community, typhoid, with its tendency to become epidemic and its brief but potentially devastating clinical course, was perhaps the more worrying. Once familiar to settlers as "colonial fever" and generally attributed by them to climatic and topographic circumstances, typhoid—or enteric fever—was increasingly regarded as an urban problem, a consequence not of climatic displacement but of closer settlement. The disease, variously defined, excited widespread fear as it rose in incidence during the 1870s, and thus it also provoked considerable investigation and disputation at the medical society. "That fearful scourge, typhoid fever, lurks in every mucky gutter, drain and cesspool," wrote a correspondent to the Melbourne *Argus* in 1878.[25] Enteric disease, characterized by a low fever, prostration, and diarrhea, was killing hundreds each year. In the 1870s and 1880s, the annual rate of death attributed to typhoid hovered between six and nine for every 10,000 inhabitants of Melbourne; in London the rate was less than two for every 10,000 people. Australian typhoid appeared early in summer and generally affected children and young adults. Its cause was increasingly contested, and preventive measures still were conjectural.[26] In 1872, Dr. J. M. Gunson expressed a lingering conventional view of causation when he assured readers of the *Australian Medical Journal* that "the weight of evidence seems to be on the side of its non-communicability by contagion." Like most of his colleagues, he was still convinced that "the special poison that causes it is conveyed in noxious gases or foetid emanations from sewers, cesspools, drains, dunghills, and all other kind of putrescent animal and vegetable matters."[27] But within a few years this environmental, or pythogenic, hypothesis would be challenged, sometimes in a strikingly vituperative manner, from within the profession.

In 1874, Dr. William Thomson, one of the leading promoters in Melbourne of the new germ theories, reported on a survey of the opinions of local medical men on the cause of typhoid. Trained in Glasgow and Edinburgh, Thomson—vain, difficult, and impossibly energetic—had arrived in the colony in 1852 and, later in that decade, became a pivotal figure in the medical society, editing the journal between 1856 and 1864. But in 1864, growing ever more alienated from his colleagues, Thomson was expelled from the medical society for calling fellow members "blackguards." Thereafter he resorted mostly to tirades in the daily papers and to self-publication.[28] The results of

Thomson's informal survey of Melbourne doctors in 1874 indicated that most of them continued to hold on to theories of filth or putrescence and to deny contagion a role in the transmission of typhoid. Thomson deplored this old-fashioned adherence to the hypothesis that "an unknown something concocted in putrescing organic, especially faecal, stuff, and diffused through air, or food, or drinking water," something quickened into action by the heat of summer, might cause the disease.[29] Having read William Budd on the causes of typhoid, Thomson favored instead the notion that some microorganism was passed from case to case—the disease did not, he thought, arise de novo from a chemical given off in decay and putrefaction. Thomson thus asserted that "a specific typhous virus, shed from diseased glands in the bowels of persons suffering from fever . . . on being exposed to dry hot air becomes crisped into a fine impalpable dust, easily borne on the air, and when inhaled, or mixing with drinking water or food, and therewith ingested, excites fever." There was no doubt in Thomson's mind that every one of the diseases present in Melbourne "has had its specific germs or seed imported." Admittedly, no one had yet identified the germ of typhoid; neither was Thomson able to explain how some people contracted the disease without close contact with other cases, or how others evaded it even when caring for its victims. Nonetheless, he urged the Board of Health to acknowledge "the discharges from the bowels of fever patients" as the only source of a specific germ of typhoid, and he demanded isolation of the sick and the disinfection of their excretions.[30] But this gratuitous instruction was not well received by the board or the medical society. A review of Thomson's tract in the *Australian Medical Journal* condemned him for his "hard-word flinging and self-glorifying" remarks. There was nothing in the book but "an exercitation of contemptuous epithets . . . an overstrained eagerness to display what he obviously desires to be regarded as his own transcendent knowledge." In a style "extravagantly tumid and pedantic," Thomson had offered no proof of the contagionist doctrine. "He is a man of possibilities," concluded the reviewer, "he is always on the point of a discovery, but he discovers nothing."[31]

A few years later, in a balanced presentation of the disputes between contagionists and anticontagionists in Melbourne, Dr. Patrick Smith lamented that doctors were no closer to agreeing on the cause of typhoid, even though the disease had carried off some 3,680 persons in the city over the past ten years. The anticontagionists—still perhaps the dominant party—argued that it arose de novo from fermentation undergone by fecal and other organic matter, whereas contagionists believed it developed after contact with specific germs excreted from a preexisting case. Both groups were now focusing on human excreta: Anticontagionists thought typhoid could derive from any excreta left out in the environment; contagionists thought it must result only from contact with the excreta of those previously infected. (Anticontagion-ists, by contrast, would claim that *fresh* stools even from a proven case could be handled with impunity.) Smith admitted he could not decide between the competing theories. In the subsequent discussion at the medical society, Tharp Mountain Girdlestone and William McCrea, from the Board of Health, favored a chemical cause, arising from putrescence; James Jamieson and many younger members were inclined, however, toward the notion that the disease was spread by a minute living being.[32]

Before long, McCrea, the colony's chief medical officer, would reveal a more ambivalent attitude toward the possible cause of typhoid. Although he had previously favored the pythogenic hypothesis, in 1879 he conceded that fur-ther studies of the "intimate pathology" of the scourge had supported the con-tagionist argument that it was "conveyed by germs and by germs only, from the infected to the healthy." Even though the actual mechanism of transmis-sion was still uncertain, McCrea had come to recommend the use of disinfec-tants such as carbolic acid and air purifiers like sulfur.[33] But this admission was not enough to satisfy Thomson, who continued to castigate the Board of Health for its failure to interrupt and thereby prevent the contagion. Although most authorities were now prepared to accept that the cause of typhoid was a "specific morbid poison," and to concede that "mere weather-kissing carrion cannot create fever without a formal seed," Thomson believed that public health officers remained unwilling to attack, and to isolate, the individuals who were spreading germs. Instead, in a quaint and old-fashioned way, they continued to prattle on about drains and sewers.[34]

An editorialist in the *Argus* was able to state in 1879 that there was "a grow-ing belief among the medical profession, and amongst scientific men more generally, that zymotic diseases are rarely, if ever, originated by the surround-ing circumstances, but are the result of the importation of germs and seeds, and these being favourably placed for development."[35] And yet a few years later, young James W. Barrett, a resident medical officer at the Melbourne Hospital, still could not entirely rule out meteorological influences on the in-cidence of typhoid. Barrett, who was to become a leader of the profession in Victoria, recalled that when he and his brother were fishing along the Salt-water (later Maribyrnong) River, west of Melbourne, they had drunk some water contaminated by sewage from a nearby farm. Though their symptoms had been different, Barrett now believed that they both had contracted the same disease: typhoid. The link to feces was obvious, but the Melbourne grad-uate remained unconvinced by the hypothesis of contagion. He had observed that "there is a distinct relation between the dryness or wetness of a season and the number of typhoid cases occurring in that season." Was it not therefore likely that summer dryness was accelerating the decomposition of sewage and giving rise to some specific poison? It would take some years for Barrett—later an enthusiast for germ theory in the northern tropics—to shift his focus from the sunny cesspit to the immured defecator.[36] But in thus hesitating, Barrett was not alone. As late as 1890, James Jamieson, ostensibly the socially acceptable champion of germ theory in Melbourne, also was still wondering about the pattern of spread of typhoid. Jamieson did not doubt that "minute organisms of bacterial nature" caused the disease, but it did not seem to be routinely contagious, in that many cases developed without contact with the sick. The seasonal fluctuations in the incidence of typhoid suggested "some affinity between it and the miasmatic diseases." Perhaps the germs found their way into the water supply and into articles of food? Perhaps they permeated "emanations from the soil, or from cesspits, drains, etc."?[37] It would not be until the late 1890s, with the gradual acceptance of the notion of the asymptomatic human carrier of typhoid germs, that microbiology and contagion became firmly amalgamated in explanations of the transmission of the disease.[38]

Thomson, not surprisingly, had wanted to utter the last word on typhoid, but his crowing proved premature. In 1882, he announced that:

> Never before did pestilence flee as typhoid fever fled at the magic touch of Germ Theory, learned by studying bacterial aetiology in man and beast in the Baconian method that amiable humanitarians deride. The fever fled from pestilent Melbourne without waiting till the noisome reeking city was drained to civic beauty and olfactory sweetness.[39]

Thomson regarded this as his own achievement because he had campaigned loudly against the dumping of nightsoil in the Yarra and the practice at the Alfred Hospital of irrigating its grounds with sewage. But alas, typhoid had not disappeared from Melbourne. And yet Thomson was surely right to suggest that older theories of the disease's causation and character were rapidly losing ground in the 1880s. "The impetuous fever reformer"—Thomson's image of himself—"would not tarry till dilatory routine in sleepy hollow snored an aetiology from medical books."[40]

Unseen Enemies and How to Fight Them

In the case of diphtheria—often known as "membranous croup" or "malignant sore throat"—a contagious pattern and a microbiological mechanism seemed from the beginning less open to doubt, though never entirely immune to questioning. Largely a disease of childhood and frequently fatal, diphtheria seemed to afflict families regardless of their circumstances and sanitary conditions.

Endemic in the colonies, it was occasionally exacerbated into epidemics, and in Victoria alone it often claimed more than 400 lives each year. In 1872, the Victorian government set up a royal commission to report on the problem. Although the composition of the commission proved controversial, it attracted a great number of depositions. Many of the older doctors still attributed diphtheria to the clearing of land, hot winds, changeable weather, damp winters, or "mephitic air," but the commissioners, led by McCrea, concluded that the disease was commonly spread as a contagion, even if some random cases did seem inexplicably to erupt into isolated communities.[41] Predictably, in an acerbic commentary on the report, Thomson took issue with the commissioners' mild and accommodating tone, with their slightly equivocal conclusion, and with much of his colleagues' antiquated evidence. He asserted that the disease was definitely the result of a "specific virus," which had come to Australia in 1858; it had never, he declared, emerged "spontaneously from atmosphere or terrene causes." Since its introduction, there had been an unimpeded "steady propagation from person to person."[42]

In concurring somewhat reluctantly with Thomson, James Jamieson argued that diphtheria, unlike typhoid, was obviously a "specific contagious disease," requiring local application of "caustics and astringents" to kill its microbial begetter.[43] A Glasgow graduate, Jamieson was then practicing in the coastal city of Warrnambool, but he later moved to Melbourne, where he became first the lecturer in obstetrics and then the lecturer in medicine at the medical school. In contrast to Thomson, Jamieson worked from within the medical society to promote germ theory, initially in a series of presentations on diphtheria and on more general aspects of bacteriology, and then as editor of the *Australian Medical Journal* from 1883 until 1887.[44] During the 1870s, Jamieson would become increasingly definite about the microbial character of diphtheria. It was, he wrote in 1873, clearly the result of the "implantation and growth of a parasitic fungus," which produced a local lesion that later gave constitutional symptoms. The rational treatment, then, was to apply dilute sulfuric acid to the back of the throat in order to poison the "minute animal organisms."[45]

In 1874, Jamieson again emphasized that the intangible agent of diphtheria must be organic and capable of reproduction—he would from now on call it a "germ." It was evident that "no close connection can be traced between the occurrence of diphtheria in a particular locality and the nature of the soil" or, for that matter, the kind of weather.[46] John Blair, a surgeon at the Alfred Hospital, agreed, pointing out that diphtheria made "its appearance under every conceivable variety of climatic and telluric condition, equally with sanitary arrangements apparently faultless, as with those most faulty." Must it not therefore be contagious?[47] Indeed, with few exceptions, the medical elites of

Melbourne were coming to regard diphtheria as a disease spread from person to person by minute organisms, well in advance of the discovery by Edwin Klebs and Friedrich Loeffler in 1884 of the responsible bacillus. Of course, many of their colleagues in the suburbs and the country, and many more of their patients, would continue to attribute membranous croup—and other afflictions—to season or to place for some time yet. But Harry Brookes Allen, a brilliant young Melbourne graduate training as a pathologist, expressed a prescient view when, in 1880, he suggested that a contagious "micrococcus," or germ, might produce a toxin, or poison, that caused the disease.[48] By 1890, informed by the latest results of German investigations, most local doctors would not dissent from this opinion. Fewer still would challenge the microbial explanation after Thomas Cherry, the first bacteriologist in the medical school at Melbourne, reported in 1895 that he had recently seen in Paris and Berlin successful demonstrations of the power of Emil von Behring's antitoxin to neutralize the diphtheria germ's toxin. He had sent back to Melbourne some stocks of this amazing substance. "I regard the remedy as having passed beyond the experimental stage," he informed his fellow doctors, "and that it is our duty to introduce it here as soon as possible."[49] As the first therapeutic achievement of microbiology, diphtheria antitoxin caused a public sensation.

Only twenty years earlier, germ theory had sounded so curious and novel. In 1876, in a pioneering article, Jamieson had claimed that "microscopic organisms play an important part in the causation of many diseases, and especially those of an epidemic and contagious nature."[50] Referring to the work of Pasteur and Lister, Jamieson had recommended to his colleagues the strange idea of a *contagium vivum*, an infectious disease organism that might reproduce indefinitely. In causing sickness, a minute germ would enter the body, and after an incubation period during which it proliferated, it would spread and wreak havoc unless killed by disinfectants. Of course, these seeds of disease required a suitable soil, or "nutritive substratum," if they were to be cultivated within the body—hence the common observation of different predispositions or immunities. Thus in order to stop the efflorescence of disease within a person, the doctor might either introduce "into the blood substances that may paralyse or kill" these germs, or try to "strengthen the system, so that it may resist more effectively."[51] Although he may have been a little tentative in the 1870s, Jamieson before long was much more confident. In 1883, he could report a shift in medical opinion, such that there was now "almost unanimous agreement" that germs "play an important, in fact an essential, part in the causation of most, if not all, contagious diseases affecting the general system." Everyone knew that cholera and typhoid, for example, would spread whenever "the specific virus meets with a prepared soil."[52] Once iconoclastic, Jamieson and other proponents of germ theories had by the 1880s become professional authorities.

Doctors and patients alike were growing more confident that laboratory scientists could detect and cultivate the invisible agents of disease in their laboratories. If Pasteur or Koch, or any of their followers who controlled a laboratory, had identified a microbe as the cause of a disease, then that nexus would hold regardless of any local circumstances. Continental rationalism was edging aside British empiricism: It was expected that the laboratory, wherever it was available, would provide more creditable answers to diagnostic and etiological queries than any amount of clinical discussion and examination. In the past, the sufferer of a disease was deemed to have special knowledge of its character and cause, with insight into the nature of the ailment that derived from unique experience and personal history. Similarly, the doctor had relied largely on local knowledge and familiarity with the family temperament to appraise the patient's story. Increasingly, however, such hard-won experience was a poor guide—clinical narratives appeared diminished, more likely to offer clues than solutions. Ultimately, one would have to be prepared to trust the laboratory man to decide which disease it was and where it came from—if it got to that point. By the end of the century most colonial health departments boasted diagnostic laboratories, and the three Australian medical schools—Melbourne, Sydney, and Adelaide—had begun to teach bacteriology. "In dealing with these organisms we are no longer working in the dark," wrote A. Jefferis Turner, a leading Brisbane doctor, in 1895. "We know our enemy and we know also his strong and weak points, and where he is vulnerable."[53] This was a standardized, even globalized, enemy. It was thus no longer quixotic to assert the "universal power of medicine"—indeed, by the end of the century, to recommend a distinctively regional medical science, as Andrew Ross and his generation had once done, was to invite ridicule.

And yet it was never forgotten that the manifestations of a disease would vary according to the individual's susceptibility or resistance. In the new explanatory framework, a place, much diminished, was thus retained for older understandings of constitutional predisposition. The seed, or agent, of a disease became ever more determinate, but the "soil" still appeared to influence the incidence and severity of the standard disease package. As Jamieson put it, the soil must be prepared to receive the seed. Proper cultivation of the land, Jamieson was telling his colleagues, was in effect less important than careful attention to an internal human soil, a soil tended and protected through custom and habit. It seemed that disease manifestation would continue to depend, in part, on the condition of the body at the time, which was the sum of hereditary endowment, life history, and environmental influence. The tenacity of notions of predisposition and resistance in explanations of disease allowed doctors to make sense of why some people exposed to a disease never developed it, as well as why cases of the same illness might differ in severity and clinical course.

How, then, did colonial doctors respond to these more objectified and universalist notions of disease causation? Mostly, they advised citizens to try to evade the external agents of disease—the germs that could be traced across a landscape and through the bodies of the local fauna, including other humans. Cities still had to be cleaned up and drained; sewage must be taken away; pure water and uncontaminated food secured; buildings ventilated; and the slums cleared. Environmental sanitation remained a focus of the colonial medical profession, even if its strategy and goals, in becoming microbiological, had changed. But in addition, medical doctors and public health officers increasingly were identifying human bodies—especially the bodies of the poor or other races—as reservoirs of recently identified disease organisms. To contain this new corporeal threat to bourgeois health, doctors urged their patients and the public to wash their hands, eat with a knife and fork, use toilets appropriately, and not to spit or otherwise spread bodily secretions. Most important of all, they should keep to themselves, avoiding physical contact with those groups most likely to carry germs: the irresponsible poor (who never listened) and other races (who couldn't help themselves). Stipulations of personal and domestic hygiene thus proliferated at the end of the nineteenth century, supplementing if not supplanting a residual interest in environmental sanitation.[54] Prevention remained better than cure, and, increasingly, preventive measures were the responsibility of the individual citizen—indeed, they came to signify good citizenship.[55] It therefore dismayed H. K. Rusden, a liberal Melbourne social theorist, when many poor people acted "as if they desired nothing so much as to spread [germs] as widely as possible," and he wondered if a medical police would be needed to regulate those without scruples, those still beyond the pale of citizenship.[56]

But what happened when preventive measures failed and someone got sick? Although most doctors in the late nineteenth century had begun to look to experimental laboratory science to provide a more specific or targeted therapeutics, their hopes generally would not be realized until well into the next century, long after many of them had retired from practice. There were, of course, a few successes, such as the use of diphtheria antitoxin in the 1890s and the discovery, in the same decade, that quinine, once used as a general tonic, was a specific treatment for infection with the malaria parasite. In the early twentieth century, laboratory scientists developed a number of chemicals, the organic arsenicals in particular, that showed promise as specific treatments for sleeping sickness and syphilis.[57] Otherwise, doctors still relied on supportive measures and moral persuasion, acting on the belief that if one could not avoid or destroy the seed of disease then at least one might try to make the soil less hospitable to it. Tonics and stimulants thus remained in vogue, and any residual interest in depletory measures was thoroughly discredited by the end of the century. After the 1870s, hygienic management and moral advice were perhaps even more common than stimulating drugs in the doctor's inventory. Nature, which was more or less exonerated in temperate regions as a direct threat to European bodily integrity, might now be called on to ward off disease or to aid in healing efforts. Doctors repeatedly advised their patients to eat well, avoid intoxication, rest, breathe fresh air, exercise in moderation, and, above all, keep clean. Of course, much of this advice was time-honored and familiar, but its goal had changed from maintaining or restoring a systemic physiological balance to enhancing a resistance to specific disease organisms. Finally, if all of these measures had failed and disease progressed, then the doctor would resort to the usual palliative and symptomatic treatments and trust, often forlornly, in the autonomous healing power of nature.

"Here, then, we stand," wrote Dr. J. W. Springthorpe in 1891, "scattered fortresses throughout the plain of existence; each with his own walls and ramparts, a little kingdom to himself." But even in the fortress "enemies may lurk, subtle, potent, and too often unseen," or else "inheritance may have built a weak and faulty structure." Outside, though, was the incessant "border warfare of sanitary science."[58] Springthorpe—known to generations of medical students as "Springy"—was the lecturer in therapeutics, dietetics, and hygiene at Melbourne, and he was warning the public, in a typically ornate fashion, about newly identified germs. "They ride like airy demons in different regiments, which we call by well-known names—the deadly diphtheria, the bothering influenza, the children's triplet, measles, scarlet fever and whooping cough, and manhood's scare, smallpox and cholera." These invisible foes could be found in food, water, sewers, drains, cesspits, and—perhaps most unexpectedly and most dangerously—in humans. "If in ordinary affairs knowledge may be held to be power, in sanitary matters it is no less true that knowledge is life." It was therefore the duty of the citizen to dispel ignorance regarding personal hygiene and, above all, to practice "self-restraint."[59] Otherwise, dread disease would as surely prevail in salubrious southern Australia as elsewhere.

A Consumptive Voyage to the Medical Society

The full meaning of the new understanding of the character and cause of disease is perhaps best appreciated when we consider the reframing of phthisis, or consumption, during this period—one might even refer to its reinvention as a new entity—"tuberculosis," a term first used in the *Australian Medical Journal* in 1880. Well into the 1870s and later, Samuel Dougan Bird and other colonial chest experts had continued to extol the southeastern Australian climate as a cure for those consumptives whose predisposition to the condition was irritated into expression by cold, damp, British weather. At a discussion in the medical society rooms in 1877, all those present, even James Jamieson, agreed that phthisis in its early stages would improve with passage to Victoria. Bird assured his colleagues that he was more convinced than ever that the dry, ex-hilarating, antipodean climate was an antidote to British consumption.[60]

But some reservations had already begun to creep into descriptions of the antiphthisical effects of Australian residence. In particular, it is striking how few of the anecdotes of regeneration and virility were set in the colonial cities. Even Bird acknowledged that social conditions and the habits of life in the more squalid parts of Melbourne might counteract any beneficial features of the climate. Of course, if chest diseases were developing in a land supposedly as inimical to them as Australia, then the sufferers must be behaving very badly indeed. Bird believed that local tuberculosis was finding root in a "large, highly-paid, consuming class," located chiefly in the cities, that indulged to ex-cess—it did not grow among "a large, poorly-paid, ill-fed, manufacturing class" as in England. Most phthisis in the colonies, in Bird's opinion, was a re-sult of "the over-prosperous condition of the hand-working classes, which has tempted them to habits of self-indulgence which they could not have practised at home." Thus imprudence could imbalance the physiological system as quickly as the climate worked to repair it. "Each of us is a walking world, tur-bulent with varying emotion," mused Bird, "and the excesses into which we plunge in prosperity, and the despondency into which we fall in misfortune, equally leave our assimilative functions deep on the verge of the mire and slough of disease." Regardless of the climate, whole classes of people "will over-strain their faculties, succumb to grief or misfortune, abuse Nature's gifts, and disobey her plainly written laws."[61] Similarly, "Medicus," who remained com-mitted to "the climate of Victoria as a specific in phthisis," forswore the temp-tation and nastiness of Melbourne. He had noticed that those who, like himself, went inland reported that "their general health considerably im-proved, the cough was almost gone, the local disease stayed, and the whole constitution had undergone such remodelling as to render them new beings, and to enable them to enjoy their life as such." But woe to those who luxuri-ated in "a fast life about town, living in close hotels, surrounded by the smoke of a thousand dwellings or manufactories, and the obnoxious odours of open drains." The consumptive immigrant required instead "a life in the open air, with judicious exercise, and no indulgence in the passions and vices so insepa-rable from our age."[62] Climate was no good without temperance, and temper-ance was difficult to maintain in an unpleasant, crowded city.

William Thomson, as usual, went further. Sending consumptives to any-where in Australia was, he declared, "a cruel imposition on the patients and a gross injustice to the climate of this country." Thomson had seen many examples where "the hapless patient is hurried to the grave some months sooner than he otherwise would have been." He condemned Bird's "falsely coloured and delusive book," and sneered at the medical society that had rejected him, claiming they "resembled so many wild savages stamping on an enemy."[63] It was obvious to him that only he was paying proper attention to epidemiological evidence. The prevalence of phthisis in Melbourne was at least as high as in London; almost one in three among the adult population of the metropolis, and one in four adult Victorians, died of the disease. Moreover, the influx of deceived consumptives was doing nothing to lower these figures. Thomson urged his refractory colleagues "to look upon phthisis in the colonies precisely as it is viewed elsewhere, to subject it to the same regimen, to observe the same means of precaution, and therefore to be entirely undeceived on the alarming delusion of a protecting climatic influence." The problem was willful violation of the laws of health, as well as personal neglect—it was, in other words, a social and moral problem, not an environmental issue. "Any idea of a climatic variation of the natural history of specific diseases is, as far as this climate is concerned, completely illusory."[64]

Like other colonial progressives, Thomson seized on new germ theories to give an explanatory depth to his interest in social and moral pathologies. He was already convinced that consumption was a problem of promiscuous social contact: In the 1880s, he could point more confidently to a microbial mechanism for the contagion. Thus phthisis, or tuberculosis, required a "transference of infecting particles," and once lodged in the body these germs might find an opportunity to manifest themselves when "the tax on vital energy" proved "too great for inherent stamina." Enhancing exposure and eroding resistance, "the circumstances of individual and social life in England or Australia alike operate to induce phthisis irrespective of climate."[65] Thomson could adduce no examples where "saturated subsoils, damp for want of underground drainage, mountain site or swampy level, dry air or moist, bad ventilation, cellar home or factory toil" had anything to do with the creation of the disease. It owed its origin to "conveyed contagion" alone.[66] The annoying contagionist, eager to apply a rational theory and move beyond "blind empirical tentative effort," therefore recommended measures to improve ventilation and reduce overcrowding: He denounced proposals for a change of climate. They change the sky, he mocked, but not the body, those who go beyond the sea. Indeed, he thought it was as a result of "the false fame the climate enjoys for curing phthisis, and the many phthisical invalids flocking hither allured by the false hope of recovery" that "the native-born, white and black, have been freely exposed to contagion."[67] Thomson was convinced that if "the active cause of true progressive phthisis be a septic germ, from whose invading growth Victorian natives, black or white, have no more immunity than her vines have from phylloxera, it follows that if contact with the destroyer were stopt the fatal effect would cease."[68]

Many of the older generation of doctors retained a considerable personal and professional investment in a geographically oriented medicine, just as many of their patients generally found it easier to affirm the significance of conditions they could actually feel than to accept an agency they had to take on trust. The depressing effects of hot winds and, by contrast, the occasional elasticity of the air were obvious and immediate; but microbes remained invisible and paradoxical. Bird, who for most of the 1880s was the lecturer in the theory and practice of medicine at the University of Melbourne, found it impossible, for personal and professional reasons, to change his mind on the subject of climate and phthisis. Before leaving England he had been given only a few months to live, but after several weeks in Victoria he had recovered, contrary to his own expectations, and he remained in excellent health. From this experience, he thus felt justified in attributing his recovery "to climatic influences alone."[69] His colleague, Dr. John Singleton, could not understand why medical opinion in the 1870s had begun to disregard the benefits of the Victorian climate for consumptives. His clinical experience had led him to believe that "even a cold climate, if free from damp and having good natural drainage, is very favourable to the prevention of phthisis."[70] Many colonial consumptives continued to hope, forlornly perhaps, that an appropriate environment would prevent a relapse of their disease. Baron Ferdinand von Mueller, the phthisical government botanist, had always felt better in the hills, and he recommended towns such as Fernshaw, in Gippsland, "to derive not only the benefit of a moderately rarified and by forest vegetation purified air, but also to get the advantage of inhaling vapours sufficiently charged with the volatile essential emanations of eucalypts, so as to give hope of thereby arresting the progress of the disease."[71]

In 1882, perhaps to the chagrin of some of Thomson's opponents, the *Australian Medical Journal* published a translation of Robert Koch's address to the Physiological Society of Berlin, in which he described the "complete proof of the parasitic nature of a human infectious disease"—the identification of a bacterial cause of tuberculosis. According to Koch, the tubercle bacillus was passed from person to person, and in the right circumstances it would give rise to disease. In the past, as Koch put it, tuberculosis had seemed largely the outcome of social misery—now doctors could concentrate on limiting its interpersonal transmission through the containment of infectious sputum.[72] Thomson believed that his preoccupation with the seed of consumption was thoroughly vindicated, but others put forward a more nuanced interpretation of Koch's discovery. Jamieson, as usual, steered the most careful course. "That organism has certainly some share in the tuberculous process," he assured his colleagues in 1883, "but it seems also, judging from clinical observation and every-day experience, that unless there is some susceptibility in the way of hereditary tendency or local irritation, there is little if any risk, in the human subject at least, of the bacillus being able to find a lodgement."[73] Many people were exposed to the germ, but few developed the disease. Whereas Thomson, like many of the new bacteriologists, was becoming more and more obsessed with interrupting the transmission of the seed, with reducing exposure to the bacillus, Jamieson and others with a more clinical orientation regarded this epidemiological approach as just one among many possible interventions. They also remained committed to making the soil inhospitable to the seed, to enhancing any resistance to the germ, whether through improved nutrition, hygiene, or even, more rarely, a change of climate. If circumstances did not directly give rise to disease, they might still modulate resistance to germs. Climate might run down the bodily system and leave one vulnerable to invisible foes; or it might perk up vital powers and strengthen the human fortress.

All the same, during the 1880s colonial doctors were ever more likely to emphasize overcrowding, poor hygiene, and imprudent behavior as key factors in the development of tuberculosis—all of them now implied exposure to the germ, though to a more limited extent they may have led to greater susceptibility too. It seemed that many conditions might facilitate the lodgment and proliferation of germs, or quicken the course of illness, and with each decade that passed fewer of these conditions were climatic.[74] Of course, some of these other factors, unlike climate, were preventable. Medical doctors urged the authorities to clear the slums and improve the working conditions of the poor; they advised their patients to behave temperately and to avoid immorality and promiscuous contact. Stipulations of personal and domestic hygiene, and behavioral injunctions, were reworked to limit the transmission of the disease agent as much as to enhance the vitality of the sufferer. Thus admission to a sanatorium was advised as a means of isolating the transmitters of tuberculosis, not simply for its recuperative qualities. Less crowding in the cities would reduce the spread of disease as well as make the inhabitants feel more comfortable and relaxed and, thus, more resistant to attack by the recently identified microbial pathogens.

While in the 1850s most doctors had concentrated on nourishing the constitutional soil, the grounding of illness, from the 1880s they paid as much attention to limiting the seeds of disease, those new microbes that so wantonly coated most people, most landscapes, and most climates. By the end of the century the major medical journals in temperate regions such as southeastern Australia gave little space to climatological theories; their pages were crawling with germs, germs, and more germs. Of course, it was suspected from the beginning that some classes and races of people might be more efficient at spreading these seeds—and such exaggerated figures, such stereotypes, would soon become the new salients in the medical war against disease.

FROM HEREDITARY SOIL TO HEREDITARY SEED

When J. W. Springthorpe offered guidance to the Melbourne public on how to fight unseen enemies, he warned, poignantly, that inheritance might "have built a weak and faulty structure," which would allow them entry and sustenance. Still mourning the early death of his wife, Springthorpe stressed "the vital importance in selecting in marriage such material as tends to build up a strong resistant fortress."[75] Similarly, when William Thomson was accused of becoming too narrowly focused on preventing the transmission of germs, he acknowledged that:

> All hygienists know that children reared amidst foul air are stunted, blanched, etiolated, sickly, melancholy, dwarfed in mind and physique; and that adults living, or rather struggling for life, in unwholesome atmospheres . . . become dyspeptic, nervous, irritable, wan, feeble, irresolute, craving for stimulants to conquer the languor of vital depression following deprivation of wholesome invigorating stimulus so amply provided in pure air by nature.[76]

Both Springthorpe and Thomson thus were able to point to elements of predisposition, whether hereditary or developing through the life span, that might alter disease acquisition and expression or would, alone, cause bodily dysfunction or degeneration. And then both turned quickly back to the more exciting business of tracking those invisible foes.

Although somewhat eclipsed by bacteriological enthusiasm in the late nineteenth century, notions of predisposition and resistance to the exciting cause of a disease never sank entirely below the medical horizon. By the end of the century, as they came to accept the new germ theories, doctors reworked their explanations of the origins of disease and altered the advice they gave on how to avoid exposure to the recently identified pathogens, but they maintained an interest in the differences in susceptibility and expression observed in practice. Evidently their patients, aware that contact with germs was virtually unavoidable, wanted to know why they sometimes succumbed and other times resisted the widely distributed pathogens. In response, doctors often resorted to variations on the notion of predisposition, which was the sum of heredity, developmental influences, and habit. The common denominator was heredity, as custom and habit, cultural style, behavioral proclivity, temperament, and capacity for civilization were all commonly reduced to ancestry.

In the past, doctors in immigrant societies had often focused on a mismatch between racial endowment, as the matrix of predisposition, and a foreign environment, which was potentially pathogenic. But after the 1870s, as temperate environments are increasingly exonerated, or as macroenvironment is taken out of the disease equation altogether, the medical understanding of predisposition is more often construed in terms of individual susceptibility to specific microbes. In southeastern Australia, where the microbes appeared to be the usual cosmopolitan ones, mostly transmitted socially, the presumed racial element of endowment was no longer a distinguishing factor in disease manifestation. But in the tropical north, with a microbial ecology as distinctive as its climate, the lack of previous European exposure, and hence adaptation, to the local pathogens would still matter, or at least it would still warrant further investigation. In the temperate, domesticated south of the continent, in contrast, one finds in the 1880s arguments for a greater *internal* differentiation of disease susceptibility and resistance, an emergent sense of the importance of persisting hereditary and developmental variation within the race that was making itself at home along the coastal fringe.

The hereditary differences within the white population were coming to seem at least as significant as the difference between the white race and its rather homely antipodean circumstances. Previously, as we have seen, doctors had been inclined to attribute disease and degeneration in immigrant societies to environmental or climatic maladjustment, to a misalliance of race and place, but from the 1880s many of them were more likely to locate pathology, infectious or not, deep within the social body. In a temperate, homely environment, such as southeastern Australia, disease and degeneration would now more often appear to germinate within the race, to arise and spread (through contact or reproduction) from subgroups with bad heredity, from those such as the urban poor, criminals, and the insane, who displayed heritable physical, cultural, and moral faults or deficiencies. In the 1870s, for example, Twopeny and other visitors to Melbourne began to complain about the larrikin pushes (or gangs) and the Bourke Street mob, dissolute criminal elements, often derived from convict ancestry, that seemed almost to take over the metropolis from within, threatening civic and moral order.[77] The problem—for comfortably settled races at least—was not by this stage so much the disease and degeneration of a whole type as the disease and degeneration that appeared increasingly to proliferate within a type.[78] It was the duty of the progressive doctor in a temperate region, then, to concentrate less on protecting vulnerable whites from alien surroundings and to work harder to regulate social conduct and to protect whites from one another—or from themselves. European civilization in the new world, and elsewhere, seemed less susceptible than ever before to circumstances and far more likely to be eroded from within or, rather, to be consuming itself from within.

This rising sense of separation, or alienation, of the body from its physical environment reflects changes in the understanding of heredity or, more precisely, revisions of the notion of adaptation, the interaction of endowment and circumstances.[79] Understandings of heredity in the nineteenth century are complex, but it is important to review them here. Assumptions of hereditary dynamism, an expectation that characteristics acquired by parents would pass on to future generations, still determined the contours of the conceptual landscape for most of the century, but such notions of a soft or pliant heredity increasingly were challenged. In the middle of the century, a few among the medical elite had argued instead for a fixed human template, a design that was either permanently fitted to its circumstances or not. By the 1880s, other experts, many of them—as we shall see—influenced by Darwin's latest pronouncements on the place of man, were coming to regard heredity as more insulated, more detached from environmental influence, than it had generally seemed during previous decades. Continuing to gather force toward the end of the century, such notions of a harder, more alienated hereditary endowment would eventually prevail.

In general, then, colonial doctors initially held to a belief in more pliant and adaptive heredity, with innate and acquired characteristics sutured together as a heritable composite, influencing physiological and pathological status. Many of the leaders of the profession had trained in the anatomy schools of Edinburgh, Glasgow, and London, where they were exposed to a French "philosophical anatomy" that was materialist and progressivist. A few, like James W. Agnew and E. C. Hobson, had even studied in Paris.[80] In their medical training they learned about Jean-Baptiste Lamarck's theory of the inheritance of those parental characteristics acquired through habit and use, through adaptation to circumstances; and they imbibed Etienne Geoffroy St. Hilaire's notions of an organic unity of composition and the serial, continuous relations of animal life.[81] Before the 1880s, most of the doctors who migrated to Australia would have been prepared to see rapid changes, modulated by habit and environment, in racial types and in the diseases to which they were subject.

The changes in racial type—not necessarily pathological—were perhaps most striking. The white natives of Australia had seemed to inherit the qualities that their parents developed or acquired in new circumstances. In the 1850s, Dr. James Kilgour had commented on the "slighter muscular system of the Australian youth," known as a result as "cornstalks." He had observed the same puny frame in local Aborigines, horses, and cattle. As the emerging "Anglo-Australian race" adapted to its new realm, its hair and eyes would become lighter in hue, its build more slender, and its skin darker. Kilgour expected that the climate would shape "a gay and temperate race like the inhabitants of southern France, preferring the wines produced by their own luxuriant vines to the stronger liquors of northern Europe: impulsive in temperament and impetuous in courage, with little thought for the morrow."[82] According to the novelist Henry Kingsley, young Australian males typically were "lanky, lean, pasty-faced, blaspheming blackguards, drinking rum before breakfast, and living by cheating one another out of horses."[83] Traveling through Australia Felix in the 1850s, Samuel Mossman and Thomas Bannister complained of the excessive heat, disrupted land, and turbulent social life; but they found, in contrast, that "the tribe of bushmen whom you encounter in the interior, present a rough and somewhat uncouth aspect, yet they exhibit more manliness of deportment than you will find amongst the peasantry of the most favoured localities in Great Britain and Ireland." According to the emigration boosters, an atmosphere transcendently pure and buoyant had produced "well-proportioned men, seldom showing any appearance of paunch, or inclination to obesity; vigorous and active while walking, with an upright carriage. They look like men who can stand fatigue." However, the transformation was as yet scarcely appreciated. "Think of that, ye maidens, who pine away in single wretchedness, the ripeness of your youthful charms."[84]

Others were considerably less sanguine about the effects of the environment on body types. Always pessimistic, Dr. Andrew Ross in 1870 lamented that the "present white native born subjects fall far short in too many instances of the standard of health, strength, durability and even longevity of their parents." The cornstalks represented a "long and attenuated form of growth," with poor muscular development a result of excessive riding.[85] When Charles Dilke, a British liberal politician, toured the colonies, he regretted that "the fitness of the term 'cornstalks' applied to the Australian-born boys was made evident by a glance at their height and slender build; they have plenty of activity and health but are wanting in power and weight." In Adelaide, he observed that the women were "small, pretty and bright, but with a burnt-up look," while the men born there were "thin and fine-featured." "The inhabitants of all hot dry countries," Dilke asserted, "speak from the head, and not the chest." It seemed that a slender, effeminate, weak-voiced type was emerging in the antipodes.[86] A correspondent of the *Victorian Review* expected that racial dislocation, the sundering of bonds of blood and soil, would thus produce an "inevitable degeneration of the Anglo-Saxon stock."[87]

While predictions of the transmutation of European bodies and constitutions abounded in the nineteenth century, a few leading colonial doctors, even during the heyday of Lamarckism, had denounced this wild speculation on physiological and pathological change of type. Such theories, and predictions, denied divine providence and challenged the Creator's original design. It did not much matter to some local luminaries whether the doctrine was attached to the name of Lamarck or, later, of Darwin—all transmutationist or evolutionary theories were equally deplorable. At the Melbourne medical school, for example, George Britton Halford, the first professor of anatomy, physiology, and pathology, resisted evolutionary incursions, from all sources, well into the

1880s. Halford, once a promising physiologist, was nominated for the post by Richard Owen, the great British paleontologist, and he endorsed his mentor's arguments for a biological science organized around fixed Platonic archetypes. Practicing a conservative Romantic anatomy, Halford taught that living forms derived from a stable, internal organizing principle, the manifestation of a higher power, not from a simple functional adaptation to circumstances. Halford condemned all transmutationists for denying this fixed organic plan.[88] It was as an ossified Owenite that he attacked the alleged deficiencies of T. H. Huxley's demonstration of human and ape affinities. In 1863, in *Man's Place in Nature*, Huxley, the chief promoter of the new Darwinian evolutionary theory in Britain, had applied his master's precepts to the question of the origin of humans, a subject not touched on a few years earlier in the *Origin of Species*.[89] Halford was incensed, and he quickly issued a tract that took issue with Huxley's specific claim that gorillas, like humans, have two feet and two hands—no, wrote Halford, they have two hands and two feet *with fingers*. It followed that man could not have evolved from apes. "Surely the intricacies of the monkey's foot were planned," exclaimed Halford, "as was also the comparative simplicity of man's. They could never run the one into the other, or, to use a fashionable scientific term, be 'developed' the one from the other." The anatomical findings of the Melbourne professor—circulated as *Not Like Man: Bimanous and Biped, nor yet Quadrumanous, but Cheiropodous*—were readily dismissed. Not surprisingly, William Thomson, a committed evolutionist and disciple of Geoffroy St. Hilaire, quickly put his boot in.[90] But Halford also found many supporters among the conservative members of the colonial intelligentsia and the medical profession: Both Mueller, at the Botanical Gardens, and Frederick McCoy, the professor of natural history at Melbourne, continued to campaign vigorously against theories that described a change in human type.

All the same, regardless of Halford's efforts, most colonial doctors had favored a vague, imprecise form of Lamarckism, a rapid adaptationism. Initially, there had been a sense of impending doom in such foreign circumstances (as physiological adaptation might mean degeneration to the local type), and then there was a tinge of optimism. After the 1880s, the local understanding of transmutation or evolution was as likely to be justified by reference to an interpretation of Charles Darwin as to Lamarck. The presumed mechanism of evolution was rarely confined just to Darwinian natural selection—the principle that nature selects for or against random variations in an organism—and commonly still included a Lamarckian inheritance of characters acquired through habit and need. After all, even Darwin often resorted to the inheritance of acquired characteristics, as well as to natural and sexual selection, to explain the emergence and proliferation of new characters. The notion of an inheritance of acquired characteristics was to prove remarkably tenacious right through the nineteenth century. The greater dynamism of such a Lamarckian mechanism, the promise of quick returns over a life span or a mere generation or two, continued to appeal to many doctors, who wanted to make observations and get rapid, yet lasting, results.

But when in 1871 Darwin finally applied his evolutionary doctrines to humans in the *Descent of Man*, he made it difficult to discern any immediate clinical relevance in his theories, arguing that the development of civilization had largely insulated advanced races from the selection pressures exerted by nature and exposed them more to the rigors of sexual selection.[91] In other words, those who were really serious about following Darwin after 1871 would have to concede that human heredity in civilized communities was, surprisingly enough, now more or less fixed, or at least there would be no major change in heredity in response to new environments, alteration in habit, or clinical intervention. When James Jamieson and Dan Astley Gresswell, both leading advocates of a strict Darwinism in the medical profession during the last decades of the century, explained the significance of natural selection, they did so largely to provide further scientific gloss to germ theory, and to the profession, not in order to guide decisions about patient management. Thus Gresswell, in an address to the medical society in 1895 on "Darwinism and the medical profession," urged his colleagues to "give what aid we can towards building up a complete Biology, as a science which must ultimately take cognisance of all conditions of life, regular and irregular, normal and abnormal, healthy and diseased." The colony's senior public health officer then discussed the evolution of diet and the selective advantages of pain sensation. But he emphasized especially the importance of using knowledge of human evolution to guide state action.[92]

Like many other popularizers of natural selection in Melbourne, Gresswell wanted to understand what the new theories of heredity and adaptation might mean for public policy. If, as Darwin had proposed, natural selection was no longer effective on humans in civilized communities, might not this explain the recent success and preservation of the maladapted, especially the urban poor, criminals, and the insane, all of whom should have been eliminated in a struggle for existence? In the past, racial degeneration had seemed to derive, through a Lamarckian dynamic, from a lamentably good adaptation to bad conditions; now it appeared that the race was deteriorating because the environment, whatever its qualities, was unable to select out the unfit from within it. As circumstances appeared to exert ever less influence, degeneration increasing came to seem a simple function of unregulated heredity.[93] An indulgent and overprotective civilization, not geographical displacement, appeared to many by the late 1890s to be the major threat to the quality of the race. Just as disease was acquiring a biological explanation that indicted certain forms of social interaction, so did degeneration separately assume an increasingly hereditarian form, which also, albeit in a different way, directed attention to social processes, especially to reproduction.[94]

It is important not to overstate the degree of acceptance in the late nineteenth century of theories that implied a more insulated human heredity, an endowment more or less unfastened from environment, nurture, and habit. The most "advanced" members of the profession were gradually coming to favor a less environmentally nuanced view of the body, a more persistent and impervious hereditary endowment. But Lamarckian assumptions still were common at the fin de siècle, and they would find advocates well into the next century, as we shall see. An older generation of doctors continued to expect that characters acquired through the habit of living in a particular place would be passed on to later generations. For them, change in habit still commonly implied a change in heredity.

Most social commentators and colonial visitors continued to argue that a change in environment would change the race. Their talk of the emergence of a new Australian type persisted, even increased, as the numbers born locally came to dominate, and a more assertive nationalism developed in the decades leading to the federation of the colonies in 1901. "The race that withers in India, and changes in America," wrote James Bonwick in 1886, "preserves in Australia the best features of its physical and mental excellence." The nation did not "become dwarfed, as in London, nor bony and straight-haired, as in the States." Currency lasses showed a "delicate bloom, a beautiful skin, a good figure, a merry laugh and a lively tongue"; while "the wiry frame, the swift foot, the nervous tension, and good humour of the currency lads by no means denote a deterioration of physique."[95] Richard Twopeny had observed in English migrants "an increased love of dram—and especially spirit—drinking; in apparel a general carelessness"; and "a roughening of manner and an increase of selfishness." But the newcomers were also turning more athletic, tolerant, and democratic and less reserved—on the whole they demonstrated an improvement in type, which Twopeny expected would be passed on to later generations.[96] Marcus Clarke, the sardonic Melbourne journalist and novelist, believed that in the south "the Australians will be a fretful, clever, perverse, irritable race," with the boys becoming "tall and slender—like cornstalks." With wry humor, he predicted that "the Australasian will be a square-headed, masterful man, with full temples, plenty of beard, a keen eye, a stern yet sensual mouth. His teeth will be bad, and his lungs good. He will suffer from liver disease, and become prematurely bald." By 1977, the average Australian male "will be a tall, coarse, strong-jawed, greedy, pushing, talented man, excelling in swimming and horsemanship." His wife "will be a thin narrow woman, very fond of dress and idleness, caring little for her children, but without sufficient brain power to sin with zest." And in five hundred years "the breed will be wholly extinct."[97]

While on the wallaby track in Victoria, the "Vagabond" suggested in 1886 that "two influences decide the future life of infant humanity—heredity and environment. Scientific authorities are not agreed as to which is the greater factor. Under ordinary conditions I really think environment . . . has the most to do with one's character."[98] But the amiable "Vagabond," like his fellow environmentalists, was by then diverging from the most advanced medical thinking in Melbourne, even if many in the profession would still have shared his views. By the end of the century, the physical environment, including climate, was largely exonerated in the latest medical texts as a cause of disease or degeneration—of any typological change at all—in the temperate south of the continent. Most doctors, informed by the new bacteriology, had come to believe that a disease developed only after infection with a specific germ—a seed spread usually by promiscuous personal contact or irresponsible behavior—although its manifestation, its expression, would still depend in part on innate and developmental influences. Racial degeneration had more or less come to appear a problem separate from disease, and the result, according to the rising Darwinians, not of a mismatch of body type with environment or climate but rather a consequence of the preservation of bad hereditary seeds, the protection of poor specimens from a struggle for existence. Thus white destiny in southeastern Australia was gradually condensing down to a matter of bad, impervious heredity—bad seeds—and the social life of germs—more bad seeds. Environmental influence was less and less a part of the problem, or part of the solution, though it was never completely expunged from consideration. In the tropical north, for example, in circumstances that still seemed terribly foreign to Europeans, anxieties about the effects of environment and climate continued to prompt calls for further investigation. Would a civilized white race in the tropics be as impervious to physical circumstances as in the south? Or could the surroundings prove so exceptionally hostile to an organism that had evolved long ago in utterly different conditions as to cause death? Or might a Lamarckian dynamic still operate and cause a gradual deterioration, a sinking to local standards? What, now, would the doctor and the scientist have to say about the destiny of a working white race in the Australian tropics?

IMAGINING THE CITIZEN

Although clinical duties tended to preoccupy colonial doctors, many of them still found time to influence public debates and to engage in a wide range of civic and cultural activities. Some of them had helped to establish major cultural institutions such as libraries, museums, and universities; many more sought to become opinion leaders in their communities. In speaking of difference and pathology, stability and change, continuity and variation, medical doctors were making available to their fellow citizens new ways of thinking about themselves and their place in nature. Biological and civic metaphors circulated between the clinic and the colonial literary salons, crossed from the clinic into the colonial public sphere and back again. This ceaseless traffic gave new inflections to words that might describe the diverse experiences of migration and settlement, health and disease, progress and degeneration.

In late-nineteenth-century Australia, a liberal, professional elite in Melbourne came to dominate debates over the character of disease, man's place in nature, and civic responsibility. From the 1870s, a rising generation of doctors, afire with enthusiasm from germ theory and evolutionary doctrine, challenged the more conservative, nostalgic beliefs of their predecessors. While Bird, Singleton, Richardson, and others from the gold-rush generation continued to seek to reestablish, or even to enhance, the bonds between blood and soil, race and circumstance, Thomson, Jamieson, Allen, and other young Turks proclaimed a certain independence from their physical surroundings, whether novel or antique. They were, in general, proudly rationalist, earnest, and liberal. Often trenchant and dogmatic, they were confident that medicine could contribute to material and moral progress in the colonies as elsewhere.[99] As freethinkers or Calvinists, they proposed to intervene in their growing communities to correct social pathologies and to treat moral infirmities; they called for more self-restraint and self-possession, for manly forbearance, in order to limit the spread of the biological seeds of disease and the hereditary seeds of degeneration. While an earlier generation had sought to master its physical circumstances, the more wowserish (or suppressive) sect that came to prominence in Melbourne in the 1870s and 1880s hoped mostly to master its own society.

Fever reform in sleepy hollow, as Thomson put it, was always a constructive endeavor. Medical thought and practice were rendering legible, and simplifying, first the colonial environment and then the bodies, the character, and the social world of the colonizers.[100] Thus fever reform built on a reframing of the southern Australian environment and a reformulation of ideas about race, sociality, and disease in an out-of-the-way place. First, doctors had charted the physical topography, documenting any pathological features; then, more commonly, they mapped the social terrain. After all, germs were biological agents only in alliance with social actors—it was social life that truly animated them. Having once urged immigrants to cultivate and domesticate the new land, doctors now sought to enroll the state in a proper cultivation of bodies and their social life, hoping to extirpate the pathological undergrowth.[101] Once primarily an environmental discourse, with some moral overtones, medical science by the 1880s had come mostly to provide a vocabulary for discussions of civic responsibility and social citizenship.[102] Medicine and public health made it possible to differentiate the irresolute subject, in need of surveillance and discipline, from the reliable, self-governing white citizen. But then, most whites, even those once engaged in promiscuous contact and dissolute behavior, might eventually learn to speak the language of self-mastery, modernity, and progress, they might pick up the lingo of hygiene, they might become health-promoting citizens. The capacity of other races for hygiene, and thus their eligibility for social citizenship, remained uncertain.

PART TWO

THE NORTHERN TROPICS

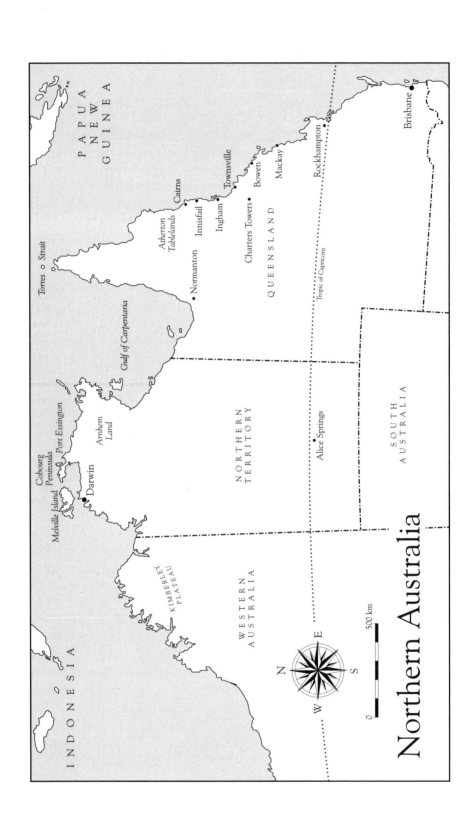

Northern Australia

INDONESIA

PAPUA NEW GUINEA

Torres o Strait

Gulf of Carpentaria

Melville Island
Cobourg Peninsula
Port Essington
Arnhem Land
• Darwin

KIMBERLEY PLATEAU

WESTERN AUSTRALIA

NORTHERN TERRITORY

• Alice Springs

SOUTH AUSTRALIA

• Normanton

Atherton Tablelands
Cairns
• Innisfail
Ingham
Townsville
Charters Towers •
Bowen
Mackay

QUEENSLAND

Rockhampton

Brisbane

Tropic of Capricorn

N
E
S
W

0   500 km

CHAPTER 3

NO PLACE FOR A WHITE MAN

AS THE SOUTHEASTERN PARTS of Australia became a domesticated British territory, the northern tropics continued to challenge even the most hardy of white sojourners. By the end of the nineteenth century, the temperate zone of the continent was exonerated as a cause of disease or degeneration among transplanted Britons, but above Capricorn heat and moisture still threatened to sap the vital forces of working white men and their dependent wives and children. Increasingly, the Australian tropics were marked off as a separate, racially dubious territory, in contrast to the more cultivated, picturesque, and innocuous southeastern crescent.[1] In medical texts, geographical reports, and popular literature, "tropical" was positioned against "temperate"; "wilderness" against "civilization"; "promiscuity" against "restraint"; and in a racial summation of these dichotomies, "colored" contrasted with "white." The sense of tropical difference that emerged and filled out during the nineteenth century came to represent an impediment to a purely white Australia.

Visitors were especially attuned to regional difference. Even in the 1850s, Samuel Mossman and Thomas Bannister, colonial adventurers, had contrasted the emerging bourgeois vigor of the temperate south with the degrading lassitude of tropical territories. North of Capricorn was not, they asserted, "such a healthy climate to reside in as the less humid regions of the south; it does not possess, generally, that pure and dry atmosphere which distinguishes the climate of Australia from all others we have experienced; and the humidity which prevails during the hottest months of the year enervates the European constitution."[2] In 1871, when Anthony Trollope arrived in Queensland, which had separated from New South Wales in 1859, the frontier colony boasted some 120,000 white residents, more than 25,000 of them in Brisbane, its southerly capital. As he went north, Trollope found that "the subject of heat is one of extreme delicacy in Queensland." Everyone admitted that whites in the northern tropics could not work the land; they relied instead on Pacific Islander, or

"Kanaka," labor.[3] Charles Dilke, a roving imperialist, also lamented that "the Queenslanders have not yet solved the problem of the settlement of a tropical country by Englishmen." Reluctantly, he concurred that colored labor, in a state of peonage, would be required to cultivate the vast tropical territory.[4]

During the nineteenth century, the boundaries between places—between regions and between climates—became ever more deeply etched into the thinking of educated Europeans. The tropics stood out most vividly, even if the defining features remained various and disputable. Some preferred a cartographic definition, referring to the region between Cancer and Capricorn; others emphasized meteorological difference and attempted to measure heat and humidity; still others delimited the place botanically, as within the "palm line." The equatorial region resisted easy categorization, but no one doubted that it represented a different type of natural order from that which prevailed in Britain, or even in southern Australia. As Raymond Williams has suggested, what is often being argued in the idea of nature is the idea of man.[5] Thus colonial scientists and others, in trying to define tropical nature, were at the same time structuring and restructuring relations of humans—whether local or alien—to the environment and to one another. In bounding a place, they were also making a race and prescribing race relations. These "tropicalisms" shaped European self-perceptions, enhancing a sense of cold-climate virility and vigor and intimately associating whiteness with civility, even as they provided opportunities for segregating or disciplining the tropical bodies that were emerging—wasteful, irresponsible, and grotesque—from the luxuriant undergrowth.[6] In the tropics, then, Europeans—assertively and anxiously—"conjured up their 'whiteness' . . . and reinvented themselves" and others.[7]

But this reinvention of self always seemed fraught with hazard. In the torrid north of the continent, specters of white degeneration and disease still passed over the landscape. Although the influence of the physical environment on health had come by the 1880s to appear quite limited in the temperate south, such concern was more resilient in the tropics. Even more than in Melbourne on a hot day, British bodies felt dreadfully out of place in a Queensland cane field, especially during the wet season. It stood to reason that a race was best fitted—whether through design or evolution—to resist the diseases of its ancestral realm and most vulnerable to those encountered in a thoroughly different place. Of course, disease might no longer appear to derive directly from circumstance, from a mismatch of racialized constitution or temperament with place, but a region as geographically distinct as the tropics might have also generated its own distinctive biological pathology. A displaced temperate race would presumably not have had any chance before arrival to develop a resistance to such peculiarly tropical pathogens. Furthermore, newcomers might find their bodily system so utterly disconcerted in new circumstances as to overthrow all their normal resisting powers, so that they might suddenly become vulnerable even to ordinary cosmopolitan germs. And if white settlers did not succumb to specific disease in the tropics, who was to say they would not still endure a slow degradation of physical and mental qualities, a degeneration to the local state of nature? Even after the decline of medical geography, a muting of older Hippocratic arguments in temperate regions, most doctors and scientists in the tropics thus retained a notional geography of disease, where disease agency was now biologically mediated, though somewhat climatically delimited, and human susceptibility still racially determined and distributed.[8]

What, then, was to be done? How should the tropics be developed along physiological lines? Could a working white race ever establish itself in perilous North Queensland and thrive? In this chapter I describe the persisting fear of white vulnerability to tropical disease and degeneration, tracing the incremental separation of these putative processes, as experts began to talk of a biologically mobile, and hence preventable, disease agency and to distinguish this from systemic degeneration, still commonly attributed to solar or climatic cause. By the end of the century, doctors could identify the specific germs or parasites that gave rise to tropical diseases such as malaria, dengue, and filariasis. They could, moreover, follow the passage of many of these microbes through their transmitters, or vectors—usually insects distributed through the tropics. They were also able to locate the microbial hosts—typically assumed to be native races, long resident in the tropics and thus presumably accustomed to these agents. Of course, as specific tropical disease is thus mobilized, and anthropomorphized, so that its link to landscape or climate appears biologically or racially mediated, then doctors might rely more on conventional methods of prevention—isolating, excluding, or perhaps cleaning up alleged human hosts and eradicating insect vectors.[9] But well into the twentieth century estimating—and enhancing—white immunity or resistance to these weird microbes would present a continuing challenge to medical colonizers. And in any case, the succubus of white degeneration, a mental or physical degradation deriving directly from climatic displacement, still lurked in the tropics. Would racial hygiene and the electric fan offer sufficient protection from surroundings potentially injurious to the race? Or would acclimatization lead inexorably to pigmentation and nativization? As we shall see in later chapters, it was not clear until the 1930s just what, if anything, was to be done about such durable tropical threats to a purely white Australia.

In entering the Australian tropics in the late nineteenth century we are shifting gradually from "British" colonies to a "white" nation. Previously, in what came to be called the temperate south, "British" had been the new settlers' preferred self-description, although "white" was used occasionally even in the late eighteenth century. A tension had appeared to pertain between

Britishness—a physical, mental, and cultural amalgam—and foreign circumstances. But by the end of the century, with increasing human mobility and autonomy, racial anxiety and assertion were concentrated on an imagined struggle for existence in the north of white against black, brown, and yellow—a tussle among races for possession of the Australian tropics.[10] Southern elites were, in effect, attempting to validate the insemination of a hitherto naturally "colored" space by "white" males. The tropical frontier had become scene of race struggle and, therefore, a crucible for the production of a virile and robust white national identity. According to Randolph Bedford, journalist and Labor parliamentarian, the fear of white degeneration in the tropics was "the prejudice of ignorance. There's not a bit of Australia that isn't a white man's country. There's no enervation—as in Java or Singapore. It's Australian, not tropical heat." As for Bedford—well, like so many other nationalists, he had found around 1901 that "the romance of world-owning caught me."[11] Before long, colonial doctors and scientists would be volunteering to promote this racial advance, offering to police the boundaries of the new white frontier—and to clean up within.

WHITE SPOTS ON THE MAP

The history of failed and forsaken settlements in the north had long haunted those, like Bedford, who proposed the establishment of a working white race in the Australian tropics. Fort Dundas was perched on Melville Island in 1824, but sickness, monotony, and disastrous encounters with the local inhabitants soon led to its abandonment. Malnutrition, scurvy, dysentery, and ophthalmia prevailed among the 120 or so soldiers, marines, and convicts; the climate seemed malignant and unhealthy, the soil sterile. By 1828 no one remained in the dreary, remote settlement. Similarly, within the first year of arrival in 1827, everyone at Fort Wellington, at Raffles Bay on the Cobourg Peninsula, had been affected by sickness, and the site was deemed unhealthy. The seventy who had struggled on, despite scurvy and fever, were evacuated in 1829.[12]

The garrison at Port Essington, established in 1838 for trade with the Malay archipelago and to deter the French, took longer to succumb to its debilitating circumstances, but once fever struck in 1840 the marines were never quite free of it.[13] John McArthur, the commandant, believed that malaria had been introduced from the swamps; he reported that had it been as bad soon after their arrival "we should have pronounced the climate to be very unfit to encounter and have rejoiced in making our immediate escape."[14] McArthur attributed the sickness in Port Essington to tropical nature alone, and even though regular contact had been maintained with the local Aboriginal population and with visiting Macassan traders, they did not intrude on his explanations of disease. His concerns were environmental. The heat was excessive, the soil sandy, the rainfall unreliable—all hope soon faded. At times, almost everyone at the isolated northern outpost was suffering from fever and ague, with the result that the garrison was crippled. In 1843, McArthur complained that "even to keep the quarters in a cleanly state is almost more than can be done." He had lost a number of men to "bilious and congestive fevers"; others suffered from "virulent fever" and "intermittent fever"; they were too unwell even to try to leave through Lombok and Singapore.[15] Some of them improved after doses of quinine and copious draughts of beer, and the convalescents seemed to benefit from the more healthful nearby environments of Port Smith and Observation Cliffs. But the fever continued to rage, and the settlement had an air of neglect and decay when young T. H. Huxley, a ship's surgeon and a keen observer of man's place in nature, visited it on HMS *Rattlesnake* in 1848. Never one to mince words, Huxley, who loathed the tropics, later wrote in his diary:

> As for the place itself it deserves all the abuse that has ever been heaped upon it. It is fit for neither man nor beast. Day and night there is the same fearful damp depressing heat, producing an unconquerable languor and rendering the unhappy resident a prey to ennui and cold brandy-and-water.

The climate, in combination with overwork and bad food, made the place uninhabitable by Europeans.[16] McArthur agreed, lamenting that "the European constitution will never exactly accommodate itself to Tropical Climates . . . the ghastly spectre of endemic disease doth stalk forth in these Regions."[17] In 1849, he and the debilitated remnants of the garrison finally abandoned their experiment in white settlement.

Immigrants had encountered slightly more salubrious conditions in the southeastern "subtropical" parts of what later became the colony of Queensland, but even around Moreton Bay, later Brisbane, it proved difficult to implant a thriving white settlement. From 1825 the site of Brisbane was simply a dumping ground for the worst convicts, those who had committed further crimes after transportation to New South Wales, but there were never more than 1,000 in residence at any one time. During the late 1820s, the miserable, remote jail—a week's sail north from Sydney—was buffeted by epidemics of scurvy, dysentery, and malaria. In 1828, drought led to crop failure and severe malnutrition; eye blight, probably trachoma, broke out and became endemic; and before the end of the next summer dysentery had killed 220 convicts. But over the next decade, health improved at Moreton Bay, and "febris intermittens" in particular (almost certainly malaria) gradually declined in incidence. The fever had been attributed to exhalations from newly cultivated ground, particularly at Eagle Farm, where the sun's rays seemed most efficiently to evolve miasma—but as the soil became stable again, and regularly cultivated, the disease eventually departed. With less crowding of convicts, better food, and a safer water supply, the penal settlement staggered on until the early 1840s.[18] Free settlers began arriving in this decade, as squatters moved overland into the Darling Downs, driving herds of sheep ahead of them. Pastoral settlement proceeded apace, and at the time of separation from New South Wales in 1859, the new colony of Queensland claimed 23,500 British residents, mostly clustered in the southeast. Brisbane had become a struggling, dusty frontier town, with a public hospital and a few dozen medical doctors. At the end of the 1850s, the local medical fraternity was finally able to report the disappearance of ague, or malaria, from the subtropical Brisbane region.[19]

With longer medical experience in the north, it became evident that ordinary ailments—typhoid, diphtheria, phthisis, and so on—still comprised most disease in the Australian tropics, even if these familiar visitors sometimes assumed odd forms. But many of the new settlers, astray in an unusual environment, also suffered from quite unusual fevers and fluxes, some of them apparently unique to the tropics. Along the sparsely settled Gulf of Carpentaria, a local "gulf fever" afflicted those who tried to reside in the area—like most colonial fevers, this was probably typhoid, though some later wondered if it had been a form of malaria. Certainly there was considerable ague, or intermittent or remittent fever, across northern Queensland. Although these malarial fevers had disappeared in southern regions in the 1850s, they continued to exact a heavy toll on life in the far north until the twentieth century, and they were not definitely eradicated until the 1920s. Along the eastern coast, those clearing the scrub came down with a variety of more obscure fevers, later attributed to typhus and leptospirosis. In the Queensland bush, until the 1920s, one might see men limping along with one grossly enlarged leg, suffering from elephantiasis—the result, as we now know, of infection with filarial worms, transmitted by mosquitoes whose range is limited to northern areas. Dengue, characterized by high fever, headache, prostration, and painful bones and muscles, and eventually recognized as yet another mosquito-borne illness, was first reported in the 1870s and since then has continued sporadically to afflict northern residents. The earliest reports of hookworm infestation date from the late 1880s, but the disease, which can cause anemia and fatigue, soon became widespread in more closely settled areas.[20] Whether one favored an environmental or a microbiological explanation of disease causation, the Australian tropics were demonstrating at least a few distinctive etiological and epidemiological features.

Despite their fears of tropical disease and degeneration, Europeans moved relentlessly northward to take up land, and later to prospect for gold. In 1846, pastoralists crossed over Capricorn and began grazing sheep along the Fitzroy River, and by the 1860s squatters and their cattle occupied the Barkly Table-lands. Later, meatworks were established at the rough tropical ports of Townsville, Cairns, and Bowen. Townsville, founded in 1864, was by the early 1880s an outpost of a few thousand people and the terminus of the railway line from Brisbane. Most of these early settlers in the north claimed British ancestry, though many of them must have wondered how long John Bull's legacy would last. Sugarcane, the most typical of tropical crops, had been introduced into northern New South Wales and southern Queensland in the 1860s; by the end of the century more than 60,000 acres of cane grew in the Australian tropics.[21] As soon as they began sugar cultivation, white planters started to import Pacific Islanders, whom they called Kanakas, to cut the crop, for natives of the tropics were deemed natural (and cheap) workers in conditions of moist heat, an atmosphere so trying to the British. As a result, toward the end of the century almost one-third of the Queensland coastal population was from Pacific islands.[22]

When gold was found in Queensland in the 1870s, the population swelled rapidly, as whites from the south left worked-out fields to try their luck along the Palmer River. Chinese miners also rushed in, and by 1874 17,000 were prospecting in the tropics, more than half the North Queensland population and 10 percent of the colony's total population. But in the late 1880s, when laws restricting Chinese immigration came into force, the proportion dwindled to 2.5 percent, only slightly more than in other colonies.[23] Many of the remaining Chinese become part of the plantation labor force in the 1880s, after the end of the Palmer River gold rush, but generally they preferred to farm fruit, corn, and rice.[24] The local Aboriginal Australians were not regarded as reliable plantation labor; they tended to be fringe-dwellers, heading, it seemed, for inevitable extinction as a result of race competition from Europeans and Asians.[25]

Without sugar or gold, the Northern Territory, administered from South Australia, would prove far less attractive than Queensland. In 1864, the Northern Australian Company had established Palmerston at Port Darwin as a farming settlement, but few Europeans were interested. No more than a few hundred whites continued to cling tenaciously to the territory, many of them, after 1877, running cattle on poor country. However, the number of Chinese—often employed as coolie labor—increased rapidly, from 200 in 1877 to more than 7,000 in 1888. From the late 1870s, Japanese were imported and used as a cheap and allegedly adaptable work force around Darwin. But all of these territory newcomers were greatly outnumbered by the northern Aboriginal people, and they would remain so well into the next century.[26] On the whole, it hardly seemed a white man's country.

A DOOMED RACE IN THE TROPICS?

For most of the nineteenth century, the tropics revealed to Europeans a disturbing scene of racial degeneracy and dissolution. The natural inhabitants of the torrid zone seemed especially lacking in vital force and mental vigor. A white race planted in this region would surely either sink to the same low level of civilization, or succumb to local diseases, or else become infertile in such alien circumstances and wither away entirely. One way or another, most experts regarded whites as a doomed race in the tropics.

The physical environment and the tropical climate seemed to generate vapors, poisons, and even germs that were especially harmful to the bodily systems of European residents. In 1866, a fatal fever had arisen in Burketown in the Gulf of Carpentaria, causing it to be abandoned in favor of nearby Normanton, which promised a more healthful site. The catastrophe stirred Dr. J. Aitken White to describe the unique fevers of the gulf. He wondered if they were all really varieties of the same "affection," merging with one another, together the result of "the inhalation, *especially at night*, of a heavy noxious malarious vapour." Unnatural geographical circumstances had led to a constitutional imbalance in the alien race. Dr. White supposed that such disorders of European bodies would be corrected, or rebalanced, only with doses of ipecac, calomel, rhubarb, and quinine—or removal to a more temperate region if all else failed.[27] Dr. Graham Browne, reporting on his medical experiences in Charters Towers, warned that "at night a miasma arose covering the flats, and hatching malarial fever; while to anyone passing between the rows of closets, the stench was unendurable." Typhoid prevailed during the wet season, its incidence "highest when there was sufficient rainfall for assisting putrefaction and fermentation in these warm months." Like many of his colleagues, Browne found it hard to distinguish all the new fevers that were emerging from the tropical environment to afflict white residents, and he regularly gave everyone calomel, quinine and salicylates.[28] Dr. Philip James, a London graduate working in Croydon, also announced that in North Queensland he had "arrived at the conclusion that it is always safe, and nearly always beneficial, to add quinine to every prescription."[29] Quinine generally seemed to act on the white constitution to counter environmental influence and thus reduce, though not eliminate, tropical fevers.

"Colonial fever" may have disappeared from a southern medical lexicon, but it still registered in the north, usually as typho-malaria. Dr. David Hardie, a Brisbane children's doctor, reported that in tropical Queensland it was uncertain "to what extent colonial fever, slow continued fever, and typhoid fever may be associated with or influenced by the malarial poison." In developing the tropical north, whites were unavoidably harvesting typho-malaria. "We know," wrote Hardie, "that malaria is intimately connected with the opening up of new country and the first approach of civilization in to any district."[30] In Hughenden, Dr. J. Sidney Hunt had diagnosed many cases of typhoid and malaria and often found it difficult to distinguish these fevers. He felt that "the tendency of a malarious soil saturated with water and sewage would be to generate a poison of the typhoid type, which would manifest itself in the prevalence of a fever having the mixed characteristics of malaria and typhoid." Hunt also remarked on "a widespread belief among dwellers in the bush and others that as a district becomes stocked up the fever dies out."[31] In Normanton, during the 1880s, Dr. T. S. Dyson noticed that malaria was still prevalent "where the dense scrubs with rich soil are found, and also in the low-lying marshy country; also wherever new or virgin soil is for the first time worked." Dyson recalled that along the Johnstone River, "as the ground became cleared, so the fevers also became of a milder type and less prevalent."[32] When Carl Lumholtz, a Norwegian anthropologist, traveled into the Queensland tropics to go among "cannibals," he found himself struggling instead with irritating flies and mosquitoes. The air seemed to vibrate with the heat, and many times a day he had to lie down in the burning sun and rest his weary limbs. "There is fever," he found, "but almost exclusively in newly settled districts, where the soil is yet uncultivated. Though sometimes fatal it is of a milder type here than in other tropical lands." Lumholtz understood that "as the soil gradually becomes cultivated, the fever disappears."[33] The question was whether the north could ever become sufficiently settled and pastoral—or submitted to stable cultivation—to suppress completely the fevers of the untamed, wild tropics.

After 1890 most whites in the tropics understood that they must watch out for germs, even if scientists had not yet identified them precisely, and that these germs would insist on lodging preferentially in the environment. Queenslanders also suspected that their constitutional struggle for existence in such hostile conditions had lowered their resistance to the local terrene microbes, to these localized pathogens. In the Australian tropics, then, germ theory remained wedded to environmental and climatic pathology much longer, and more intimately, than in temperate regions. Thus David Hardie observed in 1893 that typhoid might arise from specific germs associated with the unsanitary condition of towns; but such conditions persisted all year long, whereas the incidence of typhoid varied. This was because in summer the bacilli propagated more vigorously, and in winter whites had a more robust constitution, a result of "the stimulating properties of the weather."[34] Hardie attempted to correlate death rates from disease in Queensland with barometric pressure, temperature, rainfall, humidity, and cloud coverage. Deaths from diarrhea and dysentery, for example, tended to rise with the onset of the warm season, as "the rising and high temperature, together with the electrical condition of the atmosphere, probably

act both directly upon the nervous system and indirectly through the food supply in raising the mortality and admission rate."[35] When germ theories came to
Queensland they often left their contagionist baggage in Melbourne or other
southern cities. Everyone continued to implicate the tropical environment,
even if scientists had not yet determined its exact relation to the germs that prevailed there.

Malaria and other colonial fevers were not the only problems for whites in
the tropics. Even if specific disease was avoided, it was feared that the environment might still independently precipitate degeneration in the qualities supposedly typical of the white races.[36] In such a different climatic zone, would
not whites acquire the racial characteristics appropriate to life in that region
and then transmit them, in Lamarckian fashion, to their offspring? Was it not
inevitable that anyone living in the tropics would naturally become colored
and assume the customs and habits of colored people? Joseph Ahearne, the
first president of the North Queensland Medical Society, in 1890 addressed its
meeting in Townsville, and he warned of possible racial degradation. "We find
ourselves in the tropics," he said, "certainly a strange, if not an unnatural habitat for the European." He asked his medical colleagues the following questions: "Is our race being affected by residence in North Queensland? To what
diseases are we liable?"[37] In his own experience, malaria had become mild and
rare, and dysentery and dengue had almost disappeared. But like most northern doctors, Ahearne believed that as a consequence of exposure to new surroundings "a modification of type is in the course of formation." The
mechanism of deterioration was tropical anemia, the direct result of climate
acting on the bodily system of a displaced race. In men this led to "a pallid appearance, a wiry physique, and nervous temperament." Among women, it explained the "almost universal languor, the absence of energy, the frequent
attacks of indisposition." Repeated infusions of European immigrant blood,
and reduced consumption of meat and tea, seemed the only answers.[38] A few
years later, J. S. Hunt, a surgeon who also was practicing in northern Queensland, reiterated the concern that "our Race is becoming differentially modified." In particular, he warned that children raised in tropical conditions were
acquiring, or even by then inheriting, the characteristics appropriate to the climate and growing up unusually wiry and nervous.[39]

Ahearne and Hunt were merely repeating an apparent truism of tropical
decay. For the best part of the preceding century, biological theory and popular sentiment had mutually reinforced the fear that Europeans inevitably became lazy, degenerate, and diseased in the tropics. As usual, the ability of
white men to labor productively was the most reliable test of racial adaptation. In 1879, James Hingston reported that "the clime of Northern Australia, and that of Queensland, is inimical to the white man's labour, but

kindly to the olive-skinned Mongolian." It was therefore necessary "to en-courage the Chinese to seek work in a vast, undeveloped country, where they are so much needed."[40] In 1882, Sir William J. Sowden reported that "with regard to the effect of the [tropical] climate upon labour, there seems to be a concensus of opinion that Europeans cannot do the hewing and the drawing. That must be undertaken by coloured folk."[41] Dr. Kevin O'Doherty, a plan-tation owner and member of the Queensland legislative council, declared in 1884 that "no white man could venture into the scrub to work in it during summer without sacrificing himself"—all those who tried "would come out with utterly broken constitutions or would leave their bones in the scrub."[42] In the legislative assembly, Hume Black pointed out that for whites work un-der a tropical sun "eventually ends in their premature decay and physical wreck, even when not hastened by stimulants taken perhaps with the object of maintaining vital energy." Such failure would "involve not merely the de-cay and ultimate ruin of the industry but the physical and moral degradation of those engaged in exhaustive toil."[43]

Even in southerly Rockhampton, according to Edmond Marin La Meslée, a founder of the Queensland branch of the Geographical Society of Australasia, "Europeans find the climate too hot for outdoor work, and if North Queens-land is to be fully developed, it will be necessary forcibly to import labourers capable of standing the climate, be they Negroes, Hindus or Chinese."[44] "If tropical Australia is ever to be thickly populated," declared R. W. Dale, an im-perial booster,

> it will not be by men belonging to the great race which has erected Sydney, Melbourne and Adelaide, for they cannot endure severe and continuous labour in a tropical climate . . . Englishmen, Scotchmen, Irishmen may find the capital, and may direct the labour; but the labourers themselves, who must form the great majority of the population, will be coloured people.[45]

Twenty years later, Alfred Searcy, the dapper customs officer at Darwin, re-called that "during my fourteen years' residence there I had splendid health with only slight touches of fever." This had convinced him that some "Europeans, un-der certain conditions, stand the climate perfectly," but his wife and children had lasted only a few years before he sent them back south. Moreover, in no cir-cumstances would he "suggest that white men should actively engage in the pro-duction of tropical products on the coast, or rivers, or swamps," as "that can only be carried out by coloured labour."[46] Ecological reasoning seemed repeatedly to suggest that northern Australia was not a proper white habitat.

For white women and children the torrid zone was especially perilous. Al-though Alfred Deakin, a Victorian liberal politician and later prime minister, thought some British men could thrive when cutting sugar cane, it "involves a strain upon most of them and climatic conditions for their families which are uncongenial."[47] Robert Gray warned that "we have yet to learn whether in a climate where white women physically deteriorate, anything approaching close settlement in the true acceptation of the term can be brought about." Only with colored labor under white male supervision—with women and children left behind in the south—would North Queensland "be made a wealth-producing country."[48] The Right Reverend Gilbert White, the first bishop of Carpentaria, echoed the concern that women and children are "as a rule, unable to stand the climate, except in the tablelands, without serious injury to health . . . It remains to be seen whether the tropical lowlands will ever evolve a race of white women and children who can maintain their health there. As yet they have not done so."[49] White, who had lived twenty-two years in the tropics and always enjoyed excellent health, reassured his readers that "I am physically stronger and better than I was when I came to the north in 1885." But he found the white women of his flock "anaemic and constantly ailing" as the climate tended "to produce and intensify the diseases peculiar to women." European children in the tropics "grow too fast, and are pale and lacking in life and vigour, unless they get a change to the south."[50] In 1911, Dr. A.T.H. Nisbet, speaking from twenty years' experience of medical practice in Townsville, warned the Australasian Medical Congress that unnatural white settlement in the tropics meant that "our race is dwindling away to a few highly exotic anaemic people incapable of producing their species unless fed with a constant strain of European migration . . . Women have mammary development too deficient to sustain child rearing, they are infertile and their children are given over to convulsive seizures."[51] For Dr. Nisbet, Bishop White, and many other early-twentieth-century commentators, not much had changed since J. Langdon Parsons, the government resident in the Northern Territory, had lamented that "to the ordinary English emigrant, the bare mention of 'the tropics' is sufficient to conjure up visions of pasty-faced children, delicate women, and men with bad livers."[52]

While biological theories of man's place in nature may have suggested problems for white Australia, they had been a blessing for labor practices in colonial Queensland. As Kay Saunders has suggested, the "climatic-racial concept had provided the intellectual framework for the legitimation of hierarchical labour patterns on the estates in tropical Queensland."[53] Independent producers indentured Pacific Islanders, deemed cheap and reliable laborers, on small, relatively inefficient plantations. Poor food, inadequate housing, and medical neglect meant that the Islanders, supposedly adapted to the exigencies of a tropical climate, had a death rate four times higher than that of Europeans in the north.[54] And yet even this great disparity was not sufficient to shake prevailing assumptions of racial immunity. Matthew Macfie quoted the manager of a large sugar mill who believed that "no European with any self-respect or regard for his health would cut cane from choice. It was never intended that white should do outside manual work in the tropics. The black man has a skin provided by nature to resist the heat." A sugar planter from the Herbert River assured Macfie that the sugar industry without black labor was impossible.[55] In his presidential address to the 1911 Australasian Medical Congress, Dr. Antill Pockley, a northern practitioner, confirmed that "it is questionable if the white races can ever permanently occupy the tropics. . . . It would appear to be inevitable that if we are to hold this fine country we must either let it remain unproductive, or comparatively so, or we must evolve some scheme by which we develop it by using coloured labour."[56]

The theories of an aging generation of Australian biologists, geographers, and doctors were endorsed by many experts abroad. When Matthew Macfie addressed the Australasian Association for the Advancement of Science in 1907 on the development of tropical Australia, he could quote established local and overseas scientific opinion on the matter, all of it "in opposition to the visionary and unscientific absurdities of Messrs. Barton, Deakin, Reid, Kingston, Forrest and other self-interested partisans of the 'White Australia' movement."[57] Baldwin Spencer, the professor of biology at the University of Melbourne, had written to him to confirm that "the coastal parts of the Northern territory are not suited for white men—at least not if anything like hard manual labour has to be undertaken."[58] Macfie went on to quote Herbert Spencer, Ernst Haeckel, and other leading nineteenth-century scholars of human development in support of climatic determinism. Benjamin Kidd, the American social theorist, in his influential book *Control of the Tropics*, had summed up their arguments: "The attempt to acclimatize the white man in the tropics is a blunder of the first magnitude. All experiments based on the idea are foredoomed to failure."[59] Macfie also put great weight on the research of Major Charles Woodruff, M.D., from the United States Army, on American blonds in the Philippines. Woodruff had demonstrated that "tropical and sub-tropical exhaustion, loss of memory, tropical and sub-tropical asepsia, neurasthenia, several obscure skin diseases, and some curious fevers are due to the action of the actinic [ultra-violet] rays on a body which has not sufficient pigmentation to resist them." Macfie took this to mean that "each climate is exactly suited by natural law to the particular human racial type evolved under its influence, but cannot be adjusted to any other."[60]

A few years later, Woodruff (by then repatriated from the Philippines with tropical neurasthenia) wrote to Dr. Richard Arthur, the New South Wales medical reformer and parliamentarian, expressing his interest "in the Australian experiment in human transplantation." He confirmed that in the tropics "it is a waste of time to discuss the possiblity of the survival of any vegetable or animal form evolved to survive the vastly different factors of colder and darker climates." The white races should abandon tropical colonialism in favor of a biologically correct tropical commensalism. "The muscular labour must be done by the types of oxen, horses and men able to stand the climate, and the brain labour by northern Europeans temporarily resident." The scientific study of man, Woodruff concluded, "is a very practical matter now, and not the academic one of the past."[61]

MAKING THE WHITE RACE WORK IN THE TROPICS

But even in the nineteenth century not everyone deplored white settlement in the tropics. Some, like H. Ling Roth, a Queensland medical doctor and anthropologist, endorsed the prevailing environmental determinism yet remained optimistic, arguing that there had not yet been sufficient time to see if the climate was truly "deleterious" to white races.[62] Others, such as James Bonwick, an indefatigable rhapsodist on Australian prospects, observed in 1886 that men in North Queensland were "by no means a nervous, dyspeptic class"; rather, they exhibited a "robustness and vigour, a brightness of eye and elasticity of step, an energetic activity with an appreciation of pleasurable repose, equal to anything known in a temperate zone elsewhere."[63] Bonwick conceded that women and children did not do so well, but he insisted that the climate was generally salubrious. "Where the stock thrive so well, men can venture in safety," he wrote of Queensland. "Acclimatisation may be hardly possible in the miasmatic jungles of India, but already healthy generations of English origin have appeared in the pure atmosphere of Australian forests."[64]

Many of the early settlers had anticipated Bonwick in assessing the racial carrying capacity of the land according to its record in sustaining their European stock. If other European animals could thrive, so too should European races; or at least they should reach basic physical standards, if not high mental attainments. An overlander visiting the Clarence River country in 1857 had been convinced that "splendid pasturage for sheep and cattle insured the early success of those who took up country and settled down to steady work."[65] When W. Lockhart Morton traveled inland from Rockhampton in 1859 he was astonished to find rich soil and green grass; light breezes, not hot winds, were blowing over the good cattle country. Morton therefore recommended it for white settlement.[66] Similarly, when Joseph A. Panton visited the Kimberley District of Western Australia in the 1880s he traveled through "not coarse tropical grass, but good, short, ripe pasture, with heads full of grain," a pastoral scene that "would have delighted many of my squatter friends."[67] Nonetheless Panton held some reservations about the suitability of the Kimberley for white settlement. The natural inhabitants of the region were "a poor race physically in comparison with those of the Riverina" (in New South

Wales); and if the land was good for cattle, it seemed still more suitable for the cultivation of cotton or sugar cane, crops which naturally implied colored labor.[68] John Forrest, the explorer and politician, became even more worried when he passed through the same territory, warning "it is not a climate that one would desire to live in from choice." He could not imagine that the tropics would ever prove "a home for the Anglo-Saxon race."[69]

From the 1880s onward many more commentators were prepared to assert the naturalization of whites in the tropics, regardless of medical and geographical theories. In 1885, John Mackie, visiting the Gulf of Carpentaria, had met with "the bronzed pioneer squatter, with his easy self-reliant style."[70] Pastoral pursuits, even in the tropics, seemed to breed strong human stock. More surprising, perhaps, the sugar industry also offered opportunities for robust white labor. In 1888, the Brisbane *Boomerang* asserted that "white labour *can* be employed at sugar growing and that the presence in a country of alien or servile labour is degrading to the white workers and demoralising to the white employer." The paper's bohemian "Bystander" had no doubt that "white labour can work as well in the tropics as in the Arctic Circle *if paid well enough*."[71] Thousands of whites had begun to cut cane under the tropical sun, despite medical warnings, and they seemed no more degenerate and pigmented than laborers in the south. In 1885, "Queenslander" wrote indignantly to the *Sydney Quarterly Review* to point out that Europeans had for years "done a great deal of very hard out-door work in every part of the colony." Compared to a Pacific Islander, the white worker was better: "His muscles are more inured to steady and constant toil; he is more intelligent, and puts forth his strength to greater advantage." The experience of "Queenslander" had shown him that the Islanders owed their higher mortality rates to "the generally low vitality of the labourers, to their being, in their own islands, unaccustomed to regular and sustained labour, and to their liability to homesickness, from which great numbers of them died."[72] All the same, wrote "Killeevy" in the *Freeman's Journal*, ignorant southerners still erroneously asserted "that Queensland is a barren, scorched-up region, fit only for the Asiatic to live in, a land, indeed, of bananas and Kanakas."[73]

The demographics of the north were changing. During the 1890s, the Queensland government had restructured the sugar industry in response to the rising cost of Islander labor and the collapse of the international sugar market. The industry was shifting from labor-intensive plantation agriculture to a capital-intensive central milling arrangement. Despite medical warnings, the government encouraged white agricultural laborers to take up land to supply the mills. More white families were settling along the Queensland coast. According to Dr. Walter Maxwell, the director of the Queensland Sugar Experimental Station: "The most highly important economic and social result of this change is found in the circumstance that the ownership and occupancy embrace a large number of strong, responsible and progressive white settlers, with families of coming men and women who are being planted over the sugar growing areas."[74]

Pacific Islanders, no longer indentured laborers, had become farmworkers competing with white farmers and their families who cut their own cane, as well as with white workers drawn to the cane fields after the collapse of mining and pastoral industries in the economic depression of the 1890s. As a result, relations between white and Islander laborers were especially tense along the North Queensland coast. White workers demanded more restrictions on col-ored labor and campaigned for a halt to Pacific Islander immigration and for the repatriation of those who remained. But until the federation of the colonies in 1901, they would have little real success. Samuel Griffith, the lib-eral premier of Queensland, in 1885 had introduced the Pacific Islanders Act, which signaled an end to the labor trade in 1890, but in 1889 a royal commis-sion on the sugar industry urged its repeal, claiming that it was irresponsible to expect whites to work north of Townsville. In 1892, Griffith, in response to planter concerns and rationalizing largely in medical terms, reversed his pre-vious legislation and passed the Pacific Islanders Extension Act, which pro-longed the trade in human cargo.[75]

A growing band of radicals, labor organizers, and literary types were pro-claiming the superiority of the new white workers in the tropics. Other races often manifested diseases such as leprosy, their surroundings were deemed un-sanitary and dangerous, and they might demoralize whites with sex and opium. In general, agitators still regarded colored labor as inferior, not yet as dangerous, and as degraded and degrading, not yet as infectious—or not espe-cially more so than anyone else. The opponents of colored labor remained sur-prisingly indifferent to emerging racialized versions of contagionist medical doctrine. But they were ready to argue that Chinese and Islander laborers in the tropics, despite apparent evolutionary advantages, had become especially depraved and dissolute, to the degree that their labor power was far less than that of the robust, efficient European—according, that is, to the self-described robust, efficient Europeans. A Darwin correspondent of the *Boomerang* as-sured Queensland readers that "those European labourers you meet here are in general the picture of rude health," with fever afflicting only "a system enfee-bled by excessive and assiduous nobblerising," or drinking. The risks to white male health were alcohol, opium, and Asian prostitutes, not climate. "If a white man eschews the grog-shop and avoids the pitfalls spread for the unwary by lambers-down, and the Sirens from Nagasaki and the flowery-land, he can-not unreasonably reckon a tolerably long span of useful and laborious, but by no means unpleasant, life."[76] The language was unusually ornate, but the sen-timents were becoming widespread. As the *Boomerang*'s "Bystander" declared, "race instinct" had dictated that every stone would be "overturned in the endeavour to sustain white labour on the soil of the North."[77] In 1911, Randolph Bedford claimed that "Australia has had given to it as a sacred duty the breeding of a pure race in a clean continent."[78] By then he was not so much echoing a sentiment as joining a chorus.

When Joseph Ahearne, that pessimistic old Townsville doctor, wrote to the *Bulletin* in 1900, to warn readers that "the white race of Queensland is undergoing modification physically, morally and mentally," his views were derided. Ahearne again asserted that the local lads, in comparison to the Anglo-Saxon type, were more narrow in the chest and two inches taller than they ought to be. Furthermore, "the tropical resident of some years standing possesses less endurance than his fellow workman imported from a more bracing locality"— this was because "an intelligent God equipped Man so that he should be suitable to his environments."[79] A. G. Stephens, the wily literary editor of the *Bulletin*, had felt that the article warranted publication on the grounds that the "appeal differed from the appeals of other coloured labour apologists in that it assumed a scientific foundation. But it has been shown that Dr. Ahearne's foundation is no foundation in as much as his data are insufficient to yield a conclusion." Indeed, was not Ahearne a "Townsville medico in healthy condition with a spouting kidney and not too enlarged a liver who . . . shows none of the signs of race deterioration which he attributes to other North Queenslanders"?[80] Dr. Jack Elkington, a frequent contributor to the *Bulletin* and later one of the leaders of tropical medicine in Australia, sent in a typically pugnacious response, asserting that "the nervous savage northerner can lick the puff-muscled men from cooler climates. Damn his nerves—he can fight, and it's the fighting man who's going to succeed more than ever, the savage carnivore with alternating periods of torpor and of mad lustful, drinkful, frightful energy."[81] "Mitty from Mackay" wrote, after "a hard day's work in the canefield," to point out, rather mildly, that the white man was more than equal to the Kanaka when it came to tropical labor.[82] And S. J. Richards, the new government medical officer at Mt. Morgan, found the children there a little darker in skin color but no less robust than their cousins down south: "So welcome Federation and a White Australia."[83]

As Richards had anticipated, soon after the federation of the colonies in 1901, the new Australian parliament passed the Pacific Islanders Labourers Act, which stipulated that no more indentured laborers would be brought into the northern tropics after 1904, and those already in the country would be deported by 1907, at the end of their agreements. Part of the common—even if, for some, unnatural—aspiration to keep the whole continent for a white race, this legislation would render the sugar industry dependent on white labor.[84] Along with the Immigration Restriction Act of the same year, it comprised the legislative core of the white Australia policy, preserved more or less intact until the 1960s.[85]

Announcing the new restrictive legislation in 1901, Alfred Deakin pointed out that only a hundred years earlier Australia had been a "Dark Continent":

> In another century the probability is that Australia will be a White Continent with not a black or even dark skin among its inhabitants. The Aboriginal race has died out in the South and is dying fast in the North and West even where most gently treated. Other races are to be excluded by legislation if they are tinted to any degree. The yellow, the brown, and the copper-coloured are to be forbidden to land anywhere.[86]

The conjunction of biological thought and national policy was clearly articulated in the parliamentary debates on the Immigration Restriction Bill. Sir William McMillan expressed the general sentiment when he declared that "no matter what measures are necessary, Australia must be kept pure for the British race."[87] Similarly, Andrew Watson felt that the "racial aspect" of population policy was "larger and more important" than the "industrial aspect."[88] According to Senator Pearce, the chief objection to Chinese immigration was "entirely racial."[89] Senator Staniforth Smith noted that "all anthropologists agree that the Caucasian races cannot mingle with the Mongolian, the Hindoo, or the Negro"; the white Australia policy thus was necessary on "scientific and ethnological grounds." Smith had learned that the Chinese "cannot mix with us. We know from the teachings of science that they cannot."[90] As Mr. Wilkinson, a Queensland representative, observed: "Wherever the Asiatic congregates or hordes, there we find unsanitary conditions."[91] "What do we find as to their vile eastern diseases?" asked Mr. Page of Maranoa. "Who brought the plague to Australia? Did it not come from the eastern countries? And where did the leprosy come from?"[92] The Reverend James Roland, from Victoria, praised "the noble ideal of a White Australia—a snow-white Australia if you will. Let it be pure and spotless."[93]

But even as they were deploring the Oriental menace, many Australian parliamentarians retained some doubts about the biological fundamentals of the white Australia policy. McMillan, for example, noted that "whilst the southern parts have a climate suitable to the British people, one half of our territory is either tropical or sub-tropical."[94] Mr. Knox, the member for Kooyong in Victoria, had heard from medical men that

> a race of Australians, if forced to do heavy work under the climatic conditions which prevail in northern Queensland will breed children who, in a large percentage of cases, will have ailments incidental to tropical regions; and, further, that if there be a continuance of this work the third generation will not breed at all.

Knox concluded that "there is a class of labour in that country that the white man cannot do if he is to sustain his fibre and strength."[95] Even Henry Bournes Higgins, usually so optimistic in his nationalism, conceded that "we cannot expect children to be so healthy in the northern parts of Australia as if they were brought up in more temperate climates. I will assume that northern Australia will be totally unfit for white men to settle in." But Higgins, like many of his colleagues, "would sooner see northern Australia unused and undeveloped for a generation or two than have it peopled with Asiatics."[96]

The Boundaries of Whiteness

When J. C. Watson, who briefly had been the first Labor prime minister, visited the tropical north in 1907, he was still troubled by the question of whether "white people [can] live and work in a climate that is, admittedly, hot." But on his tour he found little malaria and few other distinctively tropical diseases among the white inhabitants of the Northern Territory. "Almost without exception they were in splendid condition, and all agreed that the climate was a healthy one." White men seemed able to endure physical labor, and even the women were in "splendid health" after many years' residence. There seemed "little reason to doubt that children can be reared without any danger of deterioration."[97] Watson's tour of the north had convinced him that whites had already acclimatized, without degeneration, to the Australian tropics—in fact, if not yet in theory.

In the early twentieth century, Watson and others were attributing the wonderful exemption from tropical disease in part to the quarantine barrier that separated the Australian tropics from the colored tropics. The would-be white continent was encircled by a cordon sanitaire that protected vulnerable settlers from the "disease centers" of Asia. With the passage of the Federal Quarantine Act of 1908, a more extensive "system of frontier defences against disease" was stretched around the new nation.[98] The quarantine service was mostly concerned to prevent the importation of smallpox, which might come from anywhere. But J.H.L. Cumpston, one of the leading advocates of quarantine, assured his fellow white citizens that "the proximity of the Asiatic endemic centres of plague and cholera, and the danger threatening Australia from these sources, is also fully recognized." W. Perrin Norris, the chief quarantine officer, went further, declaring that "the chief 'storm center' of the diseases against which quarantine is directed is the Continent of Asia."[99]

The development of a quarantine mentality in Australia during the late nineteenth century indicates a growing sense that disease was as likely to come from abroad as to spring forth from within the nation. In the 1840s, John

McArthur at Port Essington had not implicated visiting Macassan traders in the spread of the diseases that afflicted the settlement; doctors along the Queensland coast would continue for most of the century to point to the region's landscape and climate as the principal pathogenic agents; and white newcomers to the tropics still felt ill at ease, ready to believe that their circumstances were unhealthy. But contagionism does begin to make some inroads into these geographical pathologies during the 1880s. Disease agency—especially the putative cause of epidemic disease—was becoming increasingly mobile in the north, though perhaps never so much as in the southern cities. When Edward Palmer, in 1903, recalled his early days in North Queensland, he asserted that "the whole country is fitted for settlement and occupation by European races." Indeed, pioneers like him had, by living there and prospering, "proved the adaptability of the soil and climate to the wants and civilisation of the European."[100] Palmer eventually had come to believe that the occasional outbreak of disease must have derived from foreign influence. He remembered the epidemic that had struck Burketown, on the Gulf of Carpentaria, in 1866. When Palmer, toward the end of his life, came to reflect on this event, he decided that a vessel had probably "touched at some infected port in Java" and brought with it a fatal sickness that "nearly carried off all the population." Evidently, the vessel had been pathogenic—the epidemic was not, as thought at the time, the result of opening up the soil. All of the passengers had died, and infection of the town led to its abandonment. "Nothing was left to mark the spot," warned Palmer, "except heaps of empty bottles and jam tins, and some large iron pots belonging to a boiling-down plant."[101] "Bill Bowyang" was still recounting the grisly tale in the 1940s, identifying the malady as yellow fever. The lesson, once novel but by then commonplace, was that "terrible epidemics" came from overseas and endangered whites living in the north.[102]

The first colonial quarantine act had come into force in New South Wales in 1832, a response to news of a cholera epidemic in Britain, but concerns about the importation of disease did not become pressing until late in the century. Initially, the practice was to detain those vessels arriving from an infected port; but in the 1880s each vessel would first be inspected to determine whether it carried a communicable disease.[103] In earlier years, quarantine officers had concentrated on the detection of cholera, yellow fever, and typhus. They found plenty of typhus—a disease of convict and emigrant ships and one that rarely occurred on shore—but little of the others. Infected vessels were isolated and fumigated; sick passengers would also be placed apart. During the 1880s, smallpox became a major concern, a response to the outbreak in Sydney in 1881, the first in thirteen years.[104] Local fears of the introduction of smallpox from abroad added a distinctively Australian element to the development of quarantine, but then the colonies, especially Queensland, were among the least vaccinated of any modern societies and so had good reason to guard against outbreaks.[105] The special attention given to smallpox is significant, as it was one of the few diseases that everyone conceded were spread by personal contact. The detection of smallpox thus required close attention to the bodies of immigrants and travelers, whereas previously the interest in "diseases of place" like typhus had often made the sanitary state of the vessel the chief concern. Accordingly, the emphasis gradually shifted from the inspection of vessels and possessions to the examination of passengers; and from the fumigation of ships to the disinfection of foreigners. In Australia, smallpox scares gave special impetus to these changes in quarantine practice.[106]

Once aimed at checking the movement of property, quarantine by the late 1880s was increasingly directed at regulating the flow of people, especially the poor and other races. In Australian quarantine practice, the Chinese were the obvious suspects. They were selected for special attention, for the most rigorous inspection; sometimes, when other passengers were allowed to land, only they would be kept on board ship.[107] During the late nineteenth century, then, a racially focused quarantine practice emerged in parallel with restrictive immigration policies in the colonies. An environmental understanding of disease causation could, at a stretch, have been organized around notions of a presumed racial proclivity for accumulating filth and getting used to it—so that the places that Chinese inhabited might come to appear directly pathogenic. But the rising concern about contagion, the interest in the social spread of disease, would make it even easier to graft disease theory onto a racial framework. To the older stigma of unsanitary behavior was added a new sense of a likely bodily infectiousness, signaled by racial difference. By the end of the century other races, and sometimes other classes, not only seemed more dirty and sick but also were increasingly represented by medical experts as inherently more dangerous, more likely to embody a transmissible risk of disease.

Quarantine may have been a harbinger of future national health policy, but it alone was never deemed sufficient to decontaminate the nation. Alison Bashford has suggested that "quarantine assisted in the imagining of the new island-nation as an integrated whole, and in the imagining (and literal pursuit) of its 'whiteness.'"[108] But it was not enough. Behind a quarantine barrier, most doctors continued to search for local landmarks of pathology, whether environmental or social; they remained committed to biological and cultural changes that might reduce disease transmission or enhance bourgeois European resistance to disease agents. And even if they were to control specific disease, doctors still worried that the quality of whiteness might deteriorate in northern tropical conditions. Quarantine might help preserve white health, but better hygiene and morality also would be needed behind the cordon sanitaire to purify and fortify settler communities. Contagionist theories of social pathology, following contours of race and class and expressed in practices of quarantine and personal hygiene, would thus reveal to new Australian citizens the prospect of a purely white nation.

Quarantine would, they hoped, guard the borders, perhaps even establish them; practices of personal and domestic hygiene might sort out what happened behind them. Quarantine was a part of the process of setting the boundaries of the nation; hygiene would become, as we shall see, part of the process of whitening out the diseased and degenerate bits cropping up within. In mobilizing pathology in other people, as well as local fauna, the more progressive doctors, usually based in the south, hoped they would eventually make it possible for well-behaved whites to stay put in the tropics, as elsewhere.[109]

In 1911, the journalist C.E.W. Bean wrote that "Australia is a big blank map, and the whole people is constantly sitting over it like a committee, trying to work out the best way to fill it in."[110] A key problem was that the northern parts of the continent were at best a precarious habitat for the white race. The nation was committed to filling in its tropical zone with a working white race, though a few older doctors and geographers continued to cast doubt on the outcome of the great "experiment." And even though ecological bonds of race and environment might be re-formed, or rendered irrelevant, in the temperate south, some northern medicos still believed that whites in the tropics would remain matter out of place, forever nostalgic and disabled. Together even, quarantine and hygiene might not be enough. Doctors like Ahearne and Nisbet predicted that their race's struggle against the tropical climate would end either with gradual degeneration and disease or in sudden extinction. The white race would sink to the level of native races, or it would disappear entirely.

When King O'Malley, the Labor politician, argued for a federal capital in a cold climate, he recalled that he had found Europeans "in San Domingo on a Sabbath morning going to a cockfight with a rooster under each arm and a sombrero on their heads . . . We cannot have hope in hot countries."[111] After 1901 national policy had made Australia white—and yet nature, so it still seemed to many, had determined that the Australian tropics would always be colored. Thus E. W. Cole, the bookseller and controversialist, remained convinced that "there never can be a 'White Australia' because nearly half of it lies within the tropics; and wherever white people settle in the tropics, in the course of time they become coloured." Before long, Queensland would have "a population as brown as the Chinese."[112] When the *Science of Man*, a popular local anthropological journal, discussed this fate in 1911, Professor Edgeworth David of the University of Sydney reluctantly agreed that the white race in the tropics would eventually become black, but it might take many thousands of years for this to happen. In the meantime, he concluded grimly, we must be prepared to sacrifice "comfort, health and even life" to keep all of Australia as white as possible.[113]

CHAPTER 4

THE MAKING OF THE
TROPICAL WHITE MAN

IN THE EARLY 1890s, Bob and Jack, British adventurers and figures in the first Australian "science fiction" novel, *The Germ Growers*, set out gamely across the desert west of Daly Waters, in the Northern Territory. Seeking refuge after a dispute with the Aboriginal tribes, they entered a cave in a cliff that led to a hidden valley, occupied by a malign colored race, one that spoke English but as foreigners do. The locals were lighter in hue than Aboriginal people, and their technology indicated a superior—perhaps even superhuman—condition. Horrified, Bob and Jack wondered if they had come upon "some advanced guard of Nihilists, or the like, who propose to make war upon civilized society."[1] Throughout the valley were vast seedbeds, which the white intruders regarded as a "very queer-looking sort of cultivation," containing a growth "foul and offensive, and thick, filthy looking vapours floated over it here and there." Soon it dawned on them that "some substances, probably germs of one kind or another, were being examined and treated by scientific methods, and were being subjected afterwards to some sort of discriminating culture."[2] When the terrible, infectious growth was prepared, the colored people would place it in flying machines, supported by balloons, and disperse it to the ends of the earth. The science in the novel was perhaps vague and quirky, but the message was clear: Colored races in northern Australia were deliberately cultivating and distributing germs. Bob and Jack soon made a disappointingly easy escape from the germ-growers and fled to a clean, temperate part of Victoria, where they took up land together. Some time later, however, they again ventured north, to settle in Queensland. Day after day they would sit on their veranda and patiently explain the racial origins of tropical disease to ingenuous whites.

According to a new generation of bacteriologically minded doctors, disease agency was far more mobile in the tropics, and elsewhere, than previously thought. They were freeing recently identified germs and parasites from terrestrial and other physical bonds, instead animating them as biological actors in a social matrix. If there was still a climatic factor in the medical equation, it was now represented by the activity of insects and other races—the advanced guard of nihilists, perhaps—that seemed to thrive in certain conditions of heat and moisture. Patrick Manson had found filarial worms in mosquitoes in 1879 and suggested their role in the spread of the disease; Alphonse Laveran discovered the malarial parasite in 1880; and by 1897 Ronald Ross had implicated the *Anopheles* mosquito in its transmission.[3] During the 1890s, the healthy human host or carrier was implicated in the transmission of a great variety of diseases.[4] At the turn of the century, colonial governments were establishing schools for the new "tropical medicine" in London (1899), Liverpool (1899), Hamburg (1901), and Brussels (1906); and the Institut Pasteur during this period fostered tropical research in the French colonial outposts.[5] In 1893, the contributors to Davidson's *Hygiene and Diseases of Warm Climates*, an authoritative text, could still adduce an enormous variety of possible etiologies—mostly environmental or climatic—to explain the origins of the diseases that a colonial physician might encounter. But by 1898, with the publication of Manson's *Tropical Diseases*, virtually every condition now had a putative microbiological cause, whether bacterium or parasite—and the culprits allegedly most likely to host and to spread these minute pathogens were the insects and races that preferred the tropics.[6]

Equatorial fauna had evolved with certain disease organisms, so the reasoning went, thereby developing an immunological concord with them. As a result, local insects might function as efficient vectors of tropical germs, and native races would generally resist familiar pathogens unless exposed to great numbers of them—or unless especially reckless and depraved, rendering themselves immunologically incompetent. Foreigners crossing into this peculiar disease realm would, however, remain uniquely vulnerable to alien disease organisms. By the late 1890s microbiological investigation was amplifying even further the dangers of racial contact in the tropics. Increasingly, it appeared that native resistance to local germs was rarely absolute. Rather, nature had produced in equatorial races, so it seemed, only a partial immunity, enough to ensure that in normal conditions they did not become manifestly diseased, but not sufficient to prevent occult carriage of tropical pathogens. Bacteriologists began to refer to "native reservoirs" of disease organisms, fashioned over thousands of years of immunological adaptation and filled to the brim by promiscuous and irresponsible behavior. Furthermore, they assumed that such biological and cultural adaptation to local disease transmission was a racial characteristic, apparently as inherent—and now fixed—as pigmentation or skull shape.[7] In the early twentieth century, then, doctors tried to persuade white settlers up north to watch out for the meretriciously "healthy" carrier of disease, signified in the tropics by a colored skin. Trained to think in terms of typological classifications, doctors and scientists dedicated themselves, as we shall see, to fitting complex distributions of disease carriage into simplistic, and ultimately untenable, racial categories and to finding facile biological explanations for discomforting social problems. In the past, the danger for whites was imagined to derive from their transgressive presence in the wrong type of climate; now it appeared mostly to arise from transgressive contact with the wrong type of person—a colored person. The stigma of originating disease was effectively being transferred from some essential "fact" of climate to an equally essential, yet still elusive, "fact" of race.[8]

As explanations of disease causation came more to emphasize microbiological and microsocial processes, and to mute previous concerns about climate and topography, they continued to rely on a remarkably persistent framework of hereditarian assumption.[9] Heredity had once implied a temperament, a characteristic mode of response to discomforting circumstances, a special predisposition to disease, whatever the origin; now this modulating role was redefined in narrower terms of immunity or susceptibility to specific microbes. At the same time, notions of heredity were assuming a more interactive quality, contributing to explanations of disease transmission, as much as of disease acquisition. Thus it seemed that hereditary endowment, organized conventionally in racial categories, might produce a special proclivity to transport some germs, to spread them about; it might give rise to a behavioral or cultural repertoire that made a whole group of people inadvertent disease-dealers.

The influence of heredity on physique and culture came to appear ever more fixed during this period. For most of the nineteenth century, softer notions of heredity, often Lamarckian in character, had prevailed. Races might thus acquire characteristics appropriate to a new environment and pass them on to any descendants; lasting changes in resistance or susceptibility to local disease could take place; whole groups of people would acclimatize, or they and their offspring would degenerate. In the Australian tropics, many ordinary doctors and their patients continued to cling to such assumptions of hereditary dynamism. But since the 1880s a southern intelligentsia, based in the universities of Melbourne and Sydney, had been asserting new theories of a harder heredity, an endowment less prone to environmental influence, even in the torrid zone. Leaders of the medical profession in the south had mostly come to accept Darwin's argument that the development of civilization and technology more or less protected at least the "higher races" from environmental selection pressures and thus fixed their characteristics.[10] It would not be necessary to acquire pigmentation for protection from the sun if one had an umbrella; electric fans might disperse the heat; adjustments in clothing would help counteract any humidity. By the early twentieth century biologists were suggesting that the hereditary material of all races was, in any case, far more robust than previously thought, even more so than Darwin had believed. The medical elite of Melbourne and Sydney were becoming more inclined to proclaim August Weissmann's discovery of the continuity of the "germ plasm," the persistence and reliability of hereditary material, its imperviousness to circumstances. They were talking about Gregor Mendel's experiments that indicated that this hereditary material was organized in distinct, fixed units that assorted independently; they were thinking about Hugo de Vries's argument that variations arose in populations not from adaptation but from random mutation of the hereditary units.[11] It had been reassuring enough to know that Europeans could artificially protect themselves from uncomfortable environments, but now it was even more encouraging to know that such protection might be redundant.

Germ theories, notions of the "healthy carrier," racial stereotypes, and assumptions of harder heredity were woven together in the fabric of medical science at the beginning of the twentieth century, just as the colonies were federating into a white Australia. The convergence would prove propitious, reshaping understandings of race and territory in the emerging nation. Advanced medical science in the southern cities was conferring new meaning on bodies, races, and territories, and in so doing it offered a means of rationalizing, and reformulating, national aspirations. The qualities of the white race appeared more robust than once thought, so it should prosper regardless of climate and circumstance; colored races, by contrast, were now more commonly regarded as fixedly disease-dealing—germ-growers and -transmitters—and white contact with them, behind a thin line of quarantine, must forever be limited. Yet vigilance would also be unremitting within the racial fortress. Because bad behavior and intemperance might yet overwhelm even the most resilient hereditary resistance to disease, it seemed that poor whites in the tropics, and the urban centers, would require ceaseless surveillance and discipline. But this was all very good in theory. How might medical scientists in the south convince their old-fashioned colleagues in the north, and persuade their patients, that they had the answers to doubts about the naturalness of a white Australia? How, indeed, would they get the nation's leaders to endorse a medicalization of human settlement in the north, a neat suturing together of medical and civic visions?

In trying to explain the white Australia policy to an English readership in 1904, Oswald P. Law and W. T. Gill pointed out that the whole of the new nation was "unalterably resolved that the Commonwealth shall be established on the firm basis of unity of race." The future Australian race would blend British elements but must resist the degeneration that would inevitably follow a cross with "coloured people of low morality and social development."[12]

White civilization was imperiled principally by contact with colored germ plasm and colored germs: "The coloured aliens are inferior to the whites in physique and morals and low in the social scale," they introduced "scourges such as smallpox, bubonic plague and leprosy." Law and Gill expressed "a patriotic desire to secure their race from contamination."[13] "It is not so much the protection of wages that is sought . . . as the protection of blood and the preservation of society." While Pacific Islanders remained in Australia all was not yet well: "The racial taint in her blood has to be eradicated."[14] And surely doctors knew more about blood than anyone.

MEDICAL SCIENCE IN THE AUSTRALIAN TROPICS

In 1902, Dr. Frederick Goldsmith came all the way from Darwin to the Intercolonial Medical Congress in Hobart to plead for the establishment in Australia of a school of tropical medicine like those recently opened in London and Liverpool.[15] His own informal investigations in the Northern Territory had suggested that tropical disease was actually quite rare in Australia, but he feared that with closer settlement and more rapid communications the situation would soon deteriorate.[16] A school of tropical medicine, located perhaps in Brisbane, would train medical graduates in the diagnosis and treatment of the diseases of the north, and it might also supplement its teaching with scientific investigations, as did the London and Liverpool schools. Goldsmith managed to persuade the congress to recommend the establishment of a school of tropical medicine and research, at a time when the new nation still had no medical research institutes of any sort.

Whereas Goldsmith had pointed to clinical benefits, other promoters of tropical research connected their scientific interests more directly with national policy. "The most prominent arguments advanced against the colonisation of tropical Australia by a white race," declared Dr. J.S.C. Elkington, at the time Tasmania's chief health officer, "have been those of probable ill-health and racial deterioration." In 1905, the federal parliament published Jack Elkington's address on the great experiment in racial transplantation that was taking place in the north. A bellicose nationalist and Nietzschean, son of a Melbourne University history lecturer and brother-in-law of the artist Norman Lindsay, Elkington would later become the first federal director of tropical health. Tropical disease in a white Australia, he argued in 1905, was relatively rare, and its "eventual extinction" was "mainly a question of money." But the effects on a white race of an allegedly tropical climate "uncomplicated with malaria, bad diet, and other influences adverse to health and longevity, have never been thoroughly ascertained." All the same, Elkington had no doubt

that "the co-existence of a considerable native population undergoing the natural penalties of their unsanitary ways of living will, of course, increase the
danger to white residents." The connection with the new white Australia policy was obvious. "On the whole," continued Elkington, "the evidence is
against the half-caste, and the experience of other countries goes to show that
it is advisable to keep the white stock pure, particularly with respect to the
black races, and to the less vigorous brown peoples."[17]

A few years later, when addressing the Society for Tropical Medicine in
London, Dr. T. P. McDonald, a visiting Australian physician, was rather more
optimistic than Elkington. McDonald was already convinced that the defects
in white physique that many of his colleagues had described were in fact the
consequence of infestation with tropical parasites, not the result of a devitalizing climate:

> Parasitosis is the real evil of tropical lands; sunlight gives robust life to plant
> and animal; it makes children healthy, happy and beautiful, and men strong
> and active; the young stripling who grows, overgrows in fact, lanky and
> loose of limb, fills out into the proportions of a young giant in early man-
> hood, and at middle age he becomes a typical John Bull.[18]

McDonald suspected that most of his audience imagined that Queensland
was "filled with human weeds of the white race," but he assured them it was
not so, except for those sapped by the ravages of hookworm. He condemned
the "theorists who only dealt in opinions which were more or less derived from
superstitions handed down from brain to brain, or book to book." While they
claimed that color was produced by adaptation to sunlight, McDonald had established that "pigmentation of the skin corresponds to the place in time of
the race," so darkness implied a primitive state.[19] In fact, tropical disease, not
tropical climate, was the true enemy of the white race—and disease in
Queensland was readily prevented. In conclusion, McDonald startled his audience by singing:

> Hail her, White Australia, hail her!
> In the warm Pacific sea,
> Rising from the mists that veil her;
> Beautiful is she![20]

But this stirring rendition was not well received by some of the more skeptical, older tropical specialists. James Cantlie was still convinced that "tropical
Australia was a land abhorrent to mankind, black and white," and any European who settled there would degenerate.[21] Others commented that they had

always found tropical whites inferior to those bred at "home"; some complained about the unpleasantness of constant perspiration; a retired colonel kept asking if the children were rosy and healthy. Dr. F. M. Sandwith reported that flowers taken from Britain to hot countries looked sickly and anemic by the third generation. In response, a more subdued McDonald asserted again that "Australian experience exploded forever the idea that tropical climates were in themselves inimical to the white race." He still believed that one day "the white races would wake up, make for the Tropics and never come back again."[22]

But how might the white triumph in the tropics, as predicted by Elkington, and so confidently asserted by McDonald, be confirmed scientifically? Dr. J.H.L. Cumpston recalled that in 1905 as a ship's surgeon on the *Chingtu* he had spent some time with a passenger, the Reverend Dr. George Frodsham, the Anglican bishop of North Queensland, "discussing the needs of tropical Australia and the possibility of following the lead given by Joseph Chamberlain when opening the Hospital for Tropical Diseases some five or six years earlier."[23] Cumpston, a devoutly nationalist Melbourne medical graduate, later became head of the federal quarantine service and, in the 1920s, the first director of the federal health department. Strongly influenced by Victor Heiser's progressivist tropical health work in the colonial Philippines, Cumpston was an enthusiastic supporter of government activity in health matters.[24] His campaign for tropical research was soon joined by Dr. R. A. O'Brien, a Cairns doctor who had been a medical student with Cumpston. O'Brien, who would become director of the Wellcome Physiological Research Laboratory in London, also later claimed credit for recruiting Frodsham to the cause of scientific research.[25]

Frodsham, who had long been calling for a university in Queensland, began to develop plans for an institute of tropical medicine in Townsville. A man whose Episcopal presence of mind seems never to have deteriorated climatically, Frodsham had gained a reputation as a promoter of British immigration and an encourager of evangelical work among Aborigines and Pacific Islanders. In his recollections, Frodsham included a chapter on the "great colonising experiment" in northern Australia. He warned that "the whole question of the adaptability of race and environment is too obscure to allow dogmatism with regard to the suitability of the tropics to a white race." Like so many others, he drew on science to explain public policy:

> When all is said and done, the whole thing is only a big experiment. It is an experiment worth trying. Australia has seen the vision of keeping a home for the white race in the southern seas. . . . [It is] seeking to guard the existence of white civilization from being crowded out by a lower social organism. Australians desire to guard the purity of the white race.[26]

Cumpston and O'Brien had acquired an influential convert to their campaign for tropical medical research.

Frodsham set about building support for scientific investigation into whether the north was a habitat suitable to the white race. With Harry Brookes Allen, the dean of medicine at the University of Melbourne, E. C. Stirling, the dean of medicine at Adelaide, and T. Anderson Stuart, the dean of medicine at Sydney, Frodsham drew up plans for a research institute in Townsville. He solicited the support of Lord Chelmsford, the governor of Queensland, and Sir Charles Lucas, the British secretary of state for the colonies. William Knox D'Arcy of Rockhampton pledged 1,000 pounds for the new institute. The Townsville Chamber of Commerce, the hospital committee, and the Cairns Ratepayers' Association all sent petitions on the matter to the federal government. In 1907, Frodsham wrote to Lord Northcote, the governor-general, attaching a memorandum for a scheme to study tropical diseases in northern Australia. He suggested that "the Australian Commonwealth has lagged behind the rest of the Empire in this matter. It is a matter of common knowledge in the tropics that diseases now endemic are not understood nor is there any marked effort being made to understand them." An institute in Townsville would be adjacent to the diseases and climatic indispositions it investigated, and yet it could still communicate readily with the southern medical schools, thereby instilling in them a spirit of research. Lord Northcote expressed his interest in the proposal and promised to draw it to the attention of his ministers. Alfred Deakin, the prime minister, and Attlee Hunt, the head of the external affairs department, agreed that the scheme would develop local research capacity and complement Australia's growing commitment to Papua, which had been transferred from British control in 1904. Accordingly, in August 1907 the federal government offered 550 pounds for the establishment of a Townsville institute, an amount that the Queensland government supplemented with a further 250 pounds.[27]

With the help of Professor C. J. Martin, head of the Lister Institute in London, a selection committee in 1909 appointed Dr. Anton Breinl to direct the new Australian Institute of Tropical Medicine. Breinl, until then working at the Runcorn Laboratory in the Liverpool School of Tropical Medicine, was one of the leading investigators of the effect of drugs on recently discovered tropical microbes, in particular the use of atoxyl to treat trypanosomiasis, or sleeping sickness. (Paul Ehrlich, who developed salvarsan, the first effective treatment for syphilis, wrote a testimonial for him.) After graduating in medicine from Prague, Breinl had studied tropical medicine in Liverpool, where he came under the influence of Sir Ronald Ross and conducted fieldwork in the Amazon rainforests.[28] The young investigator was taught to integrate laboratory work with field expeditions and to reconcile an interest in individual treatment with the practical need for hygiene and sanitary improvement in the outposts of empire. As Breinl departed for tropical Australia, his colleagues in Liverpool and London were still debating whether they should favor the reform of native hygiene or the deferred development and segregation of colonial races. In the Australian setting, Breinl predictably would come to recommend the separation of races, through exclusion of "colored" people.[29]

Breinl arrived in Townsville in 1910, with his assistant J. W. Fielding, and soon began work in a small timber building that had been the hospital wardsmen's quarters. They had come to a struggling settlement of almost 10,000 people, with many of the men employed on the railway, at the wharves, or in the abattoir. Most of the inhabitants had moved up from the south; men still greatly outnumbered women; there were few Chinese or Pacific Islanders to be seen. With poor soil and low rainfall, surrounded by mangroves and saltpans, the place failed to convey any impression of tropical luxuriance. The local medical doctors, including Joseph Ahearne and A.T.H. Nisbet, were conservative and often allied with planters and other commercial interests. They resented the intruder with his advanced ideas and made it difficult for him to get access to the small hospital.[30] Not surprisingly, the intrepid young medical scientist from the start was eager to go bush, to leave dusty Townsville and begin mapping the diseases of tropical Australia. Within a year he had twice visited the Torres Strait, and during the next five years he would also survey the Northern Territory and Papua.

When Breinl traveled down to Brisbane in late 1910 to attend a meeting of the Queensland branch of the British Medical Association, the city doctors told him how valuable his work would be in ensuring the tropics were held by the white race. They proceeded to try to specify the diseases he should study. But Breinl assured them that he had already surveyed most of North Queensland, and he was preparing to investigate the more common, if less exciting and mysterious, diseases that he had found there, such as dengue and hookworm. He agreed, though, that it must eventually be determined scientifically whether Europeans could work in wet and hot conditions. "North Queensland is the ideal country to investigate these questions, as it is a tropical country without native servants. Does the white organism undergo any changes with regard to the composition of the blood; does the metabolism become changed?"[31] Breinl had not previously addressed these questions in his research, and he lacked the appropriate expertise to do so alone. He would need a physiologist or a biochemist at the institute to determine whether the white Australia policy made sense scientifically. "Only careful and detailed research carried on in the populated coastal districts of tropical Australia, where several generations have been reared, will indicate whether the great experiment of populating Australia by a working white community can be accomplished."[32]

MELBOURNE TO THE TROPICS

Although the Australian Institute of Tropical Medicine was administratively attached to the University of Sydney, tropical concerns were taken up most avidly by academics at the University of Melbourne. Biologists and geographers at Melbourne had been attempting for more than a decade to conduct research on race, disease, and climate, a field of study with obvious relevance to national policymaking. They had already begun to translate the project of a white Australia into scientific terms; now they were seeking government support for their investigations. If the nation intended to settle a working white race over the whole continent, then surely it must be prepared to sponsor medical and geographical research on the subject.

But research was not easily organized at the University of Melbourne. In the 1890s, Harry Allen had proposed an institute of preventive medicine, where a skilled bacteriologist might at least perform necessary diagnostic work. "Are we forever to be in treaty with institutes elsewhere for the supply of our needs?" he asked. After visiting European laboratories, Allen reported to the Victorian parliament that "in all countries public attention had been drawn to the researches conducted by Pasteur, Koch and other veterans of experimental pathology."[33] But the University of Melbourne apparently did not possess the resources for such investigation. As Frodsham was securing support for the Australian Institute of Tropical Medicine, the university was emerging from a period of neglect and financial stringency following the depression of the 1890s and the defalcations of its accountant in 1901. Repairs had been postponed, the libraries were not acquiring books, and the grounds had grown wild. Even after reducing salaries and increasing fees, a deficit remained. When the government at last provided more resources to the university after 1904, it directed these funds mostly to vocational training, not to research.[34] The academic staff complained repeatedly about their teaching loads and the lack of research equipment. Arriving to take up the chair of anatomy in 1906, R.J.A. Berry could find no specimens, no dissected parts for study, no microscopes, not even a skeleton (though he later claimed to have discovered a number of them in the cupboard). Although the equipment improved over the next decade, an increase in student numbers left faculty with little time to use it. Research, according to Berry, "was practically deleted from university work," and as a result the place was "slowly sinking to the level of a technical school."[35] In these circumstances, national concern for the future of the white race in the tropics offered at least some hope for university science.

Even as the University of Melbourne was slowly recovering from the economic depression of the 1890s, and from one of its recurrent episodes of mismanagement, academic staff were exerting a greater influence on local intellectual life than ever before. The professors gave public lectures on recent scientific discoveries; they wrote prolifically on issues of national importance for newspapers and popular journals. As the federal government was based in Melbourne until 1927, academics could dine with leading politicians and civil servants and go on rambles with them through the bush near the city. When W. Baldwin Spencer, the new professor of biology, and David Orme Masson, the professor of chemistry, arrived in 1887 there were twelve professors and twelve lecturers at the university, and 100 students had graduated the year before. In 1905, despite a long period of financial stringency, Melbourne boasted thirty-five professors and lecturers, five of them fellows of the Royal Society, and greatly increased student numbers.[36] Most of the senior staff were youthful emigrants from Britain, but some of them soon burned with the imperialist and nationalist passions ignited in Australia during the 1890s.[37] Many of them lived with their families on the pastoral campus just north of the city, not far from the squalid slums of Carlton.[38] At the medical school, enthusiasts like Allen in pathology, W. A. Osborne in physiology, and Berry in anatomy promoted germ theory, Darwinism, and the new doctrines of heredity derived from the work of Weissmann and Mendel.[39] They lectured frequently at the Medical Society of Victoria, the local Royal Society, the Microscopical Society, and the Victorian branch of the Royal Geographical Society of Australasia; sometimes they spoke at Charles Strong's liberal Australian Church.[40] They mixed with other middle-class male intellectuals, professionals, and politicians at the Melbourne Club and at dining clubs such as the Beefsteak.

To avoid the dangers of excessive "brain-work," to balance such unmanly activities with virile pursuits, the professors took eagerly to bushwalking, swimming, boomerang throwing, and other forms of outdoor exercise. Fears of the antipodean sun had dissipated a generation ago in the south. Most of them joined the select Wallaby Club, with its motto *à votre santé* (to your health), to participate in "reasonable outdoor enjoyment that would be conducive to health, conversation and good companionship." The professors went rambling with the political leaders of white Australia, including Alfred Deakin, George Reid, W. M. Hughes, H. B. Higgins, William McMillan, and the Gavan Duffy brothers. Sometimes, though, the exertion was too much for a sedentary political system (E. L. Batchelor, the minister for external affairs, died suddenly on a club walk in 1911).[41] From 1910 Wallabies could refresh themselves after strenuous climb up Mt. Dandenong at a meeting of the Round Table, a secret discussion group dominated by academics, businessmen, and politicians and dedicated to enhancing imperial ties.[42]

The work of Charles H. Pearson, the educator and politician, had stimulated interest in the tropics at the University of Melbourne. His pessimistic tract, *National Life and Character*, was a major influence on the thinking of many local academics and political figures. After a brief appointment as a lecturer in history at the university, Pearson had served as a liberal in the Victorian legislature. During the late 1880s, he was the minister of public instruction in the Deakin colonial government. In *National Life and Character*, Pearson suggested that climatic barriers would soon hinder the global expansion of the superior white races. The temperate zones had largely been taken up; and the tropics, although fertile, were inimical to whites. Tropical countries were unlikely ever to be "the homes of what it is convenient to call the Aryan race, or indeed of any higher race whatever." Instead, the lower races would move in, and thus "the black and yellow belt, which always encircles the globe between the Tropics, will extend its area, and deepen its colour with time." Lamentably, the white races now "panting for new worlds to conquer" would have their hopes frustrated and sink into a slough of "depression, hopelessness, a disregard of invention and improvement."[43]

Although Pearson's theories of race struggle were well received, many challenged the more pessimistic of his conclusions. Deakin praised Pearson's "splendid volume" for sounding the first note of alarm, warning of the "Yellow Peril to Caucasian civilisation, creeds and politics."[44] Yet he thought the dire prophecies would not come to pass. During the debate on the Immigration Restriction Bill, Edmund Barton, the first prime minister, quoted Pearson twice, but he too believed that the nation could forestall the threat from Asia.[45] W. A. Osborne recalled that he and his friend J. W. Gregory, the professor of geology at Melbourne, had regarded Pearson as "the pioneer in warning white races about losing their heritage through the pressure of brown, yellow and black races."[46] But Osborne, Gregory, Berry, and others at the university were convinced that they could harness medical science and so resist this pressure.

In 1910, James Barrett, who had become a prominent Melbourne medical academic, demanded more research on the establishment of a working white race in the Australian tropics. "Is there any reason," he asked in the columns of the Melbourne *Argus*, "to think that mere heat will cause physical deterioration? This is the question that requires answer by the experimental method. The probabilities are that life in such conditions will be vigorous, active and normal; but the experiment has never been made, or in Australia even tried, or seriously considered."[47] On behalf of the medical profession, Barrett had written to the minister for home affairs, Senator J. H. Keating. "It was in the interests of science and their own country," he claimed, "that they had asked for an attempt to be made to secure a scientific solution to a problem by no means settled. It had been said that the Anglo-Saxon race could not live in the tropics." In reply, the minister, later the author of *White Australia: Men and Measures in Its Making*, noted that the work of William Gorgas in the Panama Canal "was an object-lesson to the world that medical science properly applied to existing conditions could convert and transform them so as to make it possible for white people to continue living in places where, without the application of medical science . . . it would not be possible."[48]

Barrett commended the federal government's encouragement of the institute at Townsville, but he warned that much more would soon be required. "Great empires are developing," he declared, "and it is our business to submit this problem [of white settlement in the tropics] to the experimental test."[49] His plea came just before a parliamentary debate on the institute's funding. Sydney Sampson, the member for Wimmera in Victoria, referred to Barrett's warnings and suggested that the money available was evidently inadequate, in view of the importance of this research. "We have a small establishment at Townsville, which has done a certain amount of good work, but the investigations are not sufficiently extensive." Because the federal government would take control of the Northern Territory from South Australia in 1911, many members of the federal parliament were turning their attention to the problems of tropical development. "On the eve of our endeavour to settle a large and prosperous population in the northern parts of Australia," Sampson continued, "I know of no more important question to engage the earnest and immediate attention of ministers than the investigation of tropical disease."[50] Later in the debate, Dr. Carty Salmon, a Melbourne physician, endorsed Sampson's recommendation, suggesting that scientific investigation would prove "of inestimable advantage to us in our attempt to settle the northern areas of Australia."[51]

W. A. Osborne joined Barrett in calling for more research on whether tropical Australia was a possible European habitat. Osborne's physiological interests were closely related to the subject. He was a keen student of racial theory—regarding himself as a fine example of the Nordic type—and he saw at once the relevance of J. S. Haldane's physiological work on underground miners to an understanding of the response of working whites to tropical conditions.[52] Here was an opportunity to promote original work in physiology and race science. After a visit to the institute in 1911, on his way to the International Race Congress in London, Osborne recommended that the institute appoint more staff to conduct such research. F. H. Taylor, an entomologist, had already been appointed to assist Breinl, but there was still no qualified biochemist or physiologist in Townsville. Osborne's recommendation was endorsed by Elkington, by then the Queensland director of public health, and by the institute's board of management, which forwarded the proposal to the federal government. The government was prepared to donate an additional 4,000 pounds, but it did so on the condition that the control of the institute passed from the universities to the external affairs department. Allen and Anderson Stuart now had the authority to select more research staff for Townsville. In

1912, they appointed Dr. William Nicoll as parasitologist, Dr. W. J. Young as biochemist, and Dr. Henry Priestley as bacteriologist.[53]

With the expansion of the institute and new administrative arrangements, a formal opening ceremony seemed appropriate. In June 1913 Sir William Mc-Gregor, the governor of Queensland, addressed an assembly of white settlers and dignitaries in the grounds of the Townsville Hospital. McGregor drew on his extensive colonial experience as governor of British New Guinea, Fiji, and Nigeria and as a medical doctor who had vigorously promoted the new tropical medicine. His own career had demonstrated to him the importance of tropical research. "The policy of reserving Tropical Australia as a home for a purely white race," he declared, "is one of the greatest and most interesting problems of modern statesmanship. [But] tropical diseases, although important, occupy only a secondary place, and the main problem is whether conditions of heat and light will permit the establishment of a working white race."[54]

RACIAL PATHOLOGIES IN THE NORTH

Even before McGregor officially opened the institute, Breinl and his colleagues had been studying the diseases of northern Australia and the adaptation of whites to the tropical climate. Uncertainties in the definition of the tropics did not help their task. Just as racial types were difficult to define out of a mass of individual peculiarities, so too were the simplifications necessary in the classification of an environment controversial. Books of adventure and travel described the northern coast as a place of impenetrable jungle and unrelenting heat, yet Townsville itself was parched and barren, hardly an example of such tropical plenitude.[55] Some experts pointed to a cartographic demarcation. Thus Frederick Goldsmith, at the 1902 Australasian Medical Congress, had observed that "taking the tropic of Capricorn as the dividing line, more than one third of the continent of Australia lies within the tropics."[56] But this definition did not coincide with isothermal charts, so Breinl and others suggested that the tropical zone should be limited to the region between the two mean isotherms of 68 degrees Fahrenheit, a temperature that permitted palms to flourish.[57] Still, even this meteorological mapping presented difficulties. One geographer pointed out that "the sustained high tropical temperature of our northern areas is not that of the dangerous intensity created by the more humid conditions of the tropics."[58] So just how "tropical" were the Australian tropics? No one could agree. James Barrett, ever a staunch promoter of white settlement in the north, dismissed the geographical pedantry: "The tropics has generally been associated with a temperature of

75 degrees in winter. The whole of Australia is below 75 degrees in winter; at least two-thirds, if not three-fourths, is below 70 degrees in summer; so the region which can properly be termed 'tropical' is comparatively small."[59] Just as Breinl and his colleagues commenced work, their subject matter seemed in danger of disappearing.

In May 1910 Breinl traveled north from Townsville to assess the local burden of tropical disease. On Thursday Island Breinl found that beriberi was prevalent, "affecting mostly coloured races," and Bishop White showed him a few cases of malaria among native parishioners. In Cairns, Breinl encountered widespread ankylostomiasis, or hookworm, which "in the white man is a disease of consequence and of economic importance."[60] He also investigated some vague fevers among cane-cutters, and he reported on a few cases of malaria and dengue. When Breinl visited the Northern Territory in 1912, he found much more malaria, and he urged the locals to kill mosquitoes, dispense more quinine, and check among native and Chinese communities for human hosts of the malaria parasite.[61] As a result of these disease surveys, Breinl concluded that tropical disease was not widespread in the north, but even so, the little there was might have a considerable economic impact. Dengue fever was prevalent in North Queensland, causing great loss of money and labor; hookworm was almost universal and certainly debilitating; malaria was sporadic in Queensland scrub country and common enough in the Northern Territory to increase mortality rates; filariasis occurred frequently but was usually asymptomatic; and sprue and dysentery, both bowel complaints, now seemed rare.[62] So far, whites in the north had managed largely to resist tropical disease, but there was just enough for further research.[63]

Like so many of his colleagues, Breinl assumed that Europeans would naturally be especially susceptible to tropical ailments, whereas native races would possess a relative immunity to the diseases of their local habitat. According to Breinl, white organisms "had become accustomed, throughout many generations, to certain diseases and specific infections prevalent in temperate climates, and had acquired a relative impermeability of their living matter for certain infections." But "on transplanting the white race to the tropics this acquired immunity has become upset," warned Breinl. "The organism has become exposed to the invasion of infections to which it has hitherto not been accustomed."[64] Even as the European vulnerability to tropical disease was repeatedly asserted, native immunity to local disease had begun to appear less absolute than once thought. Evidently, some natives were behaving in so unhygienic a fashion that they contracted the local diseases that they should, in theory, have resisted. More seriously, medical scientists in the tropics had discovered a widespread, and previously hidden, disease carriage among even the apparently "healthy natives." The parasites that caused malaria, hookworm, and other tropical ailments could be found in the blood or the excreta of a majority of tropical residents. "Parasites against which a relative impermeability has been acquired by native races," wrote Breinl, "become true parasites in the newcomer, invading his organism without finding any resistance whatsoever."[65] Tropical races in the early twentieth century were thus reconfigured as natural "reservoirs" of the tropical disease organisms to which whites were still uniquely susceptible.[66]

In 1920, Aldo Castellani and Albert Chalmers surveyed recent microbiological research, including the work in northern Australia, and concluded that native races were in fact "partially immune hosts [who] act as reservoirs or carriers," enabling "the parasite to complete its lifecycle without producing marked pathological changes in the host."[67] Tropical disease would no longer permeate from the environment into white organisms; rather, it resided in the local human and insect populations. For Europeans, contact with even an apparently healthy native now seemed to carry a risk of disease and death. As the tropical environment was gradually exonerated, tropical races came to appear typically and invisibly disease-dealing. No matter how clean Asians, Pacific Islanders, and Aboriginal Australians might look and smell, they were still to be distrusted.

If evolution had fashioned these supposedly natural inhabitants of the tropics as potential reservoirs of tropical germs, to European Australians it seemed that unhygienic racial custom and habit would ensure that this pathological potential was realized. An appreciation of supposedly insidious cultural practices, especially those concerning defecation and eating, began to supplement the emerging biological understanding of tropical disease acquisition and transmission. Although the sanitary practices of Asians in particular had long been regarded as primitive and foolish, these apparently fixed racial customs were taking on a new and frightening significance. Before, these patterns of behavior had simply explained the unexpectedly vitiated physiological immunity of the race; now they suggested a source of danger for the utterly unprepared white immune system. Once merely causes for bourgeois European self-congratulation, Asian customs and habits increasingly prompted thoughts of disease transmission and danger. The belief that the "inferior, coloured races" flouted the rules of hygienic behavior was becoming more than a formalistic cultural distinction or an excuse for administrative scorn and neglect. It now appeared that nonwhites were deliberately failing to take precautions against acquiring or distributing the disease organisms that were most virulent for whites.[68]

When Dr. T. V. Danes addressed the Royal Society of New South Wales in 1910, he observed that tropical Australia was healthier than any other tropical region. But he had become concerned that "there is a numerous element of alien Asiatics, who continue to live in their most unsanitary way also in this country, and that element is to be considered as responsible if some tropical epidemics should be introduced into this continent." He no longer doubted that "Chinamen have brought the dreadful 'Beri-Beri' into the Northern Territory" and spread it among the whites, just as they had previously transmitted venereal diseases to the Aboriginal population.[69] "If the Asiatic aliens are permitted," he warned, "to live in their own highly unsanitary ways, and to have free intercourse with other elements, it is certain that in the near future tropical Australia will become much more dangerous to white settlement than is the case now." In establishing the nexus of race and disease, Dane called for a "a proper medical sanitary supervision of the alien elements, and the greatest possible restriction of their evil contact."[70]

This anthropomorphic mobilization of disease agency in the early twentieth century could elicit a number of different institutional responses, depending on colonial or national circumstances. Americans in the Philippines argued that protection for vulnerable colonial emissaries would require a more rigorous surveillance and regulation of contact with local human and insect populations: The control of personal conduct and social interaction, whether internalized or imposed, seemed to offer a prospect of limiting disease transmission in the archipelago.[71] In South Africa, medical officers more commonly urged the segregation of those races stigmatized as naturally disease-dealing, rather than their corporeal and cultural reform, as a means of protecting white settlers.[72] Breinl and his Australian colleagues agreed that there was only one way for the white pioneer to acquire the appropriate "impermeability and immunity, and this is by avoiding the infection."[73] Exposure to the Aboriginal inhabitants of the north presented few problems, as they were a dispersed and apparently doomed race; Pacific Islanders were to be repatriated; and immigration restrictions should keep out most Asians. According to W. J. Young, "Northern Australia has so far enjoyed a certain immunity from disease [because of] the absence of a large coloured population, with its attendant diseases."[74] Thus the new nation, in maintaining the purity of the white race, was also seeking to ensure its health, especially in the tropics. This medical endorsement of a quarantine sensibility meant that the white Australia policy, once a physiological impossibility, by 1920 had come to appear a microbiological necessity.

THE WHITE TROPICS

Some concerns persisted about the physical and mental effects of tropical residence on the white race. In 1915, "M. B." wrote to the *Medical Journal of Australia*, expressing his doubts on the scientific validity of the white Australia policy. The regulation of a white man's body heat was less efficient in the tropics, requiring more energy of the heart and disinclining him for muscular work. Accordingly, the white Australia policy was "poor business, bad science, and worse morals . . . the labourers in the field must have the protection of pigment." "M. B." warned that the "votaries of a White Australia claim that the white man has only gradually to acclimatise. To acclimatise is either to pigment or enervate or both."[75] But these statements spurred Dr. James Merrillees of Roma, Queensland, to ridicule the "pious opinions" of "M. B." "I am open to learn of one case," he wrote, "where a white-skinned man acquired pigmentation and passed it on to his offspring as a fixed character." Alcohol, not degeneration, was the curse of hot climates occupied only by whites; and where there was a mixture of races, "the dangers are alcohol and syphilis."[76]

Later in 1915, the *Medical Journal of Australia* published a letter from "Cosmos" in support of racial pessimists such as "M.B." "Cosmos" claimed that the "so-called science of our universities is too limited to deal adequately with the science of a White Australia." Whatever the new bacteriologists might argue, "man—black or white—is in tune with the universe when he is in that environment which called forth his characteristics. Abundant evidence exists that the people of the northern parts of Australia are coloured."[77] But this assertion merely provided R.J.A. Berry with a perfect excuse to advocate yet more medical research on the matter. He suggested that the white Australia policy "is not a policy at all, but is in reality a medical problem of the first magnitude," and as such it had not yet been put to the proper test. Berry expected a favorable outcome. Given suitable railway facilities, housing "on physiological lines," rational hours of work, proper diet, individual observation of the laws of hygiene, and elimination of the vectors of specific disease, he thought that science would prove that the Australian tropics could be settled by white laborers who would remain "white and healthy."[78] Berry predicted that local medical research would confirm that the torrid zone was no longer, if it ever had been, an inherently pathological site for the white race.

Although Breinl generally was more interested in parasitology than in physiological experimentation, he was prepared to seize any opportunity to expand the Townsville Institute's research work. Breinl had asked the 1911 Australasian Medical Congress whether a tropical climate alone might cause white degeneration. "Tropical Australia should be an ideal locality to decide this question definitely, as it is a country where comparatively few diseases are prevalent, and where the aboriginal races are practically dying out."[79] He advocated the anthropometric measurement of school children over a number of generations; making blood counts on pale individuals; and measurements of the blood pressure, body temperature, and respiratory rates of cane-cutters and wharf laborers. "Careful and accurate physiological and pathological observations must be made over a series of years, and to a less extent, over a lifetime, to ascertain such effects on the white man's constitution."[80] After Young and Priestley joined the institute, they proceeded to assess the effect, if any, of a tropical climate on the "white organism." "This is a question of vital importance to Australia," wrote Young, "for upon it depends the success or failure of the proposed development of the north without the aid of the coloured man, and the possibility of keeping the entire island continent as the undisputed possession of the white race."[81] The scale of the small laboratory in Townsville thus could shift to encompass the whole continent.[82] National policy had been translated into scientific terms: White Australia was framed as a vast experiment, the results of which only medical scientists could interpret.

The commitment of the institute to studying the effects of the tropical climate on a working white race especially pleased W. A. Osborne, who for many years had been conducting his own research on the physiology of heat regulation. In 1910, he reported on experiments on himself and a "robust country lad," carried out at his house at Warrandyte, near Melbourne. After breakfast, Osborne had first taken barometric pressure readings and recorded dry- and wet-bulb temperatures, and he weighed himself. Then, wearing a flannel shirt, serge trousers, and a waistcoat, the professor lay down in a hammock by the Yarra River for thirty minutes. At that point, he leaned over and breathed into a respiration meter to determine the volume of air expired over the next ten minutes. After an hour in the hammock, Osborne weighed himself again and recorded the air temperatures and his own rectal temperature. He repeated the same experiment on the robust country lad, who wore a climatically appropriate knickerbocker suit. On hot days, Osborne found that the respiratory rate and perspiration quickened, but as the humidity increased water loss from the skin was impeded.[83] Later, he continued his studies of the effects of the temperature, humidity, and movement of the air on evaporation from the skin, but without his young assistant.[84]

Whenever Osborne visited the Townsville Institute he brought his hammock with him. There he continued his experiments in heat regulation, seeking to provide a measure of the white man's discomfort in hot weather. "A rough and ready indication which I have come to regard as the most useful is simply the clothing that is chosen as the most comfortable when the body lies in an open-mesh hammock in a good shade and at rest." He compared this subjective assessment of body comfort with wet-bulb readings and concluded that 73 degrees Fahrenheit was the "empiric standard above which truly tropical conditions arise."[85] The wet-bulb thermometer, like human regulatory system, was sensitive to temperature and to the water content and velocity of the air. Osborne had simply added an experiential interpretation to wet-bulb readings in an effort to redefine tropical conditions in terms of Nordic discomfort. In doing so, he was reproducing and racializing the work of his mentor, J. S.

Haldane, who had measured the effect of the high wet-bulb temperatures in British mines and Turkish baths on his own heat-regulating mechanism. Haldane had found that, beyond a wet-bulb reading of 78 degrees Fahrenheit, continuous hard work in a mine became impracticable unless a fan was available. It seemed to Osborne that tropical conditions might be roughly comparable to those that a white man might encounter in a mine or a steam bath.[86]

In general, Breinl and his fellow investigators at Townsville were skeptical of Osborne's efforts to construct a discomfort scale related to wet-bulb readings. They pointed out that the thermometer was a static instrument, whereas the human body was a far more dynamic structure, producing and losing heat yet maintaining a constant temperature.[87] Still, it was undeniable that northern Australia often felt tropical, with the humidity causing whites to experience discomfort. Breinl and Young believed, however, that the intensity of the sun's rays constituted the main difference between a temperate and a tropical climate. Although they denied Charles Woodruff's theory that the rays were more "actinic" or ultraviolet in the tropics, they were nonetheless convinced that the duration of sunshine and the intensity of the light were greater nearer the equator.[88] White bodies exposed to the intense sunlight might become more heated than in temperate regions and thus more discomforted.

This heating process led the Townsville investigators to puzzle over the apparent paradox of pigmentation. Experiments conducted by American scientists in the Philippines had suggested that the body temperatures of dark-colored animals increased more rapidly than those of a lighter hue. "The dark skin of most of the Aboriginal races in the tropics," wrote Breinl and Young, "would appear to be a disadvantage, and the explanation that dark skin affords protection against the effects of the sun merely by insulating the body against the deep penetration of harmful rays must be modified."[89] Christiaan Eijkman in Batavia, the capital of the Dutch East Indies, had covered the bulbs of two thermometers with pieces of white and colored skin and found that when both were placed in the sunlight the brown skin caused the mercury to rise further.[90] The surprising possibility that color was a disadvantage in the tropics inspired Young to conduct biochemical analyses of the skin pigmentation of an "Australian Black" who had died in the hospital.[91] But eventually, Breinl and Young decided, reluctantly, that in its physiological action dark skin in the tropics was superior to white. "It absorbs a greater quantity of heat rays, warms up more quickly and reaches the point where perspiration commences earlier and the evaporation of the sweat causes heat loss and consequently effects the cooling of the body."[92] The main problem of whites in the tropics was that they just did not sweat enough when they needed to.

In choosing their topics and methods, Breinl and his coworkers were following closely the work of American medical scientists at the Manila Bureau of Science in the colonial Philippines.[93] The Townsville investigators justified the apparent repetition and redundancy by arguing that in Manila physiological observations had been limited to European males who spent only a few years in the tropics. The natural experiment of settling tropical Australia with a working white race was quite different and so might yield different results. Like the Americans in the Philippines, the scientists at Townsville studied the regulation of body heat, respiration, blood pressure, and metabolism in the tropics, but the Australian subjects included white males who had lived their whole lives in the region, as well as women and children. It seemed to Breinl and his coworkers that women and children, as well as wharf laborers, were the groups most likely to show the first evidence of racial degeneration.

For most of the nineteenth century it had been widely believed that the metabolism of Europeans increased in the tropics. John Davy, in 1839, published a number of observations made upon the mouth temperature of seven healthy young men during a voyage from England to Ceylon, and he concluded that the temperature of a European body rose when passing from a temperate to a torrid zone and that, in addition, the normal body temperature of tropical residents is higher than those who live in a cooler place.[94] Alexander Rattray subsequently confirmed this slight rise, but he based his conclusions on the mouth temperatures of a few Europeans who sailed from England to Bahia, Brazil. According to Rattray, "The tropics, especially during the rainy season, should be avoided by natives of colder latitudes."[95] Yet when Weston Chamberlain at the Manila Bureau of Science recorded 3,000 mouth temperatures at quarterly intervals from 600 healthy white American soldiers, he found that body temperature showed no appreciable variation with season or complexion. The average body temperature in the Philippines differed little, if at all, from the mean temperature of white men living in the United States.[96] In 1915, Young recorded the rectal temperatures of six healthy white men in Townsville and confirmed Chamberlain's findings—even though "Tropical Australia differs from most other places in the Tropics in that there is practically no coloured population, and the whole of the work is carried out by white people, who conform to the same working hours as in temperate climates." At rest, the rectal temperatures of Young and his colleagues were the same as they would be in Europe, but when Breinl took "horse exercise" in the morning his rectal temperature rose more quickly and decreased more slowly than in a temperate zone.[97]

The Townsville investigators also were particularly concerned to dispel the assumption that the organism's blood pressure, or "tension," would fall in a relaxing tropical environment. In 1910, W. E. Musgrave and A. G. Sison had examined ninety-seven Americans, ten Sisters of Charity, and forty Filipinos, all of them resident in Manila. The researchers concluded that a definite decrease in blood pressure had occurred after long residence in a tropical climate, with the lowest tensions recorded among Filipinos. Presumably the tropical heat had dilated the blood vessels of the skin enough to lower peripheral vascular resistance, resulting in a fall in blood pressure.[98] Despite these findings, Chamberlain suggested in the following year that a permanent change in the blood pressure should not be anticipated. He took the pressures of 992 American soldiers and established that the average tension was much the same as the accepted standard for males of the same age in a temperate zone.[99] In 1914, when Breinl and Priestley estimated the blood pressures of North Queensland children, they also could discern no marked climatic influence on the results. As Breinl and Young concluded, "a sound heart and sound arteries are adaptable to any change."[100]

A more resilient white body and a less menacing climate were similarly emerging in scientific investigations of the quality of the blood of Europeans living in the tropics. The existence of a tropical anemia for a long time had been regarded as an established fact. Visitors to the region often observed that the skin even of healthy Europeans in the tropics appeared pale and sallow. It seemed that a thinness or poverty of the blood was the natural consequence of inappropriate tropical residence and a sure sign of racial degeneration.[101] Yet it was not until the early twentieth century that the microscope had made the constituents of the blood visible in the tropics. The results were rather surprising. In the Philippines, the ever-vigorous Chamberlain performed 1,718 red cell counts and 1,433 hemoglobin estimations of 702 white American soldiers; he concluded that the figures "do not differ from the normal at present recognized for healthy young men in a temperate zone."[102] To see if these results could be reproduced in Australia, Breinl and Priestley in 1914 performed 508 blood counts on healthy white children born and bred in North Queensland. They confirmed that "there is no striking difference in the number of erythrocytes [red blood cells] and the colour index in North Queensland children when compared with the averages obtained in children of a temperate climate."[103] In most cases of anemia in the tropics, hookworm or malaria, and not the climate, was the cause, and these pathogens could be avoided if whites followed basic stipulations of hygiene and avoided insects and lower races— avoided, that is, the presumed local hosts and vectors of tropical germs.

In Manila and Townsville, medical scientists were marshaling their white subjects and ordering them into a series of scientific papers. The detailed description of methods, the deployment of statistics, and the performance of laboratory tests gave a rhetorical and dramatic force to the scientists' arguments, helping to undermine a century of pessimistic anecdote and clinical observation. Confidence in the continuity of racial type overcame fears of European constitutional decline in a depleting environment; the medical meaning of interpersonal contact became more important than the medical ecology of adaptation. Biological exchanges occurring in the space between stable, typical bodies were assuming more significance than the interactions between a body and its physical circumstances. The white organism seemed increasingly impermeable to its inorganic surroundings, or at least protectable from its circumstances, even as it appeared ever more susceptible to microbiological contamination through racial contact. "It is not the mere influence of climate which opposes colonization in tropical lands," advised Dr. Luigi Sambon, one of the leaders of the new tropical medicine in London, "but the competition of other living organisms—from man, wild beasts, and snakes to protozoa and bacteria—with which we have to struggle for existence."[104] By invoking insects and native races as natural carriers of local disease agents, and discounting the effects of a climate that was never amenable to change, medical scientists were suggesting that expert social and political intervention might yet permit the establishment of a working white race in the Australian tropics. Microbiology could thus give many nationalists a sense of purpose and a practical program for white Australia. Yet the physiological studies that demonstrated the innocuousness of the climate had also required the scientific decomposition of white bodies into pigment, eye color, blood pressure, hemoglobin, rectal temperature, white cell count, and lung capacity. The white bodies that northern settlers were told did not degenerate could scarcely have appeared to be their own.

GOING TROPPO

Even if the tropical laboratory could prove that white bodies were not degenerating physically, might not a mental deterioration still take place? Breinl and Young admitted that whites in northern Australia seemed especially prone to a mental condition resembling neurasthenia. In its milder forms, this tropical neurasthenia manifested itself "in a lability of the mental equilibrium, fits of depression alternate with states of exuberance; unwarranted irritability over trifling matters is hardly ever absent, leading to uncontrollable outbreaks of temper." After many years in the tropics, Europeans commonly found that they suffered "a loss of mental activity and power of concentration, lack of confidence and failing memory, all of which cause a decreased working capacity."[105] Whites near the equator seemed to become nervy and irresolute, their character dissolved under the strain, and their willpower failed. White bodies might survive the heat and humidity, they might even labor in the cane fields, but could white civilization thrive in such circumstances?

In the late 1860s, George M. Beard, a New York neurologist, had described neurasthenia as a novel and distinctively modern disease syndrome characterized by a depletion of "nerve force."[106] Beard had suggested that the human organism produced only a limited amount of nervous force: If the capacity was low, or the demands excessive, nervous function could become overloaded, and the system would then break down. The precise quantum of nerve force that an individual possessed was a function of a hereditary endowment organized by race and gender. The disease seemed to attack the most refined or productive members of society, the caretakers of civilization: Beard thought Anglo-Saxons and non-Catholics in the prime of life were particularly susceptible. In general, men became neurasthenic from overwork, competition, and economic acquisitiveness; and women succumbed through dissipating their more limited neural vitality in study or excessive socializing.

Beard had believed that the tropics constituted an environment so depleting that it would always be hostile to physical and mental exertion. Accordingly, neurasthenia, as a disease of civilization, would not occur there.[107] But after the U.S. occupation of the Philippines in 1898, medical officers began to diagnose a distinctively tropical neurasthenia among the American colonialists, especially among any who recklessly attempted any brainwork in such a hot and humid climate. Colonel Valery Havard, in reviewing the effects of the Philippine climate on Americans, was especially concerned that the atmospheric humidity prevented free evaporation of perspiration, forcing the white organism to reduce its production of heat in order to maintain a physiological equilibrium. The result of "this necessary tropical regime" was a loss not only of heat but also of nervous energy. "The loss of energy," he observed, "is chiefly felt by the mental faculties: there is a diminution of capacity for intellectual labor, an inability to do work requiring continued concentration." Although the tropical resident might carefully avoid the recently identified tropical pathogens, he must "resign himself to the loss of more or less of his bodily and mental activity."[108] Major Charles E. Woodruff warned "blond races" of the specific dangers of concentrated light. The actinic rays, he argued, produced "some kind of chemical breaking up which renders [the cell] paretic," leading first to a misleading sense of "stimulation" but soon followed by a chronic "low vitality of tissues." Not surprisingly, then, the poorly pigmented "blonds suffer in the Philippines more than brunets, have higher grades of neurasthenia, break down in larger numbers proportionately, and in many ways prove their unfitness for the climate."[109]

In 1913, the British Society of Tropical Medicine devoted a meeting to a discussion of the grave problem of tropical neurasthenia, or brain-fag. Sir Havelock Charles, president of the Medical Board of the India Office and a physician of the old school, reviewed the incidence of "Punjab head." Charles thought that this particular "head," and similar ones that occurred throughout the tropics, "must be attributed to the damage done mainly to the nervous system by a hot and humid climate." One could, with "despotic power," rectify unsanitary conditions, but one could not "change the heat, the sunlight, the climatic conditions, by either the power of money or the power of knowledge." Widespread and inevitable nervous exhaustion implied that "for a white race to preserve its purity and predominance in a tropical climate, and to keep that vigour, intelligence and physique which are its characteristics, fresh waves of immigration are essential to make up for the wear and tear due to climatic influence."[110] But Sir Ronald Ross noted in response that most cases of tropical neurasthenia would have been prevented with a more careful selection of recruits, a sensible diet, and avoidance of alcohol.[111] Dr. Andrew Balfour observed that "Sudan head," which caused a characteristic "marked disinclination to stoop and look for things near the ground level," was a "stagnation and regression" derived mostly from an indolent way of life. He urged the white men resident in the tropics to take up "an active outdoor life, short of actual fatigue."[112] And Dr. F. M. Sandwith commented, sardonically, that he now believed dubious cases of tropical neurasthenia "would be diagnosed more successfully if the Wasserman test [for syphilis] were tried as a matter of routine."[113] Clearly, many of the new generation of tropical experts had come to believe that with sufficient self-control one could now avoid even "tropical" neurasthenia.

Breinl and his colleagues were not so sure. They regarded some of the statements made at the 1913 meeting as "merely expressions of personal opinions, collected during a shorter or longer residence in the tropics, and often coloured by prejudice; actual data in support of these opinions were sadly lacking." Although the Townsville investigators conceded that forms of neurasthenia were quite common among Europeans in northern Australia—even among their colleagues—they found it difficult to gauge the extent to which climate was responsible. Perhaps the problem was a behavioral one, the result of a change in habit in response to new conditions of life. "The novelty of the strange environment often leads to an increased output of energy, and it is only after a time that the newcomer realises his energy capacity under the new conditions and begins to husband his strength, but often too late to avoid paying the penalty."[114] It would require more research in Townsville to establish the severity of the problem and whether its causes were climatic or behavioral. "An extensive investigation into the mental activities in general would perhaps yield figures of definite value," Breinl and Young suggested in 1920. "The applying of the Binet-Simon test for mentality to a great number of school children . . . would furnish figures of definite value for deciding the presence or absence of racial degeneration."[115]

Breinl's call for more research on neurasthenia was in part a means of deflecting the criticisms of a renegade colleague. In 1917, William Nicoll, the parasitologist at the institute, asserted that a "change of environment alone will cause radical alteration not perhaps so much in physical characters as in mental habitude."[116] In foreign circumstances, British stock was evolving into a distinctive Australian type: Its physical characteristics had diverged slightly, and antipodean mentality already had developed into a decidedly different form. Even so, this new type did not seem any more capable of colonizing the tropics than its European original. "There is not the slightest doubt that residence in the remote tropics causes much mental stasis which to those trained in mental rather than manual labour, is quite as prejudicial as stasis in any other vital function."[117] Nicoll, recovering from dengue and pining for a cool climate, discounted the results of research conducted by his colleagues at Townsville. Their technical ineptitude "made the blood run cold," and he thought that their work was a wonderful example of "assiduity combined with ignorance." Nicoll regarded Breinl's optimistic statements about the prospects for white settlement in the tropics as little more than "sententious balderdash."[118] According to Nicoll, who was perhaps writing from bitter personal experience, any talented European "will not be foolish enough to bury his energy and ambition in such a forsaken corner of creation as North Queensland." Tropical Australia, he declared, "will never under present circumstances support a permanent population of exclusively European character." White men might work and live there for a few years without degenerating, but they should return to a temperate region before their endurance fails. Otherwise, if forced, like Nicoll, to remain under tropical conditions, it would be "to the detriment of their health and character."[119]

Henry Priestley was not as intemperate and irritable as Nicoll, but neither was he quite as hopeful as Breinl and Young. In 1923, Priestley, who was then teaching biochemistry at the University of Sydney, reviewed the Townsville studies of racial adaptation in the tropics. He told the Pan-Pacific Science Congress that Townsville has a climate similar to that of Calcutta but fortunately was not "densely populated by coloured races living . . . under very unhygienic conditions and heavily infected with diseases." Indeed, with the exception of malaria and dengue, tropical ailments were rare, as there was no "large native population acting as a reservoir for disease." Yet many Australians still believed that a tropical climate would inevitably "impoverish" the blood of any whites who endured it.[120] With Breinl and Young, Priestley had investigated the blood counts, pulse rates, lung capacities, rectal temperatures, and blood pressures of white children, institute staff, and wharf laborers, and the results had been reassuring. As yet, he could "point to no striking alterations in the physiology of white persons in the tropics which could be considered the result of climatic influences." He did, however, share the widespread uneasiness about neurasthenia. At Townsville his experience had indicated that "continued and concentrated mental work is much more difficult than in a temperate climate."[121] White residents of the tropics usually succumbed to mental inertia, irritability, and shortness of temper. Women who had to work in hot and muggy kitchens seemed especially prone to tropical neurasthenia. Priestley also feared that "the almost universal discontent shown by the working man in Northern Australia may, very probably, be another aspect of the influence of climate on the central nervous system." Although definite conclusions must await further investigations, it seemed undeniable that the militant Townsville waterside workers were "much more easily inflamed by the specious arguments of the agitator. Is it not likely that this is climatic in origin?"[122]

Persistent White Anxieties

In his protean medical textbook, Dr. J. W. Springthorpe, the lecturer in therapeutics, dietetics, and hygiene at the University of Melbourne, expressed a common ambivalence in assessing the influence of tropical environments on white settlers. Few contemporary medicos were still prepared to regard the tropics as directly pathogenic; most now believed, with Springthorpe, that white bodies could more or less be insulated from the climate and local disease carriers, even if white mentality might remain vulnerable to external influences; some went so far as to exonerate the region altogether. Although "Springy" was generally hopeful that white bodily integrity would be preserved even in the harshest of climates, he expected that this achievement required constant effort and regular expert assistance. A white man "is forced to wage a daily and hourly battle in the tropics in order to maintain his normal temperature, and the endurance of his skin, heart, blood vessels and nerves is strongly taxed." In contrast, Springthorpe reported that "the coloured races, by reason of their admirable suitability to warm climates, are able to maintain their temperature without effort." All the same, he was able to tell the Melbourne students that he knew a white gentleman of eighty-two years of age who had lived in the north since 1861 and in the previous year had decided to grow sugarcane. His health and vigor were exemplary. "One day, when not feeling very well, he informed me, he had had no inclination for sexual intercourse for two days."[123] In his contribution to Springthorpe's text, Breinl's own occasional ambivalence toward the prospect of a working and fecund white race in the tropics shaded into prevarication. He reported that physiological investigations at Townsville had shown no appreciable differences between whites in temperate or tropical zones. Yet he warned that further studies might show that "minute physiological changes may take place, which will only become noticeable in the second or third, or even later generations."[124]

White bodies had come to seem more robust, or more readily stabilized or salvaged, than ever before, but they were still not completely impervious to surroundings, still not perfectly alienated from their environment. Some experts, such as Breinl and Young, were prepared to argue that physiological type altered hardly at all in foreign circumstances, provided that basic stipulations of personal hygiene were heeded. Their colleague Henry Priestley believed that even the more cosmopolitan of bacteria demonstrated an admirable stability of type in the tropics. In a startlingly analogical series of experiments, Priestley found that exposure to intense sunlight and to a variety of chemicals had not caused bacteria to mutate.[125] Why should it be any different for whites? But many older doctors, and a few of the more residually Lamarckian of the Townsville investigators' contemporaries, felt that the laboratory scientists were understating the influence of the environment on racial type. Joseph Ahearne, "M. B.," and "Cosmos" continued to assert that the white race was degenerating in the north; William Nicoll noticed distinct alterations, not all of them bad, in the physical characteristics of transgressive white settlers. Such challenges to modern scientific findings, along with the reservations occasionally expressed by the scientists themselves, merely justified demands for further research and the ever more meticulous supervision of white populations.

The major concern was mental degeneration. Tropical neurasthenia still haunted even the most confident assertions of racial triumph. White bodies might labor and reproduce in the tropics, but would the civilization so typical of the race continue to thrive in hot and humid surroundings? Mental vigor and enterprise—the most important of white male virtues—still seemed to dissipate or go awry in the depleting climate. Few were surprised when women and children became feeble-minded in the heat; but the failures of manly self-mastery and restraint—the bulwarks of British civility—presented a special concern for those who wanted to implant not just white bodies but white civilization in the north. And yet we should resist the temptation to view the widespread recognition of tropical nervousness as a destabilizing critique of white Australia. More often, a diagnosis of tropical neurasthenia signaled the beginning of a salvage operation of white identity, not its subversion; it offered a chance of recuperation and redemption, not condemnation. The notion of white nervousness in the tropics helped to keep open a space for the unremitting surveillance and disciplining of settlers in the north. As long as tropical neurasthenia elicited fear and concern, research must go on, education must go on, public health campaigns must go on.[126]

The new generation of doctors and scientists had grown up as pragmatists, acquiring as they did so a more positive view of the impact of active human effort on the environment. Gradually they were shaking off older notions of providential or evolutionary determinism, setting aside outworn assumptions of environmental constraint in favor of a new faith in human will and creative energy. Few did so with the fervor of Elkington and his relatives, the Lindsays, but most came to believe that new ideas and new technologies, the products of will and energy, could protect the white races from adverse circumstances— inasmuch as they needed any protection. Many of these doctors and scientists had read John Dewey and William James, and they were convinced that human intelligence was an effective instrument in modifying the world. They believed that at last they could use the methods of science to resolve political problems and to set national policy.[127]

In the medical schools of Melbourne, Sydney, and even Adelaide, and from the institute at Townsville, scientists were patiently explaining to politicians and the general public that human settlement and immigration policies were actually vast natural experiments. Accordingly, academics from the infant universities, and the medical doctors they had trained, would be best equipped to structure and to supervise such a biological study. "In the future," wrote Breinl, "the pioneer should not be the settler, but the scientifically trained man."[128] Politicians, he argued, ought to heed the advice of the expanding cohort of technical experts; white citizens should come to regard themselves as experimental subjects in the national laboratory and to govern themselves accordingly. "It is desirable," advised Barrett, "to arrange for several experimental stations, at which settlers could be accommodated. Each station would be under the charge of a health officer."[129] Working white citizens in the new nation, especially in its supposedly tropical parts, would require unremitting expert supervision and discipline if they were to remain working white citizens. In order to possess the whole of the continent, they would have to follow closely the doctors' orders. But obedience would be rewarded with positive governmental measures designed to foster racial well-being. In accordance with the new scientific rationalism, good behavior would earn white settlers fair labor laws, pensions, roads, railways, and restrictions on foreign economic competition.[130]

If the physiological status of whiteness in the tropics was still debatable, few of these medical experts doubted that security from infectious disease would require the exclusion of colored races from the whitening continent. When white bacteriologists found an excessive number of bacteria and parasites in the blood and excreta of other races, they generally assumed that this was because nature had fashioned natives as biological reservoirs of the germs with which they had evolved. Moreover, native culture, which then seemed as fixed a racial feature as any physical attribute, had ensured that these physical reservoirs were overflowing with germs, most of them innocuous to their hosts but deadly to vulnerable whites. Racial biology offered a more satisfying explanation of disease carriage than did any consideration of historical misfortunes.

White cleanliness and purity and self-control—the constituents of white Australia—were naturally positioned against colored disease agency and danger and promiscuity. Even apparently healthy colored people might secretly carry and distribute germs to which whites were naturally susceptible. (In a sense, the old fear that white males might acquire venereal disease from women of lower classes or other races had been generalized in the early twentieth century to cover all diseases and all forms of contact.) As environmental threats appeared to recede, whiteness came to be defined more in terms of this Manichean struggle between opposing natural typologies: white against colored; purity against danger; health against disease.

The understanding of the physical, mental, and pathological properties of race was changing, but even so race remained a potent, if still indefinite, category of analysis. Australian medical scientists were as dedicated as most other white citizens to the building of a new nation based on purity of race, so how could it be otherwise? Neither was this merely a local quirk: Until well into the 1930s the study of race persisted as a major international scientific interest, even if few academic cultures pursued the topic as single-mindedly as in Australia.[131] But if race was still everything as far as medical scientists were concerned, and as it continued to inform public health action and national policy, not all Australian intellectuals were comfortable with its simplifying biological essentialisms. In 1912, Bernard O'Dowd, the poet and socialist, addressed Victorian theosophists on the "unscientific" nature of race prejudice. He contended that "colour is one of the least important of the distinctions between man and man, that it is not a permanent distinction, and that it does not necessarily connote mental, spiritual, or even ineradicable physical differences." It was only in "comparatively recent times that men have set out deliberately to give us scientific reasons why we should hate our brothers of the coloured and other races."[132] These mutually contradictory scientific hypotheses "are held as gospel by thousands of investigators, and have even affected the students of our own Aboriginal tribes in Australasia" and given rise to "the extremely subtle and plausible and dangerous pseudo-science of Eugenics that has its influence even in Australia." O'Dowd longed for the day when "all the rich elements of all the human varieties . . . shall mingle together in one great human stream."[133] When he died in Melbourne in 1953 he was still awaiting that day.

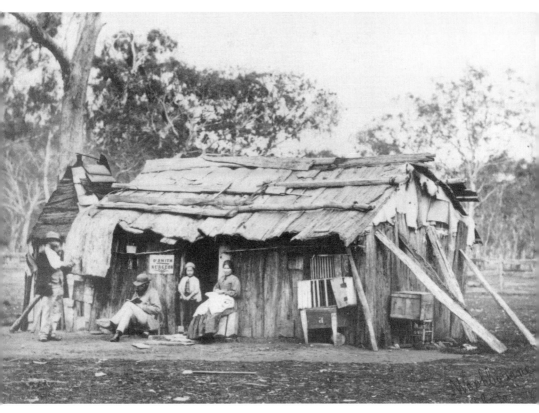

Dr. Smith, surgeon: slab hut residence, c. 1860s.
(LaTrobe Picture Collection, State Library of Victoria)

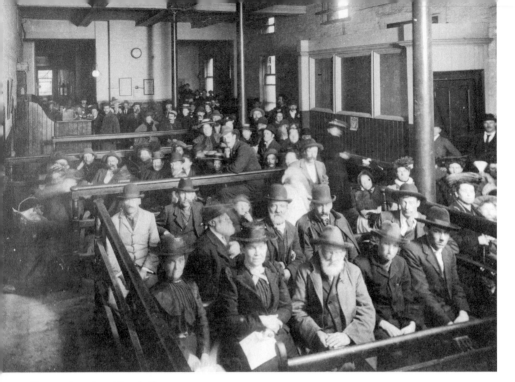

Out-patients' waiting hall,
Melbourne Hospital, c. 1900.
(Royal Melbourne Hospital Archives)

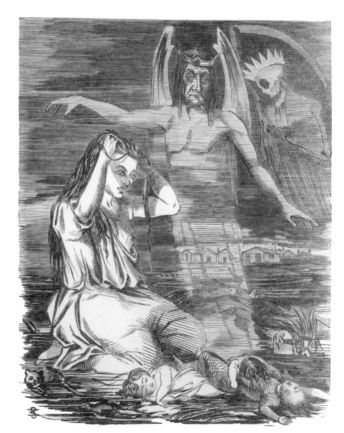

"King Fever and his
Victims," Melbourne
Punch, 9 June 1864.
(Melbourne Picture
Collection, State
Library of Victoria)

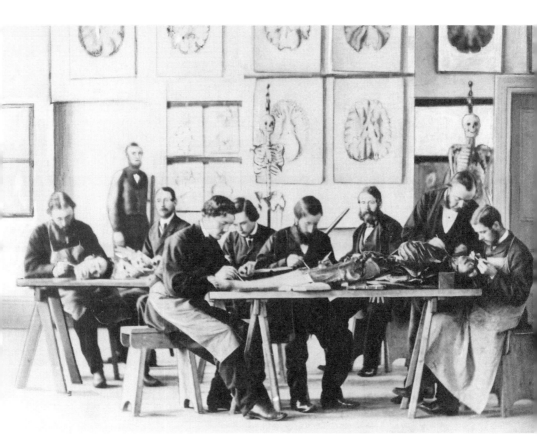

B. Halford teaching anatomy class, 1864. (Medical History Museum, University of Melbourne)

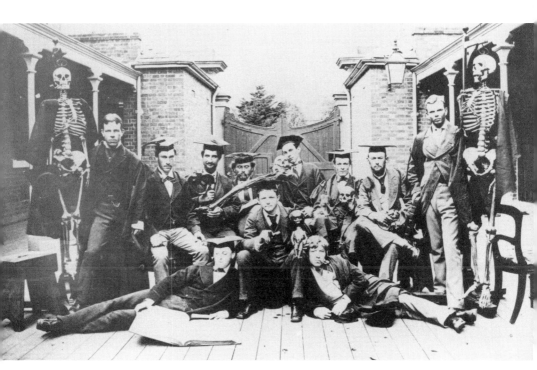

Melbourne medical students, 1878. (Medical History Museum, University of Melbourne)

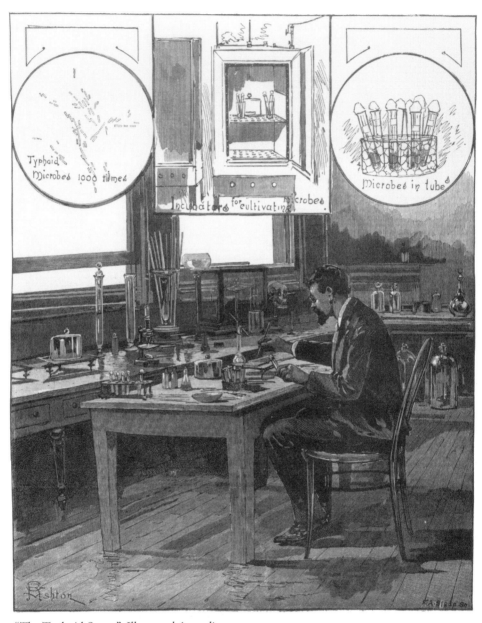

"The Typhoid Scare," *Illustrated Australian
News and Musical Times*, 1 October 1889.
(LaTrobe Picture Collection, State Library of Victoria)

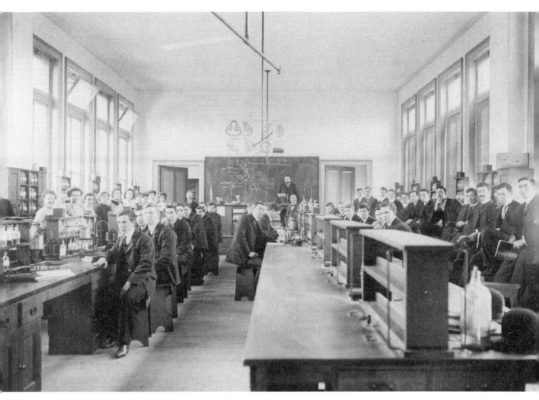

Physiology laboratory, University of Melbourne, 1902.
(Medical History Museum, University of Melbourne)

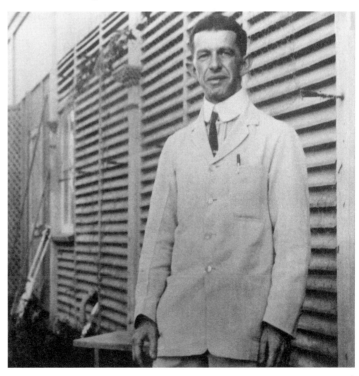

Dr. Anton Breinl.
(Rockefeller Archive Center)

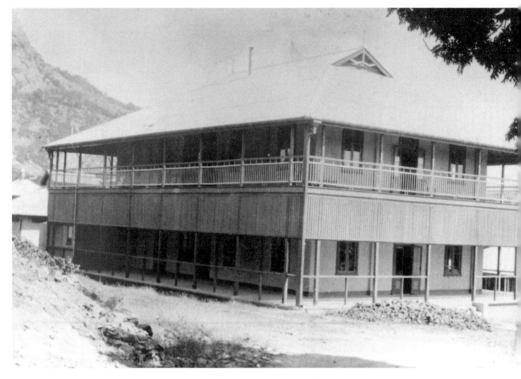

The Australian Institute of Tropical Medicine. (Rockefeller Archive Center)

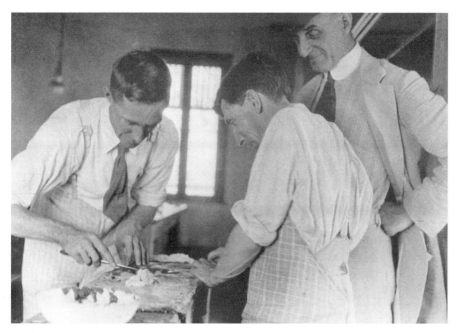

Collecting pigment at the Australian Institute of
Tropical Medicine at Townsville. Dr. Heiser looks on.
(Rockefeller Archive Center)

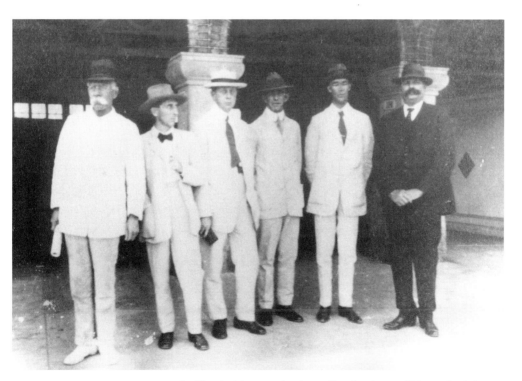

Staff and visitors at the Australian Institute of Tropical Medicine.
Young, second from left; Breinl, fourth; and Priestley, fifth.
(Rockefeller Archive Center)

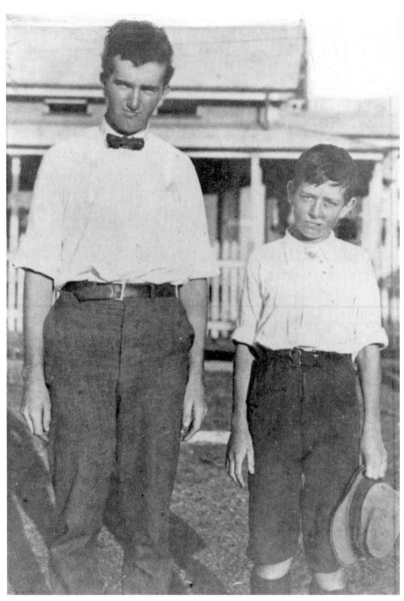

Queensland twins, one suffering from hookworm.
(Rockefeller Archive Center)

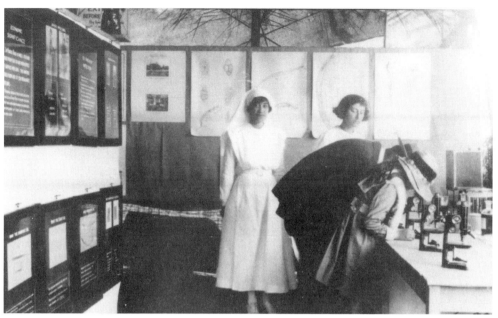

Hookworm exhibition, Queensland.
(Rockefeller Archive Center)

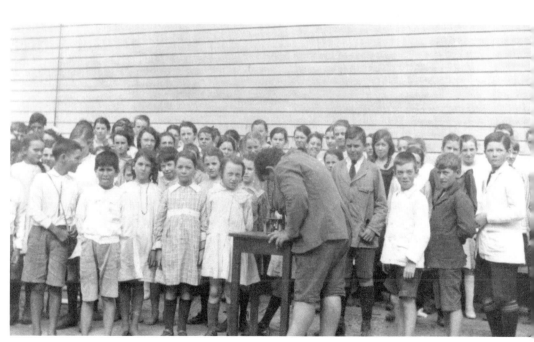

Hookworm demonstration to school children, Mackay, Queensland.
(Rockefeller Archive Center)

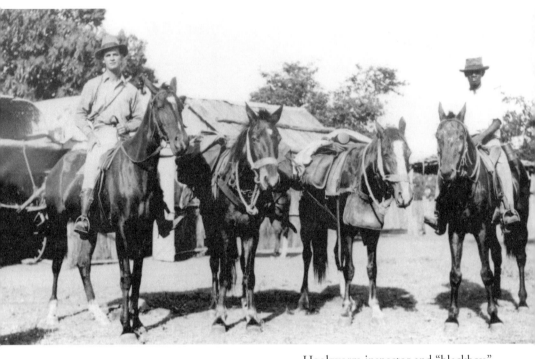

Hookworm inspector and "blackboy."
(Rockefeller Archive Center)

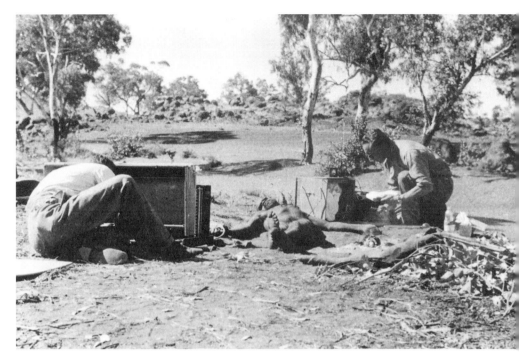

S. Hicks measuring basal metabolic rates, 1930s.
(Barr-Smith Library, University of Adelaide)

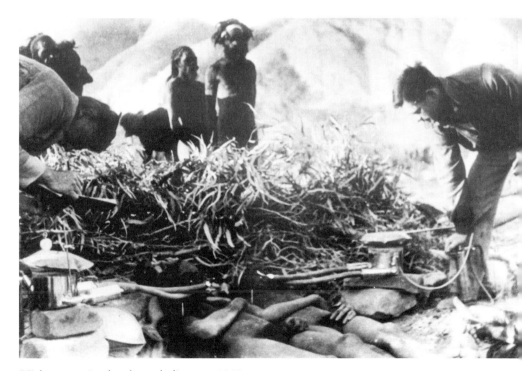

Hicks measuring basal metabolic rates, 1930s.
(Barr-Smith Library, University of Adelaide)

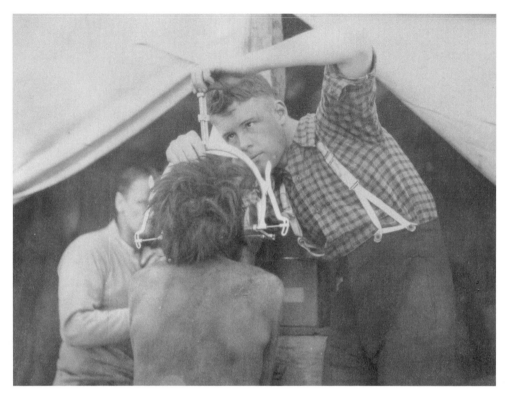

Expedition member performing anthropometry, Cockatoo Creek, 1931.
(South Australian Museum Archives)

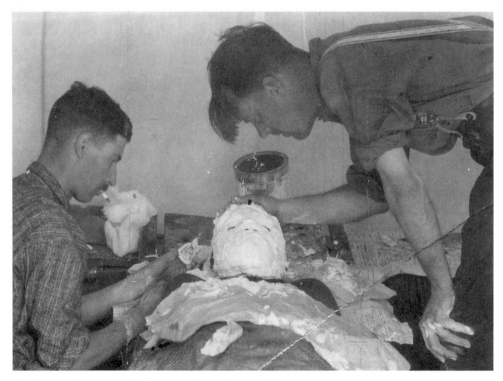

Tindale making a cast of a face, Cockatoo Creek, 1931.
(South Australian Museum Archives)

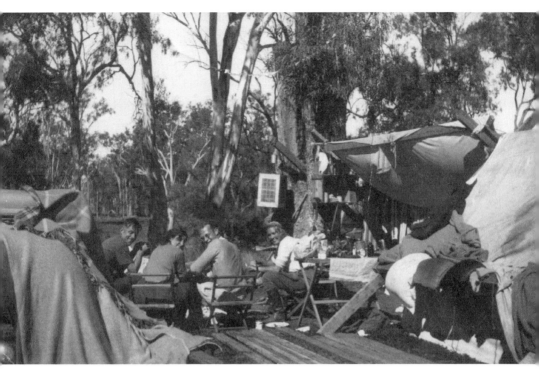

N. B. Tindale, Dorothy Tindale, Joseph Birdsell and
Bee Birdsell in Camp at Boggabilla, NSW, July
1938. "Steak and kidney pie for lunch."
(South Australian Museum Archives)

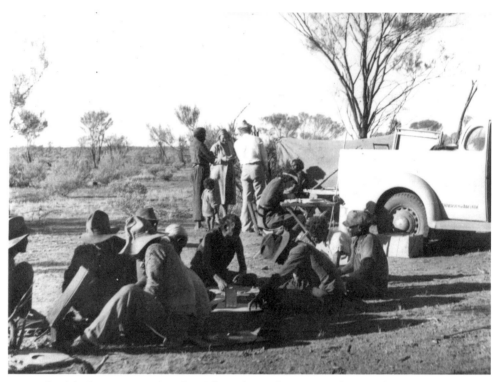

Harvard-Adelaide Universities' Anthropological Expedition at work
near Laverton, WA, May 1939. (South Australian Museum Archives)

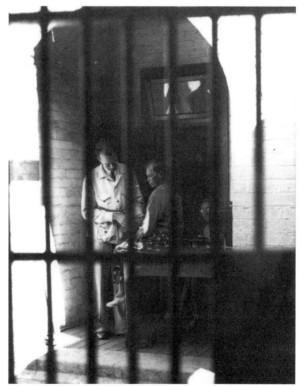

Birdsell measuring at
Colli. "In lock-up for
convenience only."
(South Australian
Museum Archives)

CHAPTER 5

WHITE TRIUMPH IN THE TROPICS?

IN AUGUST 1920, THE Australasian Medical Congress met in Brisbane to discuss pressing national concerns about "tropical Australia." After reviewing the physiological research of the Australian Institute of Tropical Medicine at Townsville, the meeting declared that "the opinion of the medical practitioners present was overwhelmingly in favour of the suitability of North Queensland for the successful implantation of a working white race." Laboratory results and vital statistics suggested no "inherent or insuperable obstacles" in the way of white occupation, and the delegates thought that, on microbial grounds, "the absence of semi-civilised coloured peoples in northern Australia simplifies the problem very greatly." Tropical settlement and development were, according to the congress, fundamentally questions of "applied public health in the modern sense."[1] Some improvements in diet, clothing, housing, and personal hygiene evidently were necessary in the north, and the congress concluded that such reforms should be based on the Townsville investigations and organized by a new federal department of health. Not surprisingly, J.H.L. Cumpston, the federal director of quarantine, spoke in favor of these recommendations and endorsed the proposal, aware that he was the leading candidate to direct a new health department. Cumpston pointed out that Anton Breinl and his colleagues, after ten years of physiological experimentation at Townsville, had detected few diseases and no signs of degeneracy in tropical whites. Immigration restriction had worked wonders, but now, in addition, a federal health department would be required to ensure constant vigilance against the introduction and spread of disease. "It is all very well to have a white Australia," he announced, "but it must be kept white. There must be immaculate cleanliness."[2]

The declarations of the 1920 Australasian Medical Congress were predicated on a medical possibilism that would have seemed hopelessly naive and utopian just fifty years earlier.[3] Most of the delegates now believed that whites either contained within themselves the biological hardiness to resist their environment or possessed the technology and knowledge of hygiene that would insulate them from otherwise pathological circumstances.[4] New theories that postulated a more robust heredity, combined with the practical advances of "applied public health in the modern sense," had allowed Europeans to view themselves as masters of their various locations, even as they became increasingly alienated from them. With medically supervised selection of white populations and careful regulation of their personal and domestic hygiene, it seemed that whites could colonize even the tropics without degenerating or pigmenting. But this turning away from environmental determinism and muting of Lamarckian theories of heredity did not mean that environment, in a more narrow sense, was deemed utterly powerless. The increasingly confident medical possibilists, such as Cumpston, Elkington, Osborne, and Barrett, never tired of reiterating the importance of diet, housing, clothing, and proper behavior. But their concern was focused on the social environment of self-possessed white bodies, an interpersonal microenvironment, not on climate and topography. They believed that it now was possible, with a scientifically managed breeding program, and, perhaps more practically, a maximizing of hereditary potential through improved nurture, to produce a stronger white race in Australia, one more pure, virile, and cleanly even than in its European homeland. Of course, until this glorious day, it would still be necessary to use immigration restriction and quarantine to protect the emergent strain of whites from unfair microbiological competition.

In 1923, the aging Sir Harry Allen, still dean of the Melbourne medical school and a tireless advocate, was prepared to praise recent Australian advances in public health administration, but he warned that much was yet to be done. Allen's views more or less epitomized the goals of post–World War I hygienists. "A general awakening of the public conscience is necessary," he wrote, "The ardent pursuit of pleasure is not the road to happiness. . . . Self-will and self-pleasing in men and women will not build up a healthy nation. There must be discipline, there must be a keen sense of duty, care for others, acceptance of social obligation."[5] The proper solution of the nation's health problems lay in "purity of life, in discipline of the body, in self-restraint taught from the cradle, in the culture of true manliness and womanliness." Government health activity must ensure that these values became the Australian standard. For this to happen, further research would have to be conducted in order to reveal unsuspected depths of public ignorance. "Give us better medical schools, build up institutes of research, popularise the theory and the methods of preventive medicine." Finally, Allen reminded his medical readers that "all our health work may but ensure the deterioration of the race, unless we find the means, with wisdom and kindness, to prevent the multiplication of the unfit."[6]

To the national hygienists, as John Powles has described them, World War I had provided a lesson in the management of populations.[7] According to Cumpston, those who returned from the war were "a body of men who have discovered what things can be accomplished by resolute men, actuated by a common impulse."[8] The rhetoric of John Masefield, C.E.W. Bean, and other artificers of the Anzac legend implied that a strong stock had already emerged in the antipodes; now Cumpston and his medical colleagues hoped to enhance this stock through means of selection or hygiene reform.[9] Drawing on military experience and a rising confidence in effectiveness of human agency in reshaping populations and their environments, the leaders of the medical profession and the public health movement in the 1920s and 1930s devised schemes to improve racial vigor and efficiency in Australia. Many of these medical doctors and scientists had trained or taught at the University of Melbourne; they shared assumptions about heredity, biological destiny, and the role of the state in national renewal. Most of these "medical materialists," to use James Gillespie's term, had been inspired also by the health activities of American progressives and the British national efficiency movement.[10] Among their early achievements, in the aftermath of the Brisbane congress, was the establishment of the activist Commonwealth Department of Health in 1921, led by Cumpston and J.S.C. Elkington and emphasizing quarantine and tropical hygiene.[11]

In this chapter, I describe the formulation of a distinctive "tropical hygiene" at the Townsville Institute during the 1920s and the efforts of its new director, Raphael Cilento, to regulate and reform white bodies and white conduct in the north to produce a corporeal white armature. Nothing escaped Cilento's gaze: housing, clothing, diet, toilet practices, sexual activity—everything was available to the hygiene reformer. From the early 1920s, it seemed that Townsville investigators would most readily get access to such intimate aspects of white social life through their participation in the hookworm program, supported by the Rockefeller Foundation and based on similar projects in the U.S. South and in the colonial Philippines. The program to detect and eradicate hookworm carriage provided an opportunity to survey all the white residents of North Queensland and to reshape understandings of bodily contact, excretion, and eating habits. But even as whiteness was being purified and cleaned up in this way, its constituents threatened to separate out at the edges. During this period, Cilento and his colleagues were confronting the issue of increasing non-British immigration, in particular the status of Italians and Jews in white Australia. For some experts, whiteness began to dwindle back into Britishness or become consolidated as the new Nordic type, whereas for others, such as Cilento, it stayed expansive, including all Europeans, though not Jews; and for others still, the category might be stretched into Caucasian and potentially include even the Aboriginal inhabitants of the country. It was never easy to delimit the boundaries of white Australia. In any case, Cilento's attention kept shifting to new colonial possibilities, to health responsibilities in the territories of Papua and New Guinea. Ultimately, neither the focus on hygiene reform of tropical white residents nor colonial health administration would prove sufficiently attractive to the federal government for it to continue to invest in research at Townsville. By the end of the decade, the nation no longer regarded the tropical white man as a distinctive burden requiring special medical investigation and treatment.

PROBLEMS AT TOWNSVILLE

After Cumpston's plea for an ever more pure and cleanly white Australia, Breinl painstakingly took the delegates at the 1920 Brisbane congress through the findings of the Townsville studies. He pointed out again that the heat regulation, metabolism, blood pressure, and blood composition of tropical whites all resembled temperate standards. The northern birthrates were high, and infant mortality was lower than in the south. Breinl had found that tropical diseases, with the exception of hookworm, were "only scarce and easily controlled."[12] He concluded, of course, that a working white race could thrive in the north. Professor W. A. Osborne, the Melbourne physiologist, rose to congratulate Breinl on his work and agreed that the tropics were not "unwholesome" for the working white man, even though some of his colleagues still wondered if they gave rise to an "irritable heart" or to a neurasthenic condition.[13] But there were a few skeptics present at the congress; among them was Dr. A.T.H. Nisbet, a second-generation tropical physician. Nisbet believed that his women patients were especially prone to deterioration in the oppressive heat. He warned the meeting that as white women gave up tidiness and took to wearing kimonos, we would "breed degenerate generations willing to live on rice and bananas," a race not "British but North Australians resembling the Levantine in type."[14] Women were succumbing to neurasthenia and debility; children became unusually pale and languid and inclined to convulsions. But Nisbet's anecdotes of climatic evil and constitutional decay merely provided a rather antiquarian contrast to the shimmering array of vital statistics and laboratory findings presented at the congress. Few delegates paid much attention to him.

Later, in a more formal address to his medical colleagues, Osborne discussed the physiological factors in the development of an Australian race. "We are a white population and intend to remain white," he declared. "We hold this island continent as the citadel of the Western Pacific where momentous issues charged with destiny for the white man may one day be decided." Although Charles H. Pearson had once discounted any further progress of the race, Osborne now was far more sanguine. "May we look," he surmised, "to improved conditions and eugenic safeguards rejuvenating the white races and starting a new epoch in their progress."[15] The abundance and high quality of local food had already benefited the Australian physique; but the understanding of the effects of climate was still uncertain. Temperate conditions, such as those prevailing in the south, undoubtedly were advantageous; however, more research was still required to exonerate the tropics completely. Osborne conceded that in moist and hot conditions the heat generated within the body would take longer to escape, but a physiological difference of this sort was not always pathological. Moreover, appropriate clothing and the use of cooling fans might circumvent any environmental discomfort. And even if whites continued to feel uncomfortable in the tropics, they at least enjoyed in Australia "a singular immunity from the worst tropical diseases." Predictably, Osborne believed that this advantage was the result of "the absence of a large native population, for such always acts as a reservoir of infection from which epidemics spill over into the surrounding white population." The vigor of the Australian race thus depended on continuing immigration restriction, rigid quarantine, and the further development of "preventive medicine." "The white Australia policy may become more difficult," the physiologist reflected, "but it will become more desirable."[16]

A few months after the Brisbane congress, an editorial in the *Medical Journal of Australia* congratulated Breinl and his colleagues "on the thoroughness of their research, on the care and patience they exhibited and on the earnestness of the attempt to provide data for the elucidation of. . . the physiological problems associated with the white Australia question."[17] In the opinion of the editorial writer, North Queensland was no less healthy than any other part of Australia, but there was still, even after the congress, insufficient data to settle the matter. This was a serious concern:

> Unless an affirmative reply is given within a relatively short time, this vast, wealthy, inexhaustible land will neither be safe for those who have struck the first cord [*sic*] of a wonderful national melody, for those whose blood and sweat has been given in the pioneer stage of the making of a great nation, nor retain the characters which have compelled him to hold it dearer than any other. White Australia is at once a sentiment and a necessity for all of us.

The *Medical Journal of Australia* expected that "true and direct experiment alone can yield an unequivocal reply" to any questioning of white Australia.[18]

Those who had long opposed white settlement in the north were less impressed with the findings of the congress. Dr. Richard Arthur, a politician from New South Wales, reported that he was not even permitted to speak in

Brisbane. It was all part of a "put-up job." But "a day or so later all the newspapers of Australia were appearing with editorials announcing to a credulous public that the problem of tropical Australia had been settled once and for good. All the doubts and fears had been dissipated." Arthur, a great supporter of British migration and measures to improve the birthrate, was astounded that it was now supposed that "it only remained to persuade the Anglo-Saxon to enter into this 'Land of Promise' and multiply and replenish the earth there."[19] Certainly, Arthur and other critics felt they were in a censured minority. Before long, most experts were adducing the findings of the Brisbane congress to demonstrate that white Australia was indeed a physiological fact. G. L. Wood, for example, pointed out that the conclusions at Brisbane had come as "a shock to orthodox opinion." But they convinced the Melbourne political economist that "the careful researches of the Institute failed to reveal the slightest evidence that the tropics had any deteriorating influence on life and growth."[20] Similarly, a few years after the congress, Senator Lynch, speaking on the future of northern Australia in the federal parliament, could approvingly cite the medical conclusions reached at Brisbane. "Thus we have it," he said, "on the authority of our own scientific men who have studied the problem on the spot, that the settlement of tropical Australia offers no insurmountable difficulties."[21]

For the next twenty years or more, few advocates of white settlement in the tropics would fail to mention the conclusions of the Brisbane congress. Sir James Barrett was typical. In 1922, Barrett assured his fellow imperialists at the Royal Colonial Institute in London that the Australasian Medical Congress had found that in northern Australia "a vigorous white race is being developed in spite of defective housing and sanitation."[22] A few years later, he was explaining to students at the University of Melbourne that "the deliberate opinion of the vast majority of medical men and physiologists is that, so far as climate is concerned, there is nothing whatever to prevent the peopling of Australia with a healthy and vigorous white race." He reported that the medical congress had determined that tropical diseases were no threat so long as colored migration was prevented. In other tropical countries there was "a large indigenous population, extensively infected with tropical diseases, to some of which the native population has become partially immune. On the other hand, the white man is not immune, and is frequently infected with disastrous results." But the striving for white racial purity in northern Australia had prevented such pathologies.[23] And as late as 1938, at a geographical congress in Amsterdam, Barrett was harking back to what he had heard at the Brisbane meeting in 1920, arguing that the medical profession had agreed that "if Australia possessed an infected indigenous population on a large scale, tropical diseases would give much the same trouble as in other tropical countries." It was fortunate, Barrett assured his audience, that Aboriginal Australians were too few and too dispersed to represent a health problem for whites.[24]

The Brisbane congress proved conclusive in another sense. Breinl's research career was sputtering to a stop, and the meeting on tropical Australia became its terminus. If the war had shown Cumpston and his resolute colleagues how they might organize and discipline a population, its effects on Breinl and his fellow scientists at Townsville had been less than salutary. Breinl decided to take over clinical duties at the hospital; support for research evaporated; and Priestley left for Sydney in 1918, followed by Young, who took up a position at Melbourne in early 1920. Moreover, it seems that Breinl's interests gradually were shifting from laboratory work toward more lucrative private practice, especially after his marriage in 1919. Breinl, a protozoologist, may also have found it increasingly difficult to meet with any enthusiasm the constant demands of the committee of management of the institute for yet more physiological research. The committee, dominated by Elkington, repeatedly advised Breinl that his priority should be an inquiry "into the various matters likely to affect the permanent establishment of a working white race in tropical Australia."[25] To ensure the appointment of another physiologist, Breinl grudgingly agreed that "the whole question of the physiology of the white man in the tropics is far from being solved," and the research work of the Americans in the Philippines was "open to a great deal of criticism." North Queensland, "where a second and even a third generation is growing up and where coloured labour is absent," would make a natural laboratory for such a study.[26] (Indeed, it had already done so.) Yet Breinl was not trained in physiology, and Priestley and Young were moving on from tropical matters, so even a positive response to his forced entreaties could scarcely at this stage of his career have offered him much personal satisfaction. In October 1920, soon after his success at the Brisbane congress, Breinl resigned from the Australian Institute of Tropical Medicine, though he remained in Townsville, building up a large private practice to support his young family.[27]

Breinl's replacement was Philip A. Maplestone, a mercurial young expert on parasitic worms. Maplestone was already convinced that any effort to do tropical medical research in Townsville was futile. For a start, he had no doubt that whites could flourish in North Queensland. A few years before, in a breezy lecture addressed to students at the University of Melbourne, the helminthologist had recalled an outback ball that he attended with his fellow tropical residents, "an evening quite as strenuous and, to them, enjoyable as any ever experienced in southern Australia." This was despite the fact that such a dance occurs "irrespective of the season of the year, and that it takes place within the latitude of that 'dread' tropical belt of Australia where it is alleged by many southern experts—medical men and others—that the white man cannot live and work." If tropical whites could dance so often and so strenuously, what was the point of further physiological experimentation?[28] Neither did he find much of great pathological interest at Townsville. In 1921, Maplestone told a meeting of the committee of management of the institute that there was "very little tropical disease in Australia and consequently he doubted whether the existence of the Institute in its present form was justified." When he further irritated his overseers by suggesting that the new physiologist, E. S. Sundstroem, would never find volunteers for the proposed experiments, they instructed him to secure "persons in gaols and such institutions" for physiological studies.[29] A month later, Maplestone sent the committee a memorandum, repeating that the institute was "in the wrong place" and should either be moved farther north, where there might be more tropical disease, or reestablished at Sydney, where there would be more intellectual stimulation. He regarded the institute's record as dismal since "with the exception of a few physiological facts nothing really new has been added to pre-existing medical knowledge."[30] In a parting shot, after his resignation in 1922, Maplestone urged the medical profession to "cease for a time at any rate to make poor tropical Australia appear a hot bed of dread diseases for the purpose of trying to stimulate into effectual life a moribund institute."[31]

As Maplestone predicted, Sundstroem, who previously had studied the diet of more cooperative Scandinavian workers, did have trouble in finding volunteers for his Townsville investigations. But he managed nonetheless to conduct a series of physiological and dietary studies of tropical whites before he took up a position at the University of California–Berkeley, even if occasionally he had to resort to using himself and his family as experimental subjects. Surprisingly, Sundstroem identified a few physiological alterations in the white bodies he investigated. The basal metabolic rates for his twelve subjects were lower than temperate averages; their urine was more alkalotic and concentrated; their blood contained more nitrogenous metabolites and chlorides; and the children grew faster than expected. But Sundstroem was able to boast that "personal experience has convinced me that the brain, even in the very hot months, is able to function quite as capably as in a cooler climate." His own reaction times met temperate norms. But what did all this mean? It was apparent to Sundstroem that on the whole "the Townsville climate is capable of altering, often to a considerable degree, physiological equilibria established in cooler climates."[32] All the same, the changes in metabolism, acid-base equilibrium, and chemical composition of the blood that he had discerned were not likely to be pathological. In particular, he pointed out that a lower basal metabolic rate did not imply "lower vitality." Moreover, any slippage from temperate standards might be avoided by improvements in house ventilation, lighter clothing, proper diet, and physical exercise. Significantly, Sundstroem referred not to a working white race but to a "white working race."[33] Far from avoiding manual labor and physical activity in the tropics, white men now were enjoined to exercise vigorously and labor hard in order to restore their physiological equilibrium and to concentrate their minds. Hard work would preserve their whiteness and make them good citizens.

The Whitest Man in the Tropics

The new director of the Townsville Institute, Dr. Raphael Cilento, was another tireless advocate of increasing white productivity as an antidote to degeneration. Cilento had grown up in South Australia, the son of an Italian-Australian station master who converted to Anglicanism and became an anti-Catholic zealot. But such family adaptations did not prevent Cilento from being called a "dago" in his youth, a pejorative label he spent a lifetime attempting to erase. After completing a medical degree at the University of Adelaide, where he had come under the influence of Frederick Wood Jones, a physical anthropologist with strong Lamarckian inclinations, Cilento had been posted at the end of the war to the new Australian territory of New Guinea. There he became interested in tropical medicine, acquiring an appreciation of the importance of nutrition in maintaining health. On returning to Adelaide, Cilento decided that he would make his career in tropical hygiene and proceeded to find a medical position in Malaya. In 1921, not long after Cilento and his wife, Phyllis, another medical doctor, had begun to acclimatize to Lower Perak, Elkington, by then the director of tropical hygiene at the new Commonwealth Department of Health, visited the couple. Elkington invited Cilento to take up the post of director of the Townsville Institute, provided he undertook further studies at the London School of Hygiene and Tropical Medicine, with the support of the International Health Board of the Rockefeller Foundation.[34] The Cilentos and Elkington soon found they had much in common. They shared an understanding of the state as an organism—in Australia's case a white organism—and an interest in developing the fitness and efficiency of the individual body and the national body. Raphael Cilento came to regard Elkington as a friend and patron, referring to him as *tuan* (master) and regularly engaging with him in boxing matches and other muscular contests. And in Cilento, Elkington finally had found an apostle of white physical culture and national efficiency.

Cilento lacked enthusiasm for original research, but he possessed a genius for publicizing the work of others and giving it effective form. From 1922, under the new director, the institute gradually shifted away from scientific investigation in order to concentrate on more practical activities, including the provision of diagnostic laboratory services to local practitioners and the training of health officers for the new Pacific colonies.[35] Cilento became a brilliant promoter of white settlement in the Australian tropics. In *The White Man in the Tropics*, he bragged that Australia "has the unique distinction of having bred up during the last seventy years a large, resident, pure-blooded white population under tropical conditions."[36] But Cilento lamented that this national achievement was not yet fully appreciated:

> To the great majority of inhabitants of temperate climates the word "tropical" conjures up visions of sweltering mangrove flats, the haunts of the crocodile; of rank and steaming forests that exhale the musky odour of decaying vegetation and conceal within their murky depths "miasmic" swamps; of deadly snakes and of the skulking savage with his poisoned spear.

But most of the Australian tropics did not resemble these preconceptions. In particular, there was "no teeming native population riddled with disease"; rather, it was a place "occupied by many thousands of pure-blooded European settlers."[37] Indeed, Cilento wondered if he should stop referring to northern Australia as "tropical," retaining such a derogatory term only for "countries within the hot belts of the earth which have a teeming native population riddled, as most such populations are, with diseases against which white people have little immunity." It had become, he mused, "a mental hobby that I fear I ride to death."[38]

Using the laboratory findings of Breinl, Young, Osborne, and Sundstroem, and deploying vital statistics for the whole state of Queensland, Cilento summarized the likely physiological consequences for whites of tropical residence. It was becoming a litany of environmental exoneration—or perhaps, rather, one of white triumph over ecological adversity. In any case, the outcome was generally benign. Body temperatures kept within temperate norms; the blood was scarcely affected; and white children might grow faster than expected, but they were not weedy. If the excretory system was more likely to become clogged, it was the result of faulty living habits, not climate; similarly, the evident increase in venery was a consequence of greater opportunity and license, not simply a function of the weather. Overfeeding, lack of exercise, faulty daily routine, indulgence in excesses, parasite diseases—not climate—together gave rise to "tropical" neurasthenia. Cilento conventionally regarded this nervousness, even though it was rare, as the major impediment to white settlement in the north. In white men it manifested as a loss of mental ability and self-confidence and the development of an "unresponsive memory." "Fits of exuberance alternate with states of depression; there is an unwarranted irritability over trivial matters, or even bursts of fury." Their wives, in contrast, would suffer "melancholia" and "extraordinary occasional exhibitions of ostentation or immodesty," craving the sensational or eccentric in dress and manner. "She talks too loudly, she drinks too much, she is over-intimate in her dancing, she displays transient amorous attachments."[39] According to Cilento, the only way to avoid such a baleful condition was to exercise and work harder and to engage more fully in family duties. He cited approvingly Sundstroem's prescriptions of physical activity (even though in private he deplored the Scandinavian's "uncouth" writing style and was pleased that he had left for the United States).[40] Laboratory studies had shown that "far from being an impossibility for the white man, work is the factor which will render it ultimately possible for him to adapt himself entirely to his new environment."[41] All a white man needed to thrive in the tropics was physical exercise, hard work, preventive medicine, and "purity of race." "The nation that admits native labour," Cilento declared, "abandons its birthright."[42]

Unlike many of the Melbourne experts, who argued for a harder and more stable transmission of hereditary features, Cilento had retained some Lamarckian sympathies, perhaps as a residue of his Adelaide training. "Climate and environment," he wrote, "undoubtedly modify considerably racial types."[43] But his Lamarckian assumptions did not lead him into the pessimism of many earlier environmental determinists. Cilento was convinced that the peculiar Australian combination of European stock, a tropical environment, and modern preventive medicine would ultimately produce a superior type of tropical white man, not another native degenerate. A definite type of "tropical-born Australian" had emerged in only a few generations:

> He is tall and rangy, with somewhat sharp features, and long arms and legs. Inclined to be sparely built, he is not, however, lacking in muscular strength, while his endurance is equal in his own circumstances to that of the temperate dweller in his. This North Queenslander moves slowly, and conserves his muscular heat-producing energy in every possible way. One can pick him out in the street by the fact that, as a general rule, he walks more deliberately . . . The hair colour is darkening, black, dark-brown, and red-hair is becoming increasingly frequent in long-settled localities. There is, moreover, a pallor of the skin . . . which produces most perfect feature-types in dark haired women, though it is unkind to the fair-haired, and gives them a freckled and faded appearance. The race is in a transition stage, and it is very apparent that there is being evolved precisely what one would hope for, namely, a distinctive tropical type, adapted to life in the tropical environment in which it is set.[44]

Whereas Osborne and R.J.A. Berry, the Melbourne anatomist, continued to argue for a preservation of the temperate type of white man, Cilento discerned the emergence of a higher type of tropical white Australian.

Cilento was not alone in charting the development of a new tropical white man.; neither was he the first. When E. J. Brady, a literary nationalist, visited Townsville in 1912, he had found that the 14,000 or so whites were "healthy and prosperous looking" under perpetually blue skies. "They will not listen to disparaging remarks about their climate," he wrote. "Their faith in northern Queensland is firmly fixed." After talking to the scientists at the institute, Brady predicted the emergence of "a European type of leisurely habit, resembling in character the southerners of the United States." The Australian tropics "must naturally evolve a people less robust, but more volatile and swarthier than the natives of either Geelong or Hobart."[45] They would still count as a healthy white race in Brady's Australia Unlimited. A few years later, Dr. Ronald Hamlyn-Harris, the president of the Royal Society of Queensland and an associate of the Townsville Institute, also proclaimed his belief in:

> The formation of a type of human beings specially adapted to live in Tropical Queensland. The type would be based on British blood and be so sustained and nourished, and be British in sentiment, but would be amended by the sun and soil in appearance, physique, speech and temperament.

It was the responsibility of tropical scientists and anthropologists to cultivate "in the rising generation year after year a vision of greatness and a dream of a great unifying force at work producing a single Evolutionary unit . . . a new race, bred of sun and soil."[46] It was this coming man, a form of whiteness renewed in the tropics, that Cilento would spend the rest of his life extolling.

The work of Cilento reflected his desire for a muscular, virile white male body and a modest, pliant white female body. Each of these ideal types would be productive in its way, the man in agricultural labor, and the woman in the house, especially in the kitchen. Each would behave energetically and with propriety, avoiding indulgence and excess and maintaining purity of race. In the tropical medical regime, white bodies were enclosed on themselves, separate from the contaminating influences and promiscuity of other races, insulated even from irresponsible sensuous contact with other white bodies. Representatives of the new type of white Australian occasionally might fail, becoming unmanned or unwomanly, but the national hygienist had the tools to recuperate their identity, their self-possession; the tropical environment might still exert a relaxing or depleting influence on whites, but dutiful citizens now knew how to resist it, perhaps even how to harness it to improve the race. Cilento assumed that the body of the retentive, productive citizen, once forged, would be available in mass for further racial and national development. It would become the subject of unremitting surveillance, discipline, and mobilization across a landscape that "preventive medicine" had rendered more or less innocuous. No wonder, then, that Cilento became an admirer of Benito Mussolini, sharing his fantasies of massified, armored bodies in the service of the state.[47]

As Cilento was not committed to laboratory work, he was able to spend long periods of time away from Townsville. In 1924, he was seconded as director of health in New Guinea, and he remained there another three years while Dr. Alec Baldwin acted as director of the Townsville Institute.[48] When Elkington resigned in 1928, Cilento left Townsville to succeed him as director of the Division of Tropical Hygiene in the Commonwealth Department of Health, still based in Melbourne. During the 1930s, Cilento organized the first national fitness campaign and, with wife Phyllis, fought for improvements in the national diet. After his appointment as the first director-general of health in Queensland, in 1934, Cilento began to reform the state's health care system, helped to establish a medical school at the University of Queensland, and contributed to setting the priorities of the new National Health and Medical Research Council in nutrition research and physical education. In 1937, he became the professor of social and preventive medicine at the University of Queensland, developing the first Australian program in social medicine, even before John Ryle in Britain had charted the field.[49] When not preoccupied with administrative or teaching duties, Cilento continued to promote white settlement in the tropics. In his history of Queensland, written in 1959, he was still praising the first "successful colonisation of a tropical and sub-tropical land by a population almost entirely white." Of course, the achievement had depended on "the absence of any teeming native coloured population riddled by endemic diseases" and on medicine's "increasing capacity to control introduced diseases." In the last paragraph of *Triumph in the Tropics*, Cilento congratulated himself on succeeding in "the struggle to establish a tropical consciousness in Australia."[50] But his struggle was not over. In the 1970s, Cilento welcomed an opportunity to speak at a League of Rights meeting, urging his listeners "carefully and repeatedly" to "examine the purity and dilution of our racial blood." The abandonment of the white Australia policy would lead to the arrival of diseased and degenerate immigrants. Indeed, there was "more danger from Indonesian germs than Indonesian arms." National health required continued immigration restriction, the selective breeding of the existing white population, and the eradication of multiculturalism, which seemed to him nothing less than another Jewish conspiracy.[51]

THE PHYSIOLOGY OF WHITE CITIZENSHIP

Cilento spent most of his career campaigning for what he believed were the necessities of white tropical living: a good water supply; housing that provided "a maximum of shade, a slow rate of heating, and a free circulation of air"; efficient disposal of waste; and "personal prophylaxis," which included looser clothing, better diet, and the avoidance of insects and natives.[52] In Cilento's persistent affirmation of white Australia, one finds the culmination of a century of more of physiocratic doctrine, the conviction that Australians must be governed, and govern themselves, along physiological lines if they were to be accorded the rights of citizens. Only the trained medical scientist could guide incipient white citizens along the correct path, assay their compliance with the rules of race hygiene, and discipline those who strayed into pathological excess and abandon. Cumpston called it preventive medicine, Cilento knew it as social medicine, and many still referred to it as public health or national health; but as a whole the medical profession agreed that society should be organized according to the biological principles that they had discovered and that social problems would usually have biological solutions.

Like other national hygienists, Raphael and Phyllis Cilento were preoccupied with nutrition, with enhancing the diet (and therefore the development) of their white charges. They argued that tropical whites must reduce the amount of protein they were eating in order to limit heat production. It was important to replace protein with fat and to drink more water. The Cilentos strongly criticized the tropical white family's reliance on tinned and canned foods. "People fail to recognise," Raphael Cilento complained, "how great a percentage of the lassitude, the lowered energy and the lowered disease resistance is directly traceable to the vitamin-deficient but handy preserved or canned foods and their attractive labels."[53] The perils of alcohol also were frequently denied by northern whites. There was still a common belief that gin and whiskey would stimulate the white constitution in such trying circumstances—but grog was in fact "a depressant to the body-resistance to diseases." Raphael Cilento was tired of listening to the "gin-sodden beachcomber, who announces with enthusiasm that only plenty of alcohol has kept him alive 'these twenty years.'"[54] The old gin-and-tonic, an allegedly stimulating combination of alcohol and quinine that was concocted in India a century earlier, ought to become anathema to the new tropical white man and woman.

Tropical clothing also had long fascinated physiologists and hygiene reformers. Because the natural inhabitants of the tropics possessed a dark skin, a few doctors had proposed that dark-colored garments would be ideal. But it was found, in Townsville and elsewhere, that dark clothes absorbed the heat too efficiently, thus promoting sweating while also providing an obstacle to the evaporation of sweat from the skin. Breinl and W. J. Young had learned from bitter experience that "the dress material becomes more and more impregnated with moisture, and the meshes of the fabric clogged with water, and the degree of saturation between skin and clothing exaggerated."[55] They had suggested that tropical clothing instead should be white to reflect heat rays, have the capacity to absorb moisture, and be sufficiently porous and lightweight to allow air to circulate over the skin and speed evaporation, as long as modesty could be maintained.

The American experiments in the Philippines with colored underwear had not impressed any of the Townsville researchers. Believing that orange-red underwear might mimic skin pigment and thus exclude damaging "actinic" or ultraviolet rays, James M. Phelan had conducted a practical test on blond and brunet soldiers in the Philippines. He supplied 500 soldiers with orange-red underwear and compared their well-being over the course of a year with another group less colorfully attired. But such pigment envy had proven misguided. Those wearing orange-red underwear did worse, with falls in body weight and hemoglobin and blood pressure; they complained incessantly of discomfort and itch; and many of them discarded the underwear before the end of the experiment.[56] Breinl and Young regarded the whole enterprise as slightly ludicrous, but neither did they intend to follow the common-sense advice of one of Phelan's colleagues, H. D. Gibbs, who simply recommended a large white umbrella lined with green—and no clothes at all.[57] Rather predictably, and somewhat unfashionably, Breinl and Young decided to don light-colored suits, and they advised white Australian laborers to continue wearing khaki trousers and absorbent flannel shirts.[58]

Raphael Cilento added little to his predecessors' opinions on the matter. He concurred that although the ideal for cooling was "a naked skin and an umbrella," for practical purposes tropical garb should have a loose texture, a light weight, and a capacity for reflecting sunlight. "The problem for a woman in the tropics," he mused, "is how to wear the fewest clothes and yet appear in public." He recommended a loose but modest blouse.[59] But his wife Phyllis thought this was inadequate instruction and sought to develop special guidelines for women's clothing in the tropics. "Every woman knows," she confided to the Townsville Women's Club, "that she is comfiest when lounging at home in a princess petticoat, or loose one-piece house frock without her corsets." She recommended light, loose clothing that provided sufficient protection from the sun, bearing in mind that "our objective should be always to look attractive, sometimes dignified and occasionally to apply supports to various parts of our bodies to suit special requirements." This justified the continued use of stockings, bras, and petticoats, but corsets and garters were forbidden. Surprisingly, she had acquired a belief in the value of colored underwear, with a preference for black, but outer garments should be white or pastel. Hats, sunglasses, and parasols were obligatory out of doors. Just before the "dainty afternoon tea" was served, Phyllis Cilento reminded her audience that "the future of North Queensland lies mainly in the home and the kitchen, and that we, who in the final analysis are the determining factor in the nation's growth, should use every endeavour to preserve our health and comfort."[60]

If physiological standards of dress often proved difficult to determine, housing seemed to offer far richer opportunities for biological adjustment. The basic principles of tropical housing were not disputed. A suitable dwelling would protect the interior as much as possible from the direct rays of the sun and at the same time provide sufficient ventilation for cooling. Yet most of the houses in the tropical outback were little more than shacks of termite-proof galvanized iron without verandas or any insulation. In towns, most dwellings were raised on piles and boasted a narrow veranda on the front, and sometimes on the sides, but the roof generally consisted of galvanized iron sheets, often without an inner lining, and the kitchen was invariably a detached small cubicle of galvanized iron only. Breinl and Young pointed out that "a galvanised iron 'humpy,' without verandah, is the most unsuitable structure to reside in a hot climate."[61] Raphael Cilento thought that cooking in a galvanized iron cubicle gave rise to the "kitchen neurasthenia" that afflicted so many white women in the tropics.[62] He campaigned for a regulation tropical dwelling that would be painted white; elevated on piles to allow effective ventilation; surrounded by a wide veranda for shade; and covered by a roof slightly raised from the walls, with ventilation in the top gable. A few older, high-set houses already met these criteria, but Cilento urged the public and local councilors to ensure that the model became standard.[63] He knew his task would not be easy. "The ordinary man in Queensland," he lamented, "is exceedingly pig-headed in this respect and would far rather live in some little humphy [sic] adapted to the arctic conditions of a Scotch or Irish bog than live in any house (however well adapted to tropical requirements) that differed in the slightest from what he had been accustomed to, or from what his neighbours used."[64] Evidently, hygiene reform in the tropics would be a constant struggle, even among whites.

GERMS OF TROPICAL LAZINESS

Adjustments of diet, clothing, and housing might help to improve the white race in the tropics, but how would settlers be protected from any residual disease in the region? Immigration restriction and quarantine seemed to present the main bulwarks against new infection, but even so, a few germs still lurked in the Australian tropics, ready to attack vulnerable whites. Of all the conventionally "tropical" microbes, hookworm was the most significant and common white infection in northern Australia. Cilento regarded it as "a stultifying disease" that explained much of what passed as tropical neurasthenia and fatigue, whereas others referred to the ankylostome as "the germ of laziness."[65] The parasite enters humans through the skin, usually through bare feet, eventually reaching the intestines by way of the trachea, esophagus, and stomach. Once in the duodenum, the worms fix themselves to the intestinal walls and feed from the bloodstream, in time causing a marked anemia. Blood loss might produce the symptoms of pallor, tiredness, and fatigue. The infected person is meanwhile excreting thousands of ova each day, and if deposited on warm, moist soil, the eggs generate infective larvae that seek another host. At the turn of the century, Dr. T. F. Macdonald, practicing at Innisfail, found the "insidious enemy of health . . . deeply rooted and flourishing among the inhabitants of the Johnstone River district." Nine of every ten children were infected, many of them displaying an extraordinary appetite for eating earth "not in casual manner, but under the impulse of an irresistible craving"; such children soon became pale, disobedient, cunning, dishonest, and immoral. Affected adults did not eat earth but "developed abnormal delights in pickles, curries and alcohol" and progressively became more lazy and fractious. Predictably, Macdonald had become convinced that Pacific Islanders, "Arabians," and Italians were the sources of infection—affiliation with one of these races was prima facie evidence of worm carriage and of worm shedding during defecation. But even as Macdonald "became animated with the desire to stamp out the scourge," which he saw "plainly was sucking the heart's blood of the whole community," he claimed he had received little support from the Queensland government.[66] Before World War I, Breinl had also detected widespread prevalence of hookworm in white communities in North Queensland, especially between Cardwell and Cairns, and in the Northern Territory. He had urged a house-to-house examination, with sufferers compelled to undergo a thorough treatment with the latest specific, thymol, notorious for its nauseating taste and smell.[67]

The problem was not properly addressed until 1916, when the International Health Board of the Rockefeller Foundation began to cooperate with the federal and state governments on a survey and eradication campaign, which continued until 1924.[68] Regarded by Cumpston and Elkington as a means of committing the federal government to public health activities, the Australian Hookworm Campaign followed the pattern that the International Health Board had already established in other tropical regions. The Rockefeller Foundation provided fieldwork teams, initially led by American experts, and it supplied most of the financing. The first stage, based in the north at the Townsville Institute, was a survey of the prevalence of hookworm, followed by the selection of limited areas where teams would locate and treat all those affected. During this process, officials in the hookworm campaign attempted to educate the general public about the disease and the means of preventing it, advising parents to ensure that their children wore shoes, and stipulating that everyone was fastidious in the use of water closets, avoiding "soil pollution" and "promiscuous defecation."[69] In these circumstances, health education meant inculcating in whites a fear of waste matter, especially the excrement of other races and the poor, and a distrust of an environment that might secretly be contaminated, especially, again, by other races and lower classes with slacker cultural standards. (Even so, at the polluting pole of this binary typology, poor whites usually seemed more reformable than natives, who conventionally were assigned a hereditary obstinacy.) The implication was that the tropics were not dangerous until rendered so, until contaminated; and the typical culprits in this dirtying of an otherwise pure, white place were irresponsible, disease-dealing natives, many of whom, quite duplicitously, appeared healthy. Potentially, the region was innocent and innocuous, as long as lazy natives and poor whites were not allowed to pollute the land.[70]

In assuming that the presence of worms in a fecal specimen meant that a white carrier would be symptomatic, the hookworm campaign tended to exaggerate the social effects of hookworm. In white communities, hookworm carriage was common only among children, miners, and inmates of institutions, and rarely did it manifest as disease. Yet the campaign made sure that most communities lived in fear of infestation, thus amplifying its health education message and ensuring better compliance with preventive measures. J. H. Waite and I. L. Neilson, a hookworm survey officer and his nurse assistant, warned that 40 percent of schoolchildren between Cooktown and Townsville suffered from this "blighting disease," which was "stamping serious mental, physical and sexual degeneracy" on many of them. It was easily prevented, but if unchecked it would lead "toward the obliteration of the race through the unsexing of its victims and reducing individual resistance to acute infections."[71] In *Smith's Weekly*, H. C. McKay parroted the hookworm propaganda, warning his readers of the "earth-eaters of Queensland" who had sunk "nearly to the level of the animals." Infected children were shorter, lighter, and weaker than normal and were always mentally deficient. He declared that "if we wish to remain a virile, healthy, alert-minded nation and not a collection of 'poor whites,' it is our duty to take our tropical plagues seriously. . . . Otherwise a leering Asia may one day not far distant point the finger of scorn at our native-born—the 'white trash' of Asia." Promiscuous soil pollution was leading to nothing less than the degeneration of the white race.[72]

Occasionally, the survey officers encountered individuals who refused to supply a fecal specimen, even at the risk of obliterating the race, but usually they were overwhelmed with large volumes of suspect excrement, much of it delivered unsolicited to the Townsville Institute. Fear of hookworm was far more widespread than the disease itself. In 1925, for example, a mother from Home Hill wrote to the institute, concerned that "two of my children are very weak and puny. I thought it possible they were suffering from hookworm."[73] A Bowen woman pleaded for hookworm medicine as "my child has not been well since a week's holiday in Kuranda last year in September."[74] A resident of a hamlet outside Townsville wrote to the "Hookworm Office" because "I have a little brother living with me that had hookworms before and I am afraid he may still have them as he is not as healthy looking as I'd like him to be. I have five children of my own will you send me six little tins to see if any of them have hookworms."[75] From Ayr a father sought advice about his daughter: "She is a fat, healthy, active child, weight 24lb, but has a perfect mania for eating dirt. I dare not let her off the verandah for a moment, she will fill her mouth with dirt, will even lick the mud from our own shoes if she can get them." But in this case the results were negative.[76]

Hookworm surveys indicated widespread carriage of the parasite in Aboriginal communities: At Yarrabah the infection rate was 100 percent; and at Palm Island, near Townsville, it was close to 75 percent.[77] In 1922, when he replaced W. A. Sawyer, an American, as director of the hookworm campaign, Cilento quickly realized that he had located a native population "riddled with disease," if not quite "teeming." Here, at last, was the legendary "native reservoir" of disease, spilling over to contaminate the white population. Cilento urged that the racial threat remain segregated, but he also insisted, unusually, that Aboriginal communities received mass treatment, if only to protect vulnerable whites.[78] Previously Aboriginal ill health had not often been recognized as a problem even for whites because the original inhabitants were widely dispersed, and it was assumed they would soon disappear. Now Aboriginal ill health, especially the prevalence of infectious disease among "half-castes" in shantytowns, was recognized as imperiling adjacent European communities, but still not as a problem in its own right. Cilento wanted to bring the Aboriginal body out of the anthropology museum and into the biomedical present, where he might display it, and treat it, as a modern disease threat, not as a mere primitive specimen. But he showed little concern for Aborigines as sufferers of disease, and he continued to attribute their infection to racially modulated customs and habits, to biological destiny, rather than tracing the social and economic causes of the problem.

Whereas Europeans were tested individually and treated only if infected, Aborigines usually received mass treatment. Cilento was keen to document the extent of infection, so he advised his survey officers to obtain as many specimens as possible, but then to treat everyone. Dr. R. E. Richards was one of his more vigorous collectors. In 1923, Richards toured the Gulf of Carpentaria collecting blood and fecal specimens from Aborigines and whites: Apart from the "natives" at Mitchell River, who were "most insolent," everyone was polite and obliging. Richards thought that most of the Aborigines were "very thin and anaemic looking, although the white men tell me they are fairly strong and seem to have few ills other than fever." On this occasion he found few positive specimens among the dispersed communities, and no one was treated.[79] But when he visited Palm Island that year he detected hookworm in most of the fecal samples. He reported to Cilento that he had arrived "per dinghy, one nigger power," only to find that there were "680 niggers," not the 400 he had expected. Nonetheless he took specimens from most of them and treated them all.[80] Cilento later thanked him for his "interesting and breezy epistle."[81]

In attending to "native reservoirs" of hookworm, Cilento was participating in an exchange of medical ideas and practices between the settler colony and nearby sojourner colonies. His experiences in Malaya, northern Australia, and New Guinea would influence his work at each subsequent site. If most of his Australian medical colleagues felt more comfortable dealing with fellow whites, segregating themselves and their patients from stereotypically diseased natives, Cilento had learned in New Guinea and Malaya how to begin to drain the "native reservoir." To a considerable extent, Cilento's enthusiasm for mass treatment of segregated Aborigines derived from colonial practice, where quarantine methods alone were inadequate to ensure the health of white colonialists. Just a few years before in Papua and New Guinea the International Health Board had worked out procedures for hookworm control that might be transferred unchanged to Aboriginal communities. In describing mass treatment of plantation workers and the development of an effective latrine system to prevent soil pollution, Waite had implied that it might be necessary to resort to coercion. Cilento, Waite, and other white hygienists believed that if education had a role at all among such ignorant and refractory races—wherever they were located—it was a minor one.[82] Later, in treating New Guinea plantation workers for yaws and hookworm, and stipulating improved rations for them, Cilento sought again both to protect adjacent whites and to develop native labor power. It amounted to a generic program of "developmental medicine," focusing on white protection and native industry and largely ignoring maternal and infant welfare among indigenous populations.[83] In pursuing this program in Malaya, Australia, and New Guinea, Cilento rarely resorted to educational campaigns in indigenous communities, assuming that colored peoples had inherited only a limited capacity for lasting behavior change. In contrast, he believed that white men, women, and children in North Queensland would usually heed medical advice and respond to guidance toward civilized standards of personal hygiene. "The conditions in a native country," he wrote, "are closely akin to those that must obtain during a military campaign [except that] the medical sanitary officer in New Guinea is dealing with irresponsible natives."[84] Cilento would always seek thus to treat New Guinea natives and Aboriginal populations alike.

SHADES OF WHITE

Even as Cilento was proclaiming a white triumph in the Australian tropics, the character of that "whiteness" was in dispute. During the 1920s, some 300,000 migrants came to Australia, swelling the population to more than 6.5 million by 1930. Many of the newcomers had set off from southern Europe. In 1923, fewer than 1,000 Italians had arrived, but within three years, as a result of stricter entry requirements for the United States, almost 7,000 were disembarking in Australia each year.[85] Because the protected sugar industry was thriving, many Italian, Greek, and Maltese migrants went north and found themselves competing with British-Australian workers. In 1924, *Smith's Weekly* reported that "the foreign element in the [sugar] industry represents only 11 percent, the remaining 89 percent being Australian and British, but unfortunately the foreigners are concentrating in a few districts, such as Innisfail, South Johnstone and Babinda, where they form 50 to 75 percent of the cane cutters and farmers." Sections of the labor movement, and the Returned Services' League, campaigned against such "alien penetration," disparaging the "foreigners" for an ethnic clannishness and ability to survive on low wages. But not only workers feared Mediterranean contamination and competition. As early as 1907, when there were only a few hundred Italians in North Queensland, Gilbert White, the Anglican bishop of Carpentaria, had declared that such foreign elements were nonwhite and inassimilable, and he therefore questioned "whether we are wise in introducing a large Italian element into our population."[86] At all social levels, it was assumed that if southern Europeans were white, they were only marginally so.

In 1925, the Gillies Labor government in Queensland reluctantly established a royal commission to inquire into "the social and economic effects of increase in the number of aliens in North Queensland," headed by Thomas A. Ferry, a public servant. Ferry visited most of the sugar districts to investigate non-British labor in the sugar industry. He concluded that the best workers in the tropics were British, followed by northern Italians, who were more readily absorbed than their southern brethren. Sicilians, Greeks, and Maltese generally made undesirable immigrants, as they subsisted at a low standard of living and tended to dwell in towns rather than cultivate the soil. Ferry condemned Greeks because they "add nothing to the wealth and security of the country" and had "even displaced the Chinaman from his China Town." Sicilians were often illiterate and "more inclined to form groups and less likely to be assimilated into the population of the state."[87] Ferry urged state and federal governments to select more carefully any potential immigrant, to subject applicants to a rigorous medical examination, and to prohibit ethnic clubs and other barriers to assimilation. Some "racial stock," such as those from the Mediterranean littoral, should be excluded altogether, in favor of those "that will assist rather than hinder the building up of superior social and economic conditions in the state."[88] But the federal government in Melbourne, led by S. M. Bruce, hesitated in responding to the report. Provision was made to impose a quota

on migrants from the Mediterranean, but by the end of the 1920s so few
southern Europeans were leaving for Australia that any restriction soon became unnecessary. During 1927, Mussolini limited emigration from Italy, and
in 1929 no more than 1,500 Italians migrated to Australia.[89]

Those who were prepared to accept southern Europeans into white Australia insisted that most, if not all, of the "foreigners" were acceptably white
and, therefore, absorbable and candidates for citizenship. Cilento, for example, proposed that Italians—like his own ancestors—might contribute to
the evolution of the higher type of tropical white man. True to his origins,
Cilento argued that the white race was singular and broadly European. But
even Cilento, who claimed a specifically northern Italian ancestry, had to draw
the line somewhere, so he chose to exclude "foreigners" such as Sicilians and
Greeks from his relatively broad definition of "whiteness." Evidently there still
were limits to the plasticity of the white race. Most of the local Italians, however, were of "Teutonic or mixed Dinaric origin from Lombardy, Piedmont,
etc.," and Cilento protested that the common suggestion that these types
would "react differently to the English, Scotch, Irish and Welsh argues a faulty
acquaintance with ethnology."[90] Others were not so sure. Although southern
Europeans were commonly criticized for their clannishness and refusal to assimilate, the underlying concern was that they might infuse bad blood, and
thus bad customs and habits, into a biologically homogeneous nation. In not
being assimilible, they came to appear to many as a contaminating and degrading element in the body politic. Some experts on race and population policy, especially those in Melbourne, therefore sought to limit whiteness in
Australia to those of British origin or to those of Nordic type. When Osborne,
for example, spoke of the white race, he meant British or Nordic like himself—not even Alpine Europeans passed muster. Reflecting on the racial debates of the 1920s, K. H. Bailey, a professor of law at Melbourne, recalled that
some Australians reverted to looking on themselves "as an outpost, not merely
of the white race, but specifically of the British race." Even in 1933, Bailey observed, the desire for purity of subtype was strong, and it was "opposed to the
European as well as the Asiatic."[91]

In 1927, Jens Lyng, a statistician and the Harbison-Higinbotham scholar
at the University of Melbourne, published his influential book, *Non-Britishers
in Australia*, a major contribution to the reshaping and delimiting of ideas of
whiteness in Australia. Lyng was responding to debates over the proper composition of white Australia, the degree to which it might shade into a variegated whiteness. Like others at the University of Melbourne, he postulated a
hard heredity and rigid racial categories. Thus racial characters "are at best
subject only to modification by environment during a long period of time."
Lyng agreed that 98 percent of Australians might be classified as white, but

how much of this population was Nordic, or Alpine, or Mediterranean? Nordics, like himself, typically displayed "restless, creative energy"; Alpines were "a sturdy, tenacious race, very stable but apt to be stolid and unimaginative"; Mediterraneans inevitably were "passionate and excitable, loving and hating intensely."[92] Assuming that most Celts and Anglo-Saxons were Nordic, that Germans and northern Italians were Alpine, and Greeks and Sicilians were Mediterranean, Lyng had calculated that 82 percent of white Australians were Nordic, 13 percent Mediterranean, and 5 percent Alpine. Queensland was more Mediterranean than the other states, which supposedly explained its political instability and turbulence and deficiency in discipline.[93] Most of the Italians migrating to Australia were Mediterranean, unfortunately, and therefore their ancestors had already suffered "an infusion of inferior African and Asiatic blood."[94] Lyng believed that eventually Mediterraneans might be absorbed biologically into white Australia, but they must remain a small part, almost undetectable, of the mixture.

A strange, racialist harbinger of multiculturalism, Lyng thought that "the best result is not obtained by racial purity but through a mingling of different human strains." It was the duty of population experts, such as himself, to monitor and guide the composition of the white population and to organize its reproduction to optimal effect. Australia did not need a more Mediterranean whiteness, but it would benefit from a greater Alpine element. In order to develop "a virile and numerically strong body of cultivators," the country required a type of white "to whom toil is a pleasure and who, if need be, is content with a lower standard of living than that to which the Nordics of today readily submit."[95] White Australia needed Nordics and Alpines, not citified Mediterraneans:

> The Nordics are dynamic pioneers, innovators of new ideas and methods, good organisers and progressive farmers. The Alpines are frugal, patient, hard-working plodders, who possess that intense love of land which makes them cling to it in rain and sunshine, generation after generation, without which the growth of rural tradition is difficult and a stable rural population an impossibility.[96]

According to Lyng, whiteness could be differentiated and disaggregated into fixed biocultural types and then arranged in different combinations, depending on state inclination. Some like Cilento might continue to speak in general terms about a dynamic whiteness while conceding its particulate character; others like Osborne would choose to emphasize just one fixed type of whiteness.

With the decline of southern European migration in the late 1920s, the concern about the proper typological composition of white Australia became less pressing. In 1931, the Commonwealth Sugar Inquiry Committee expressed only muted concerns about "alien penetration." It was "disposed to resist the gregarious tendency of certain foreign races to congregate in self-contained communities" and found it disturbing that Italian laborers were benefiting from tariff protection designed to encourage white workers. But the committee believed that this was just a "transitory stage," and the new restrictions on Italian migration would eventually allow the aliens to assimilate into white communities, without increasing the Mediterranean component of the population too greatly.[97] In 1939, when A. Grenfell Price, an Adelaide geographer, wrote his survey of white acclimatization in the tropics, he conceded that "the living standards of the aliens, the greater part of whom are Italians, were lower than those of the Australians," and "the Italian works harder and for longer hours than the British-Australian." But he had become convinced that the next generation "rapidly acquires Australian characteristics" and contributes to a homogeneously white Australia.[98]

FROM NORTH TO SOUTH

During the 1920s, the Townsville Institute increasingly looked toward the Pacific. Cilento and, for a time, Cumpston hoped that the institute would become the base for an inland and island tropical health service, training medical doctors for work in northern Australia, New Guinea, and other parts of the Pacific. Just as in 1911 the ceding of control of the Northern Territory to the Commonwealth had stimulated the growth of the Townsville Institute, the acquisition of New Guinea in 1914 led Australia to assume greater responsibilities in the Southwest Pacific after the war. Cumpston deplored the weakness and inefficiency of native plantation labor, urging that Australia should attempt, without delay, medical measures for "the conservation of native races" and establish, with other colonial powers, a Southwest Pacific quarantine zone "to prevent inter-island exchange of infection."[99] Cilento took advantage of the nation's increasing interest in the Pacific to offer a short course in tropical medicine for district officers, plantation managers, and missionaries, as well as a longer course for medical graduates leading to the award of a diploma in tropical medicine.[100] The Townsville Institute, which had done so much to stigmatize Pacific Islanders, now proposed, belatedly, to investigate and treat their diseases. But it was not prompted to do so merely to relieve their suffering; rather, its primary goal was now the extension into the Pacific of a safe and productive empire, supervised, if not settled, by whites.[101]

And then, toward the end of the 1920s, many of Australia's colonial and tropical health ambitions faded. Financial constraint and political opportunity were leading Cumpston to consolidate the health department's activities in temperate urban areas. A shift in emphasis was already evident in 1925, during the hearings of the Royal Commission on Health. Cilento, who was then the acting director of health in New Guinea, told the commissioners that in North Queensland one could find "white people carrying out what is probably the biggest experiment in acclimatisation that there is in any part of the world." There were more than 100,000 whites along the Queensland coast "unaware of the fact that they are performing a scientific miracle, and that they have been doing so, in some families, for three generations."[102] This was possible only because the native population was "negligible," although some on Cape York "may act as a reservoir of disease," and nearby pathogenic New Guinea represented "a serious menace to all Australia."[103] But it was by then all so predictable. Cumpston instead chose to signal his interest in refocusing medical research in Australia. The director-general of health agreed that more training in tropical medicine was required for doctors in northern Australia and New Guinea, but he thought this might better take place in a school of public health in Sydney. "There has been difficulty in getting an adequate staff for the Townsville Institute for some time past," he dryly reported. "The amount of clinical material at Townsville has been distinctly disappointing."[104] Elkington attempted to defend the Townsville Institute, insisting that it should continue with "systematic investigation and recording of local disease prevalence." "It would be a serious loss to tropical Australia if an institute carrying such useful and varied activities were terminated," he warned the commissioners.[105] But they, like Cumpston, had clearly become more concerned about internal threats to a virile white Australia—the problem of the degenerate urban poor already seemed acute, and with the onset of the Depression it would come to preoccupy Melbourne and Canberra policymakers.

Cilento and Elkington complained bitterly that Cumpston was abandoning the white race in the tropics, and in so doing he was curtailing or impeding their own careers in tropical hygiene.[106] But it was also evident that the Townsville Institute had become a victim of its earlier rhetorical and political successes. After 1920 few medical doctors doubted the viability of the white race in the tropics, even though some of the more obdurate geographers continued to express misgivings. There was not much left for the Townsville scientists to do: Their investigations had more or less normalized the region. Research seems almost to have evaporated, and the institute was degenerating into a combination of laboratory service, hookworm clearinghouse, and propaganda unit. The training program stumbled along, weak and ineffectual. In 1925, Elkington had accused Alec Baldwin, the acting director of the institute, of "marking time," neglecting tropical research and education. "We want initiative," he wrote. "Anyone can carry a job on sufficiently to keep it in existence, but it needs a man's whole soul to get the most out of it, and the job of direct-ing the Institute so as to get the most out of it is as important a one as there is in Australia today."[107] When Elkington proposed a study of the "medical anthro-pology" of the Aborigines on Palm Island, Baldwin protested that routine work left him little time for research.[108] In 1928, Cilento complained that the insti-tute was also neglecting its "propaganda work" and had let the hookworm cam-paign fall into disarray, though he commended some of the recent research in protozoology and helminthology.[109]

Such counsel had come too late. Prompted by Cumpston, the Royal Com-mission on Health of 1925 recommended the transfer of the Townsville Insti-tute to Sydney and its incorporation into a school of public health and tropical medicine.[110] In 1930, Dr. Harvey Sutton became the first professor of preven-tive medicine and director of the new school, with Baldwin as his deputy, in charge of tropical medicine. Sutton's appointment officially confirmed the closing in Australia of the tropical frontier and signaled a renewed attention to the problem of the urban child in the temperate south. If the fortress of white Australia was being undermined from within, it was no longer the climate or topography that was at fault but rather the proliferating urban poor, spreading germs and reproducing inferior germ plasm.[111]

CHAPTER 6

WHITENING THE NATION

IN STUDYING THE NATIONAL frontier, scientific experts on tropical Australia were also constructing a scene of race struggle, at first pitting an ideal of whiteness against the strange environment, and then opposing it to other, "colored" races. By the late 1920s, medical scientists had assayed and approved the white race that emerged, virile and hygienic, from the tropical crucible. But in the cities along the southeastern coast, already thoroughly whitened and domesticated, another threat to racial integrity and health had been growing, and it was to this perceived internal problem—to the degraded poor of the urban slums—that scientists would increasingly direct their attention. Jack Elkington and Raphael Cilento were still out on the tropical frontier, unswerving in their efforts to fend off allegedly pathogenic colored races; but other national hygienists had turned southward to deal with the supposed threat from within, to suppress the bad seeds, the diseased and degenerate elements, that were sprouting up inside white Australia. Even in the 1870s, contagionist doctrine had implicated the degraded habits of the urban poor in the transmission of germs; at the end of the century, notions of a more insulated, or harder, heredity seemed to suggest that physical and mental degeneration also would emerge from deep within the social body, not from a mismatch of race and circumstances. Many doctors and scientists feared that in civilized areas natural selection was failing to weed out inferior and degraded types from the white race. Indeed, a few of the national hygienists in Melbourne and Sydney had always regarded tropical investigations as a distraction, as little more than an opportunistic attempt to attach medical research to national policy. Their focus had never shifted from the dangerous urban white child, and for them the aftermath of World War I, and the onset of the Depression of the 1930s, served only to magnify a longstanding concern and to recruit others to the cause.

Professor R.J.A. Berry was one of those race scientists who grudgingly supported tropical research while their real commitment was to the study of an internal, urban degeneration of the white race. In 1917, as president of the Victorian branch of the British Medical Association, the Melbourne anatomist condemned "the decline of the birth-rate of each of the abler and more valuable sections of the community, and the increase in numbers of the actually feeble-minded and less effective and profitable citizens."[1] Berry reported on the work of Karl Pearson, the British eugenicist and head of the Galton Laboratory at the University of London, a scientist convinced that the state should intervene to encourage the breeding of the "fit" and to limit the reproduction of the "unfit." The birthrate was falling in Britain and Australia as middle-class women limited the size of their families; meanwhile, in the cities, the thriftless and dirty classes, even though manifestly unfit, continued to proliferate. For Berry, this was "a question on which the whole future of our race depends," but Australian politicians, transfixed on the tropics, did nothing about it. "Modern democracy," opined Berry, an irritable and bitter man, "would appear, like Sodom and Gomorrah, to be doomed to destruction, and for the like reason—there are not ten righteous persons within it."[2]

In 1925, the royal commission on health gave tropical research just enough attention to allow it to recommend the closure of the Australian Institute of Tropical Medicine at Townsville: The commissioners were far more interested in maternal and child health, mental deficiency in children, venereal disease, and relations between federal and state governments. Testimony to the commissioners was dominated by accounts of the mentally defective child. "Cerebral underdevelopment is applicable all over Australia," Berry warned them. "There is no question about that."[3] He wanted a population survey to assess the full extent of the problem, and he demanded that the state assume control over feeble-minded children to rescue them from their degenerate parents. Idiots and imbeciles were not the dangerous ones, as they were easily identified. Rather, he feared the higher-grade morons and the feeble-minded who may appear normal until scientifically measured. "That is the class of case in which there is danger, and the class of case which, if left to itself, on the streets of our big cities becomes a real menace." Like all other authorities, Berry accepted heredity "as a potent factor, on the Mendelian principle that feeble-minded parents will produce feeble-minded children."[4] Dr. William Ernest Jones, the inspector-general of the insane in Victoria, thought that at least 1 percent of state schoolchildren were feeble-minded and should be segregated. "Inasmuch as the defect is an inherited one and capable of transmission, it is obviously desirable that in the first place only those people who are healthy in mind and body should be allowed to mate." Although sterilization seemed most effective, Jones felt that "we are not sufficiently civilised and educated to tolerate the restriction."[5]

Dr. Harvey Sutton, at the time the principal medical officer in New South Wales's education department and a lecturer in preventive medicine at the

University of Sydney, suggested to the royal commission that "marriage should not be allowed between hereditary mental defectives of an unmistakable character." Segregation was needed, and "in certain cases it would be a benefit if mental defectives and epileptics could be sterilised"—but he would not recommend compulsory sterilization.[6] Sutton was especially disappointed in the quality of white schoolchildren in the southern states. Bad heredity, poor diet, unventilated rooms, and infectious diseases had produced poor physical and mental specimens. He estimated that 20–30 percent of school entrants in Melbourne showed some signs of rickets, a disease of vitamin deficiency. Dedication to national hygiene prompted Sutton to recommend the medical examination of all schoolchildren, a thorough system of physical training in schools, and the charting of the history of every child from the beginning of life to adulthood. "I am very interested in statistics," he told the commissioners, "and I try to get hold of all the statistics I can."[7]

They were all very interested in statistics. Maintaining and enhancing the health of white Australians required an endless registration of bodies and social facts; citizens must be measured, swabbed, tested, classified, and then checked again; urban spaces required careful, and repeated, assessment and planning. Medical science, even as it was improving health, thus could inform a larger state project: the modern attempt to render legible, and to simplify, the body of the citizen and its interactions.[8] Some involvement of medicine in the calculation, the assaying, of population—the construction of a national body and of the problems within it—can be discerned in the late nineteenth century in Melbourne and Sydney. Once a minority enthusiasm, this effort by the 1920s had become a medical commonplace and well-organized. Many doctors and scientists—and others among the progressive middle class—were strongly recommending governance within an ostensibly physiological, and therefore racial, framework. After World War I, state and federal governments became ever more readily persuaded that a knowledge of physiological standards—not just a reckoning of disease outbreaks—should inform public administration, helping them to define and to manage growing populations. With increasing self-confidence, physiocratic advisers, such as Berry and Sutton, urged the state to intervene in social life in order to maintain the racial standards they had developed. Generally, they favored a pragmatic mixture of hereditarian and social interventions against the evils within the national body. A few, like Berry, chose to emphasize the supervision and regulation of reproduction, calling this "eugenics."[9] Others, such as Raphael Cilento, clustered around the farther pole of microenvironmental facilitation, demanding improvements in nutrition and physical activity that might fulfill white developmental capacity or even, rarely, enlarge hereditary potential. Ever more assertive, national hygienists, most of them combining hereditarian and environmentalist prescriptions, expected to reconstruct personal conduct and everyday life according to biological ideals; they were insisting on a biomedical reframing of citizenship in the modern white nation.

But medical possibilism was not the only way of imagining, or managing, white Australia. In the 1930s, it became clear that even if environmental determinism and racial pessimism might briefly be repressed, they would surely return, or at least hang around nearby.[10] Though geographical anxieties were largely reconfigured in medicine—to be expressed more optimistically as social and racial fixations—geographers and new experts in "population policy" were emerging to argue that environment might yet set limits to the modern white nation. White bodies were perhaps not so autonomous and alienated that they could be settled down in any place, in any numbers. The conceptual framework of geographers such as T. Griffith Taylor and Ellsworth Huntingdon still included racial doctrine and physiocratic aspiration, but their geographical studies would support a far less robust national edifice than the medical possibilists had envisaged. Geographers too wanted a modern, racialized Australia, but for them, as we shall see, it would never become an unlimited white nation.

From the White Race in the Tropics to the White Child in the Cities

After his appointment as head of the new School of Public Health and Tropical Medicine in Sydney in 1930, Harvey Sutton became the unchallenged leader of academic public health in Australia, shaping population health research and training for generations. Graduating in medicine from the University of Melbourne in the same year as J.H.L. Cumpston, Sutton had been awarded a Rhodes scholarship, which enabled him to study at Oxford with J. S. Haldane—whose physiological work had inspired W. A. Osborne—and to run for Australia in the Summer Olympics in London. He returned to Melbourne as a medical officer with the Victorian Department of Public Instruction, committed to transforming the state school into a venue for preventive medicine and racial hygiene. He had little time for the tropics. For the rest of his career, Sutton worked to strengthen the body of the white urban child, promoting personal and sexual hygiene, good posture, balanced diet, exposure to fresh air, temperance, and physical education in the slums of Melbourne and, later, Sydney. His prescriptions for urban race improvement consisted of a conventional amalgam of hereditarian and environmentalist solutions. As a member of various eugenics societies and the Family Planning Association, he sought to discourage the breeding of the physically unfit and feeble-minded, and he recommended sterilization for hopeless degenerates. As an educator and athlete, a founder of Health Week, and an active member of the Surf Life Saving Association and the National Fitness Council, Sutton also endorsed environmental intervention, especially improvement in nutrition and physical fitness, as a means of developing a superior Australian type.[11] With other leaders of the medical profession, including Sir James Barrett in Melbourne and Cilento in Queensland, Sutton therefore favored the expansion of infant welfare centers, kindergartens, playgrounds, and garden suburbs; and with his fellow national hygienists, he ensured that when the National Health and Medical Research Council was established in 1937 it would concentrate initially on nutrition and physical fitness.[12]

Even before World War I Sutton had observed that "much popular attention has been directed towards the Australian and his characteristics," with self-appointed experts "prophesying either ridiculous failure or superlative supremacy for the Australian and the Australian nation." Yet no one had properly evaluated the emerging type. In Victoria, Sutton began systematically to measure the Australian-born schoolchild, and soon all children in the state would have their dimensions and intelligence quotients recorded on separate cards. In this way Sutton hoped "to determine at the earliest possible moment what influence the environment of southern land and skies is having on our race." He called for a wider "systematic investigation of the child-life of the various states—a veritable stocktaking" of white Australia.[13] Yet almost twenty years later, as he assumed his duties at the school of public health, Sutton was still complaining that "we are in the completest ignorance of the physical and mental characters, growth and development, progress or degeneration of our race in its new Australian environment." Again, he recommended a classification of children by "racial stream," indicating the degree of Australianness and a "national stocktaking." But with his new institutional responsibilities, he seems also to have awakened to the call of the tropics, even though the recognition of it would prove sadly evanescent. "The settlement of Australia by the British section of the white race is an experiment," he declared, and "when we consider that five-thirteenths of the continent is in the Tropic zone—a daring and novel experiment for which we have no parallel elsewhere." Predictably, this new prospect led Sutton to urge yet more anthropomorphic study of the schoolchild, just as he had for the temperate south.[14]

Measurement of the growth, development, and intelligence quotient of schoolchildren would become a national obsession, but the calibrators disagreed on the meaning of the results, and no one was quite sure what to do when deficiencies emerged. As early as 1902, Christian Bjelke-Petersen, an expert on physical education, had wanted to learn more about the development of Tasmanian boys and to compare them with other "races." His preliminary investigations suggested that on most measures Tasmanians compared favorably with other whites, although the Scandinavians usually surpassed them, and the chest girth of Hobart boys was distressingly small, an especially lamentable finding because "we all know that a large chest increases the individual's vitality and reserve powers."[15] Elkington also had recommended medical inspection as a means of identifying defective children, deploring the "ocean of ignorance and indifference which envelopes the body of young Australia." The amateur boxer urged his medical colleagues to "give young Australia as good an opportunity as we can to grow up a broad-chested, keen-sighted, hard-fisted race, respecting its body, and better equipped mentally than is at present possible."[16] Dr. Mary Booth, an early votary of eugenics, added to these calls for anthropometry in the schools. The collection of information on height, weight, head circumference, eye and hair color, vision, hearing, and intelligence would permit

> a stock-taking of the physical fitness of the nation and an estimate of the hereditary and environmental factors at work on the whole or sections of society. . . . The eugenicist, in conformity with modern thought that science has its highest sanction when it is of service to man, makes use of the data of anthropometry for his study of what the race may become.

Careful measurement would show "the modifications (if any) which the new environment or Anglo-Celtic admixture of our population is producing."[17] To further this investigation, Australian results might be compared with the information that the British Anthropometric Committee and the American Association for the Advancement of Physical Culture had already assembled.[18] Such pleas for more scientific research on the Australian child body prompted the Australasian Association for the Advancement of Science to appoint an anthropometric committee, which included Berry, Cumpston, Elkington, and Booth. In 1913, the committee published standards for the periodic measurement of Australian schoolchildren, emphasizing the need to be meticulous in recording chest girth, that perpetual Achilles' heel of Australian youth.[19] But it seems, on the whole, that teachers did not respond with the alacrity that the medical profession had expected.[20]

In one of his many proposals for school anthropometry, Sutton had cited the work of Franz Boas, an anthropologist at Columbia University who had investigated the changes in head shape of children of immigrants to the United States. Sutton speculated that in Australia too "there is every possibility that measurements may demonstrate a new national type on the side of physical development."[21] And yet even as he expressed these environmentalist sentiments, he was also prepared to advocate the sterilization of the irredeemably unfit. The combination of environmental analysis and hereditarian prescription was an awkward, but not uncommon, one in the early twentieth century.[22] A few medical experts, such as Berry and Booth, argued for a genetic determinism that implied a singular policy of race advancement through selective breeding; others, such as Ramsay Smith, the Lamarckian director of public health in South Australia, regarded most eugenic enactments as naive or futile, proposing instead a more thorough program of education and preventive medicine.[23] But most national hygienists, like Cumpston, Sutton, and Barrett, were more pragmatic than these purists, favoring a mixture of sterilization and segregation of the manifestly unfit, encouragement of the breeding of the indubitably fit, and improved nurture and training of those in between. Sutton, for example, was convinced that "mental deficiency is a public health as well as an educational problem, for from mental deficients are recruited many of the social parasites of our civilization—the unemployable and thriftless, prostitutes, delinquents and criminals." But while it was worth trying to prevent them "from perpetuating their defect," benefits would also come from slum clearance, free kindergartens, and the provision of urban playgrounds.[24] Cumpston, more cynically, suspected that advocacy of sterilization laws, no matter how advisable, would be simply a waste of time in Australia, so he concentrated on environmental reform. If a consensus—or least objectionable position—emerged, it was that the fit, especially among the middle class, should produce more children and the environment should allow all citizens, regardless of class, to make the best of their genetic potential. Of course, everyone, whether on the hereditarian or environmentalist poles, agreed that schoolchildren should be measured, and measured again, to determine the success of any program of racial advancement in Australia.

The desired outcome of national hygiene was clear to all, whatever the preferred means to this common end. Sutton expressed the racial ideal perhaps most vividly when he imagined a future white body "fully trained, free from defects of posture, upright, elastic, vigorous, alert, the responsive and capable instrument of the will."[25] It had long ago become evident that the greatest deviations from this model were found among larrikin youth in southern cities, not among laborers in the Australian tropics. From the 1870s, physicians and novelists had been documenting the physical and mental degeneration of the city-bred child, an ever more weedy, sallow, fatigued, and delinquent specimen of the white race. By contrast, children raised in pastoral regions, and even those growing up in the tropics, had come to appear more robust and virtuous. Not only did the large southern cities concentrate disease and degenerate types; the character of the urban environment—its inadequate ventilation, lack of open space, dens of vice and immorality—seemed directly to produce a physical and spiritual deterioration in the children of the poor.[26] In 1907, C.E.W. Bean, that influential patriotic journalist, warned that "as soon as a nation begins to shut itself up in cities it begins to decay. First its bodily strength, and along with that its moral strength, declines."[27] Perversely, the fall in urban mortality rates since the 1870s did not help to exonerate the urban environment but, rather, suggested to middle-class professionals that their society was aiding the proliferation of city-bred defectives. A supportive, soft civilization had rendered natural selective processes obsolete: The social problem was thus, at its root, a biological predicament. Sir James Barrett, "the leading spokesman and organisational pivot of progressive reform in Melbourne," responded in typical fashion, urging the voluntary sterilization of the more profoundly defective, a promotion of middle-class reproduction, and the development of infant welfare, kindergartens, playgrounds, Scouting, temperance, sexual hygiene, worker education, and a system of national parks.[28]

Medical fears of the proliferation of urban defectives complemented a widespread, and longstanding, uneasiness about the decline in the middle-class birthrate. Doctors expressed dismay that since the 1890s the more talented and better-educated members of the white community had taken deliberate measures to limit their fertility. In Victoria, Barrett deplored the use of contraception and abortion to restrict family size: Rather than take "pride in the propagation of a branch of the Anglo-Saxon race," selfish middle-class Australians had resorted to a form of "race suicide."[29] In New South Wales, the state government established the Royal Commission on the Decline in the Birth Rate in 1903, chaired by C. K. Mackellar, a medical doctor and politician.[30] Good, quality white immigration was declining, so if the more vigorous and talented classes of white citizens did not increase their numbers, it was felt that the whole nation might be vulnerable to foreign invasion—not just the discomforting tropical north, but even the more providential temperate regions.[31] Accordingly, even those medical experts who disagreed on the relative value and effectiveness of breeding policies and environmental reform maintained during this period a policy of middle-class pronatalism.

Although microenvironmental reform remained the more common prescription for Australian social problems, a trend toward eugenic solutions emerged more forcibly in the 1920s and 1930s, led by middle-class professionals in Melbourne and Sydney.[32] Birth control clinics and popular eugenics societies were established in the major cities.[33] R.J.A. Berry, who was perhaps the first to teach Mendelian genetics at the University of Melbourne, became increasingly strident. He was vigorously professing theories of hard heredity that largely discredited the effects of environmental change on human types while preserving a limited, and strictly individualized, developmental role for education and nurture. With Stanley Porteus, who developed a simple, and allegedly universal, "maze test" for intelligence, Berry attempted to correlate mental capacity and skull size.[34] Berry, a short man with a large skull, persisted with craniometry long after Karl Pearson in Britain had abandoned efforts to relate intelligence and brain capacity. From his psychometric laboratory in the department of anatomy, Berry and his colleagues recorded the skull dimensions and intelligence of mental defectives and criminals, urging restrictions on the reproduction of such small-headed people, either through voluntary sterilization or segregation.[35] In 1929, after his return to Britain to assume the post of director of medical research at the Stoke Park colony for mental defectives, Berry's eugenic sentiments would become, if anything, even more fierce.[36]

In the late 1920s, W. E. Agar, the professor of zoology at the University of Melbourne, took over the teaching of genetics to science and medical students. For the next twenty years or so, his stance on heredity and environment influenced new generations of doctors and scientists. Agar told them that August Weissmann had identified the role of chromosomes in heredity and postulated a continuity of the germ plasm, its insulation from external influence; Gregor Mendel, whose work was rediscovered at the turn of the century, had studied the statistics of assortment of discrete hereditary units; and William Bateson, C. B. Davenport, T. H. Morgan, and others were now exploring the patterns of inheritance and location of the these units, or genes. A new understanding of heredity was accumulating gradually, but its relations to Darwinian theory were not fully established. In the prior few decades, biologists had demonstrated that most diversity within and between populations arose from different combinations of genes, not from exposure to different environments. According to Agar, this meant that the potential for evolutionary change was more limited than Darwin had believed, for mutations of the genetic material were rare and often disadvantageous. Yet Agar thought that the balance of evidence was definitely opposed to a Lamarckian inheritance of acquired characteristics, much as he would have liked a more teleological, and less mechanistic, scheme of development than the "genotype theory" allowed.[37] The environment would merely allow "inherent potentialities" to become manifest during the lifetime of an individual. Agar thus drew sharp implications from theories of hard heredity. With higher birthrates among the poor, it was evident that the intellectual capacity of the white race would soon decline, leading to national disaster. Like Berry, Agar recommended that the state limit the breeding of unfit members of the population, encourage the reproduction of the talented middle class, and select only "a good class of immigrant," especially those of Nordic ancestry.[38] In particular, he advocated "sterilisation for eugenic reasons on a voluntary basis" for mental defectives and the insane, those failures of natural selection. Australia was falling behind Germany, which since 1933 had already "introduced measures to improve the eugenic quality of the nation."[39] According to Agar, if a new type of white citizen were to emerge in the antipodes it would be the result of a state-directed purification and reassortment of northern European genes, not as a response to a new environment or a consequence of advances in preventive medicine.

Even as Agar and Berry and their Melbourne acolytes continued to propound eugenic solutions to racial deterioration, scientists in Britain and North America had begun to challenge formalist taxonomies of race, attempting to repudiate a century or more of typological theory in biology and medicine. Inconsistency and doubt plagued racial classification; each type shaded into another; culture seemed increasingly to be separable from biology and to derive more from local historical settings.[40] A few anatomists, like Sir Arthur Keith in London, continued to assert that historical development was secondary to racial qualities and rivalries, but many more were now prepared to disassociate race and culture.[41] Indeed, the actual biological premises of race seemed increasingly dubious. In Britain, statistical attempts to establish coefficients of racial likeness had failed, throwing into doubt the classificatory value of a vast heritage of anthropometry. Skull size did not correlate with pigmentation; eye color did not overlap significantly with nose dimensions.[42] In the 1930s, a radical group of British biologists was assailing the crude efforts of physical anthropologists and medical doctors to recuperate an anatomical basis for racial categories. The underlying weakness of most racial classifications was that they were derived not from genotypes but from the study of adult structures and appearance, or phenotypes, to which both heredity and environment had made recondite contributions. In the United States, Franz Boas had suggested that even a feature as apparently fixed and hereditary as skull size might change over a generation in a new environment, so how could it be useful in genealogical classification?[43] At the London School of Economics, Lancelot Hogben, the professor of social biology, questioned the genetic basis of any racial typology, arguing that genes were distributed through a population and clustered geographically, not according to ideal types.[44] In *We Europeans*, an extraordinarily influential book, Julian Huxley and A. C. Haddon condemned the "vast pseudo-science of 'racial biology'" that served "to justify political ambitions, economic ends, social grudges, class prejudices." Although at times even they could not resist acceding to an older classificatory impulse, Huxley and Haddon repeatedly emphasized the "relative unimportance . . . of purely biological factors as opposed to social problems in the broadest sense." They recommended that "for existing populations, the word *race* should be banished, and the descriptive and non-commital term *ethnic group* should be substituted."[45] The notion would prove influential in Australia, but not until after World War II.

Australian biologists and doctors were perhaps slower in separating out society and biology, but even as they continued to adhere to a sociobiological amalgam they were usually more inclined to look for environmental solutions, not hereditary interventions, for any defect or deficiency. Despite the efforts of a few Melbourne intellectuals, the segregation and sterilization of the unfit remained a minority taste. If Australian scientists tended to hold on to racial typologies longer than some elite British and North American colleagues, the categories they continued to affirm were generally more plastic—more subject to environmental modulation, for better or for worse—than the harder notions that were discredited more rapidly in the Northern Hemisphere. Racial thought grew vigorously in Australia, but it was perhaps a more variegated crop than elsewhere. Berry and Agar may have sought to introduce the eugenic enactments that had proved so popular, a generation earlier, in Europe and the United States, but most Australians seemed to regard even poor quality whites as better than none in an underpopulated continent. Usually, the hopeful proposals of Cumpston, Sutton, and Cilento, for improvements in race hygiene through education and preventive medicine, had prevailed. The nation had to do its best with whatever white material it had, wherever it was found.

From Medical Geography to Population Policy

An optimistic racial meliorism had emerged in Australia after World War I, drawing strength from advances in preventive medicine and education, occasionally even appealing to eugenic interventions. With careful hygiene and perhaps even with selective breeding, there seemed no limits to the proliferation of whites over a landscape once so thoroughly disparaged. Thus E. J. Brady, in *Australia Unlimited*, praised the continent from end to end, observing that "to the sane, healthy native-born, it is a mother of everlasting youth and beauty, and the freest, richest, happiest land on earth." European stock, whether agricultural or human, was thriving in the new territory as well as it had ever thrived in the Old World. By the time of federation, "a new type of colonist had come into being, evolved by over a century of new conditions. It represented the best of the Anglo-Saxon, the Scot and the Celt, with a dash of the best of Europe and America to give it tone." Even in the tropics the race was flourishing. Native white Queenslanders might be tall and tanned by comparison with southern Australians, but Brady had found nothing anemic or unhealthy about them. In Townsville, he had seen "sturdy wharf labourers work after the strenuous manner of wharf labourers in colder climates," and "the young girls are fresh-complexioned, active, vivacious, apparently not unduly affected by the climate." It was perhaps the richest land under the sun, and he predicted a future tropical population of more than 50 million whites.[46]

A few polemicists continued to challenge such great expectations. In 1926, Fleetwood Chidell suggested that northern Queensland would never become wholly white:

Here we have a realm endowed by nature with a great capacity for production in response to the world demand for cotton, sugar, coffee, tobacco and other tropical growths. Is there any prospect that the white man will succeed in obtaining returns from these regions at a level with those which the yellow or brown man could obtain? It must be admitted that there is no probability of such a return.

Chidell argued that colored labor under white leadership was necessary to develop the Australian tropics. A line might be drawn north of Brisbane, and the land above that boundary could be reserved for colored races.[47] But William Morris Hughes, the former wartime prime minister, was appalled by the notion, arguing that color would soon seep downward through the continent. Australia was "a white island in a vast coloured ocean," and as such it needed to "build dykes through which the merest trickle of the sea of colour cannot find its way." The "little digger" cited the racial research of Sir Arthur Keith that proved the danger of the mixing of human types. "Racial purity pays in the long run," Hughes assured his readers. "A certain percentage of the people of some European countries can be absorbed into our community, but we cannot assimilate these coloured people; their ways are not ours." Hughes, who became the federal minister of health in the 1930s, had a vision of 100 million or more thriving and pure whites populating the whole continent.[48]

But some geographers, economists, and political scientists still expressed skepticism toward medical possibilism and literary hyperbole. In the second series of *The Peopling of Australia*, P. D. Phillips, a lecturer in international relations at the University of Melbourne, suggested that "statistical exuberance" had led scholarship into "the delusive realm of far distant prophecy." He called for "an economic survey of every aspect of national life and of the varying nuances of political feeling and practice." Like many other contributors to that volume, Phillips also felt that the environment remained "relatively permanent and relatively intractable, and as such is the chief conditioning factor in population absorption." In particular, Phillips feared that in the north there were "certain geographical and climatic controls which made the area economically sterile."[49] The environment might not be inimical to whites, but its white carrying capacity was severely limited, far more so than Brady and Hughes had proclaimed.

T. Griffith Taylor was one of the more prominent of the geographers who continued to argue that environment and climate would determine racial destiny. Trained in geology at the University of Sydney and in paleontology at Cambridge, Taylor went on to establish departments of geography at Sydney (1920) and Toronto (1935) and taught at the University of Chicago between 1928 and 1935. He consistently claimed that the environment was more influential than heredity in shaping character. "As the environment changes," he wrote, "so does the civilization wax and wane, and so different races rise to eminence and then sink into oblivion."[50] In *Environment and Race*, Taylor reviewed earlier confused efforts to classify the races, concluding that skin color, language, and nationality were unreliable indices of racial difference, but skull measurements and hair texture could provide more consistent distinctions between human types. Although no one had yet identified a single factor that might differentiate the races, Taylor suggested that a number of "harmonious combinations" were obvious. Thus "broad-headed folk nearly all have white to yellow skins, wavy or straight hair, and live in temperate lands," and "very long-headed folk, broad-nosed, nearly all have dark skins, very frizzy hair, and live in the tropics."[51] Taylor was convinced that some races were superior to others, and he attributed their position in the human hierarchy not to an inherent and fixed biological quality but to the character of their environment. Accordingly, the "broad-headed folk" who had been exposed for generations to the stimulating circumstances of their temperate environment were superior in mentality to the "long-heads" in the enervating tropics. But with migration, this would change, the natural consequence of "a climatic stimulus acting on the plastic human organism."[52]

Taylor believed that advocates of white settlement in the north had understated the region's detrimental tropical character. He demonstrated that the Australian tropics are hotter than anywhere else in the world, except for parts of the Sahara. Comparing a range of meteorological statistics, Taylor claimed that "it is in southern and central India that we get parallels to most of our tropical regions, and any student of Australia's future will do well to ponder on all that implies."[53] By plotting monthly averages for wet-bulb temperatures and humidity readings for each locality, Taylor derived a twelve-sided polygon, which he called a climograph (see Figure 6.1). When plotted on the same chart, the positions and shapes of each climograph could be compared. Thus Darwin's climograph was limited to the "muggy" quadrant, whereas Melbourne's straddled both the "raw" and the "muggy" quadrants. Taylor combined the readings for "the chief centres of white settlement in both hemispheres" to form a composite climograph that indicated ideal conditions for the white race. The closer the overlap of a local climograph with this composite, the more suitable the place would be for future white settlement. Thus Melbourne proved more suitable than Sydney, and Sydney was preferable to Brisbane, but "none of the tropical towns in any way resembles the average conditions of the centres of our race." Indeed, Townsville possessed the "homoclime" of Calcutta, and Darwin boasted the meteorological conditions of Lagos.[54]

Taylor was convinced that the climatic discomfort implied by such a mismatch of actual and ideal climographs would lead inevitably to the degeneration

178

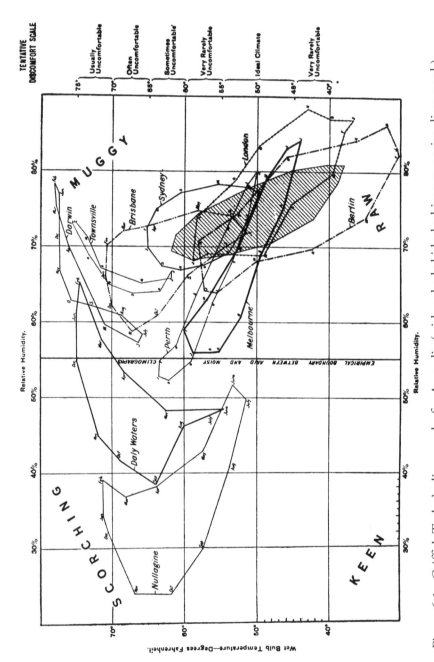

Figure 6.1: Griffith Taylor's climographs for Australia (with a shaded ideal white composite climograph). (*Proceedings Royal Geographical Society of Queensland*, vol. 32-3, 1918)

of any pure white race in the tropics. Cilento and his medical colleagues had been far "more optimistic . . . than the facts warrant."[55] It might be true that tropical diseases were rare, but the continued discomfort of whites in an alien environment inevitably would lead to degenerative forms of tropical neurasthenia, to "depression, irritability, loss of mental activity, and power of concentration."[56] White women and children were especially vulnerable. "How the struggling white farmer's wife is to rear her babes, handicapped by a tropical climate, and probably only assisted by ignorant black gins, is a problem of which no solution is at present obvious."[57] Improved housing, electric fans, and refrigerators might mitigate tropical discomfort, but a laborer's family could not afford these luxuries. Settlement of northern Australia by "inferior races" had been ruled out; and a policy of "race fusion," which Taylor favored, was politically inconceivable. The only hope lay in an expensive and "slow migration from cooler to warmer regions accompanied by generations of gradual acclimatisation."[58] Even so, Taylor did not expect future white generations to resist the tropical climate forever.

In determining optimal population densities for Australia and other "available" regions, Taylor was projecting northern Europe onto the rest of the world. The carrying capacities that he calculated were bourgeois European carrying capacities. Much of his work was prompted by one question: "How will the white population of the world be distributed when the empty continents are occupied to the extent that Europe is at present?"[59] In order to determine future white settlement, Taylor attempted to plot the assets and characters of the various regions, thus obtaining a sort of contour map in which the contours, which he called "isoiketes," represented degrees of "habitability." He listed the factors controlling white settlement, estimated their order of importance, and then assigned a weighting to them. Temperature, rainfall, and agriculture each contributed 15 percent to the locality's score; coal, timber, and health (principally a function of the climograph) each determined 10 percent; and pasturage, communications, and current population each were worth 5 percent.[60] The total score of each locality could be plotted and lines (isoiketes) drawn through points of equal value. Using the current population density in Europe for each isoikete as the criterion, Taylor was then able to predict the future white population of the available parts of the rest of the world. Although the Atherton Tablelands in North Queensland received a score of 82, suggesting "great potentiality," most of the Australian tropics had a low white carrying capacity, and Taylor predicted a population of no more than 1.4 million whites, most of them slowly degenerating.[61] He believed that the optimal white carrying capacity of the whole of the continent was 10 million, with an upper limit of 62 million (see Figure 6.2).[62]

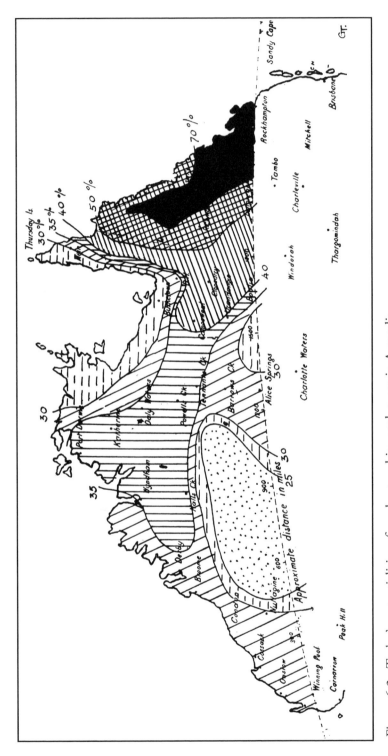

Figure 6.2: Taylor's potentialities of moderate white settlement in Australia.
(*Proceedings Royal Geographical Society of Queensland*, vol. 32-3, 1918)

Other geographers shared Taylor's skepticism toward white Australia. The work of Ellsworth Huntington, a professor of geography at Yale, perhaps marked the high tide of such climatic determinism. In 1915, he proposed a "climatic hypothesis of civilization" as the basis for the "new science of geography." Huntington argued that "human character as expressed in civilization" could be mapped onto physical and organic phenomena in order to determine the relations of man and his environment. It was a truism that "the nature of a people's culture, like the flavor of a fruit, depends primarily upon racial inheritance which can be changed only by the slow processes of biological variation and selection"; but it seemed to Huntington—a staunch environmentalist— that the role of climate in the selection of race culture had been understated. (Although he admitted that it had been "generally agreed that the native races within the tropics are dull in thought and slow in action.")[63] From his analysis of the records of hundreds of white U.S. males, Huntington found that "mental activity reaches a maximum when the outside temperature averages 38 degrees Fahrenheit, that is, when there are mild frosts at night." From this data he drew a map showing how human energy was distributed throughout the world. The tropics were defined as an "unstimulating environment" where it would be impossible to sustain "European and American energy, initiative, persistence, and other qualities upon which we so much pride ourselves."[64] Not surprisingly, Britain, northern Europe, New Zealand, and the Pacific Coast of the United States had ideal climates for civilization; the chief defect of California was that it was "too uniformly stimulating," a factor in generating "nervous disorders"; and the level of white energy in Australia was generally dismally low. "Man," according to Huntington, was "much more closely dependent upon nature than he has realized." Huntington concluded piously that "if we can conquer climate, the whole world will become stronger and nobler"; but he dismissed any hope for progress in the tropics. The climatic impediment to white civilization was simply too great in the torrid zone.[65]

When Huntington visited Australia to attend the second Pan-Pacific Science Congress in 1923, Griffith Taylor showed him around the temperate southern capitals. They compared notes on the baleful effects of tropical environments. But on his return voyage to the United States, Huntington rashly disembarked at unstimulating Townsville, where he found "white people of British stock . . . carrying on an experiment which is of vital importance to the whole world." He thought that Townsville was "a bare struggling little town," with streets that were "drearily broad, dusty and treeless." "As I looked at the sad front yards," the American visitor recalled, "I could not decide whether this desperate attempt to keep up the good old British ways aroused more pity or admiration." Huntington went to visit the Townsville Institute—"one of the most creditable and far-sighted of the many good things done by the Australian government" but by then overwhelmed with routine work—hoping to talk with Cilento.[66] "We looked at the subject from such different standpoints," Cilento later reported, "he from a geographer's, and I from that of a medical man, that it was difficult to find a common basis for discussion."[67] But Cilento was able to show Huntington a number of healthy third- and fourth-generation white children. The American geographer was taken to admire the white cane-cutters and observed that "fair-haired, red-faced young fellows with a strong British accent hew the juicy stalks with quick firm blows of a long knife day after day from June to December." On the docks Huntington saw "good Anglo-Saxons tugging at heavy bags of sugar, bales of wool, and carcasses of beef." His views changed, but only slightly. Huntington still believed that Henry Priestley had been correct in identifying the underlying climatic causes of neurasthenia and trades unionism, and he continued to suspect that children born in the north showed less "physical vitality" than southern Australians, but he was now prepared to admit that "a most strenuous and persistent selection of the right types of people" meant that the white settlers of Queensland had resisted the climate better than he had predicted.[68] But how much longer would they last?

Not all geographers endorsed the environmental determinism of Taylor and Huntington. J.W. Gregory, the professor of geology at Melbourne (and later at Glasgow), had learned about tropical settlement prospects from W.A. Osborne and other friends in the Melbourne medical school. When he was appointed in 1900, Gregory was already well known for his book that had demonstrated a great rift valley through eastern Africa. His exploratory zeal led him to spend as much time off the beaten track as in the classroom, and from one of these excursions came his popular book *The Dead Heart of Australia*. As a result of his study of Australian conditions, Gregory confidently predicted that the whole of the country would eventually be occupied by a healthy white race. In 1910, from Glasgow, he had written that even in tropical Queensland the white children were "not weak anaemic degenerates, while the increased output of sugar since the deportation of the Kanakas shows that white men are willing and able to work there."[69] Of course, this great white achievement had required isolation from inferior tropical races. Later, in his tremendously influential treatise *The Menace of Colour*, Gregory would expatiate on the dangers to health not from a foreign environment but from contact with disease-dealing colored races.

Like his idol, Charles Pearson, Gregory saw the emergence of "a struggle for existence between the white and coloured races," with civilization "endangered by the rising tide of colour." He conceded that no exact classification of race was yet possible, but he remained immensely satisfied with a crude division of mankind by color. Each color decreed a certain way of life and a capacity for civilization, with whites at the top and African blacks at the bottom of the hierarchy of potentiality. It was clear to Gregory that Australia was "the last continent available for the white race" and therefore the last place left for the spread of civilization.[70] Yet many other geographers, including Taylor and Huntington, had claimed that the northern parts of the continent were inhospitable to civilized whites. Gregory disagreed, citing medical evidence, including the findings of the 1920 Australasian Medical Congress, in favor of white settlement in the Australian tropics. He also pointed out that colored races, such as Eskimos and American Indians, could live healthy lives in temperate or cold regions; and black laborers in the tropics frequently were sicker than white residents in the region. Ignoring the effect of living conditions, Gregory observed that "life in tropical Queensland was . . . more fatal to these carefully selected Kanakas than to the white population." It seemed, therefore, that nature had not determined that the tropics were colored. With better housing and clothing, the geographer could imagine "no physiological reason why the white man should not live and work in the tropics, and . . . medical opinion is becoming steadily stronger in favour of that possibility." But it was imperative that white workers were protected from infectious disease and from the unfair competition of colored people who had inherently lower standards of living. Some doctors still speculated on the direct effects of the tropical climate on the white nervous system, but Gregory understood that psychological ailments were "notoriously intangible, and often depend on social conditions." Indeed, "nervous strain is more likely due to inter-racial friction than to climate."[71] Thus, according to Gregory, medicine and geography were converging in support of white Australia. Taylor had suggested a hybridization of superior Asians and whites to provide preadapted tropical settlers, but Gregory denounced this promotion of miscegenation. Science had demonstrated that race-mixing produced mentally and physically unsound offspring. So, yet again, Gregory concluded "the co-residence of different races should be avoided in the interest of the future of mankind." If the white man secured the Australian tropics, and removed all color from the region, he could, "for the benefit of all, continue to conquer the forces of Nature and thereby strengthen the broad foundations of civilization."[72] Thus Gregory, like Brady and Hughes, could discern no limits to white Australia.

TROPICAL COMPROMISE

In the 1930s, a popular compromise eventually emerged between the theories of Taylor and Gregory. With careful selection, or self-selection, of settlers and a combination of immigration restriction and preventive medicine, the Australian tropics might support a limited white population, perhaps not the tens of millions that Brady and Gregory had predicted, but more than the few sad sojourners that most geographers were prepared to forecast. In 1930, G. L. Wilkinson reviewed many of the projections of Australia's future white popula- tion, discounting the grandiose prophecies of Gregory and Hughes in favor of the more modest proposals of Huntington and Taylor. Wilkinson had calcu- lated that the rainfall over the continent would permit no more than 23 million residents if contemporary living standards were maintained. Like Gregory, Wilkinson extolled purity of race and warned of the consequences of race- mixing. Interbreeding between closely related human stocks might confer ad- vantages, but it was clear that "miscegenation between peoples far apart gives bad results which are not eliminated, but rather are accentuated, in successive generations." Wilkinson therefore supported continued immigration restriction and the further segregation of Aboriginal Australians. He deplored the sugges- tions of Chidell and others that colored laborers might be confined to the trop- ics, and he was sure that "no proposal for allowing a large non-European population into any part of Australia, and segregating it there, is ever likely to be advocated by responsible people in the Commonwealth."[73] On the question of whether Europeans could live in the tropics without degeneration, he ac- cepted the advice of Gregory, Cilento, and the participants in the 1920 Aus- tralasian Medical Congress. "That modern sanitation, and the removal of a native population that would not or could not adopt sanitary ways of living, can transform a European's health in the tropics is now well-established," he wrote. But Wilkinson still wondered if some of the doubts of Taylor and Hunt- ington had merit, if eventually some "enfeeblement" would occur, causing Queensland whites to "lose their will to work." But "there were many factors which will help in delaying the effects of tropical climatic disabilities in north- ern Australia; and these factors may operate sufficiently long to allow many habitable parts being fully developed and fully populated by Europeans." Even if they became somewhat enfeebled, limited numbers of tropical whites "will still have the same civilisation and ideals as others in Australia."[74]

In his comprehensive survey of white settlement in the tropics, the Ade- laide geographer A. Grenfell Price also drew on both the geographical insights of Griffith Taylor and the medical possibilism of Raphael Cilento. Writing in the late 1930s, Price conceded that criticisms by Haldane and Huxley re- cently had rendered suspect the category of race. But although Price admitted "the difficulty of discovering any satisfactory terminology or classification" for either race or climate, such inexactitude would not impede his willingness to generalize. Racial thought was simply too important to let the quibbles of British socialists stand in its way. For Price, the principal of an elite Anglican college at the University of Adelaide, "white" clearly meant the "white races of northern European ancestry," not Mediterraneans; and he defined the "trop- ics" by the annual isotherm of 70 degrees Fahrenheit, even though several di- verse climates occupied this belt. Price described the poles of a debate on the white race in the tropics where medical optimists felt "certain that the whites can now defeat sickness, particularly if they exclude or rigidly control coloured races of a lower standard of life" and where geographical pessimists postulated "external and unchangeable factors that will always prevent white acclimatisation." But he thought that statistical information was not yet sufficient to compel a conclusion, and the laboratory research of scientists like Breinl and Young had produced results that "are indefinite and contradictory and touch but the fringe of the problem."[75]

On the whole, Price was optimistic about prospects for white settlers in the Queensland tropics. He followed Cilento in welcoming that fact that in Australia "there are no teeming millions of coloured people to absorb white settlers." This happy state had come about because "the young Australian nation saw the dangers to the economic status and health of her white citizens and carried out a long and difficult purification." Thus in Australia white settlers had managed to "keep to themselves the results of scientific progress" and make sure that advances in preventive medicine did not serve merely to increase the numbers and mobility of colored folk.[76] Along with Gregory and Wilkinson, Price condemned those who, like Taylor, might advocate adaptation through race-crossing. Scientists, he claimed, had shown that "hybridisation may be dangerous between extreme racial types such as those which so frequently make contact in the tropics." On medical grounds, then, "the 'White Australia' policy may have a sound biological basis." Indeed, if "a century of experiment has proved that northern white males can survive in these wet-dry or arid tropics and maintain fair standards in the face of isolation and other difficulties," their success was due to the preservation of racial purity and the willingness to engage in hard manual work. It seemed that "work" and "purity" had become the watchwords of white Australia.[77]

Price still shared some reservations with other advocates of white settlement in tropical Australia. Much of the white male population of northern Queensland was migratory, or else it was Mediterranean in origin and therefore dubiously white. Few white males of any provenance had managed to settle in the extremely arid or the monsoonal regions of the Australian tropics. Price suspected that such country was "totally unsuited to the intensive settlement of any human race." This meant that large tracts of land had been left to scattered groups of Aborigines, so that "despite the 'White Australia' policy a great part of the continent is black Australia still."[78] And even the more hospitable Queensland coast, which supported a large population of white male laborers, still seemed a bad place for white women and children. Price feared that white "women age rapidly, lose vitality, and in the drier areas suffer from dehydration of the tissues"; whereas the children "develop rapidly and are of good physique, tall, highly strung, excitable and sexually advanced."[79] Elsewhere, Price amplified his concerns, noting that "how far the climate affects mentality is not yet known, but 'tropical memory' certainly exists, and many North Queenslanders are doubtful as to whether white children develop in mentality after the age of sixteen as satisfactorily as do children in temperate climates."[80] But these mixed results might yet improve with more careful selection of residents, better housing and diet, and the avoidance of alcohol. Thus, according to Price, even in 1939 it was still too early to be sure of the endpoint of the great white experiment. Would a thriving white race establish itself in the Australian tropics, or would Capricornia become a dumping ground for a few nervy, isolated white sojourners? "In the hands of scientific workers," Price piously concluded, "lies the solution."[81]

THE PHYSIOCRATIC STATE

Pleas for further scientific research in the tropics proved futile: Southern public health officials and medical academics were turning away from the region to focus on the supposedly more pressing problem of urban degeneration. White settlement in the tropics may have become a great racial "experiment," but there were few scientists after the 1930s who could be bothered to monitor it. At the new medical school at the University of Queensland, and later at the Johns Hopkins University, D.H.K. Lee was converting his physiological studies of white adaptation into more general investigations of human fatigue and "climatic stress."[82] In the 1950s, at the Sydney School of Public Health and Tropical Medicine, his former colleague R. K. Macpherson studied principles of housing design in the tropics, but with the generic goal of improving human comfort, not specific racial conquest of the torrid zone.[83] Studies of racial adaptation to foreign environments, once the sum of medical research in Australia, were neglected; a specifically "tropical" hygiene, formerly a pillar of public health activity, almost disappeared in the 1930s. Thus the legacy of Breinl and his colleagues was not so much the establishment in Australia of a medical specialty in tropical medicine as the permeation through all levels of society of an assumption that most political problems—tropical or otherwise—have biological causes and solutions and that medical scientists were social experts. As G. L. Wood put it, to have the problem of population policy "lifted from the arena of party politics to the laboratory of the scientist is a very real contribution to an ultimate and successful solution of our greatest national problem."[84] But if the laboratory was not in the arena of party politics, it was still, as we have seen, generating its own sort of politics: The elevation of an issue into the heady realm of science would not imply the transcendence of self-interest or of other interests.

Medical scientists and geographers had managed to translate the complex and uncertain political problem of the settling of Australia into a technical idiom; the task of nation-building had become a vast experiment; all white citizens were assuming the status of research subjects. Experts in the universities and government bureaucracy hoped that individual behavior in the cities and in remote regions would henceforth concord with a new scientific grammar, whether hereditarian or environmentalist in inflection. National hygienists would stipulate the correct way to eat, drink, dress, sleep, reproduce, and work—wherever one was located. They knew the scientifically proven mode of inhabiting a place, cultivating it, and taking permanent possession of it. According to health educators, women should be modest and compliant, good mothers and homemakers; men ought to be strong, virile, and hard-working. All whites were enjoined to regulate bodily contact in a fastidious manner; temperance and propriety were to oust promiscuity and irregularity. Even a cursory observation of ordinary behavior in the developing nation reveals how successfully these ideals of hygiene were internalized and came to shape many people's conduct and sense of themselves. And yet it is also clear that no one could always live up to these standards, and some never really tried. This simply meant that the performance of hygienic, responsible white citizenship would have to be supervised, not licensed, even after scientists left the scene, or lost interest, and research institutions had crumbled. In the endless pursuit of Cumpston's "immaculate cleanliness," the family, schools, and workplaces would become venues for low-grade health education and intermittent inspection and discipline.

Scientists, geographers, and national hygienists had shared the goal of stabilizing, or settling, whiteness in Australia, though they often differed in their definition, or bounding, of the race, as well as in their understanding of its robustness or plasticity. Some experts, as we have seen, focused on a vaguely white race, some on Europeans, others on Britons or Nordics, still others on Caucasians. In general, scientists from Melbourne and Sydney had come to believe that the race, whatever it was, wherever it was, would stay much as it was, so long as it obeyed the principles of hygiene, temperance, and industry and eliminated the unfit. Many geographers, we know, held on to the old ethnic moral topography for far longer, arguing that whites would degenerate if outside of their proper place, that the tropics might consume European bodies and character. By contrast, a few national hygienists, like Cilento, predicted that whiteness would be enhanced in the tropics, that a new virile type of tropical white man would emerge from the cane fields. Such variation in forecast should not blind us to the assumptions that these experts held in common. They all, with the partial exception of Griffith Taylor, valued whiteness above any other human quality—and even made a fetish of it. It was just that white Australia might be limited, as the geographers claimed; or it might stay normal, nothing exceptional, given proper attention to nurture and breeding, as Sutton stated; or it might be as unlimited as Brady, Cilento, and other boosters trumpeted. Moreover, whether these authorities thought the character of the race was robust or plastic (for better or for worse), they all assumed that whites, especially poor or marginal ones, would require relentless supervision and discipline if they were to live up to their responsibilities in the new nation. All these experts naturally expected that their own scientific work should continue to inform and guide public policy and everyday life. And to a great extent, if not completely, their expectations of influence were met.

Not surprisingly, it was the biological utopianism of Cilento and his coterie that resonated mostly loudly outside the medical profession and health bureaucracies, as it appealed especially to those political radicals and bohemian writers who were trying in the 1930s to distinguish a new national character.[85] A leading literary nationalist, P. R. "Inky" Stephensen had grown up in Brisbane, met Jack Lindsay—later a British Marxist novelist and litterateur—and became an admirer of his uncle, Jack Elkington, the tropical hygienist and boxing Nietzschean.[86] Stephensen had learned that "physiographic factors work slowly, and are only slowly defined in their effects upon a people. Ultimately the Australian race will be quite different from the 'English' race, and hence Australian literature will be quite different from the merely English literature, of England."[87] An evolution of the sort was becoming apparent. "Our background, such as it is, is operating upon us subtly to produce a new variety of the human species." Like Cilento and Elkington, Stephensen predicted the emergence in Australia of a hard, vigorous type of male body and mentality. "In a new and quite different environment from that of those damp British Islands," white Australians were evolving their own cultural forms.[88] For Stephensen, as for so many others, racial hygiene and racial expression were inseparable, together giving rise to a virile, white national culture—to an "Australian legend," as it would later be called.[89]

PART THREE

ABORIGINAL AUSTRALIA

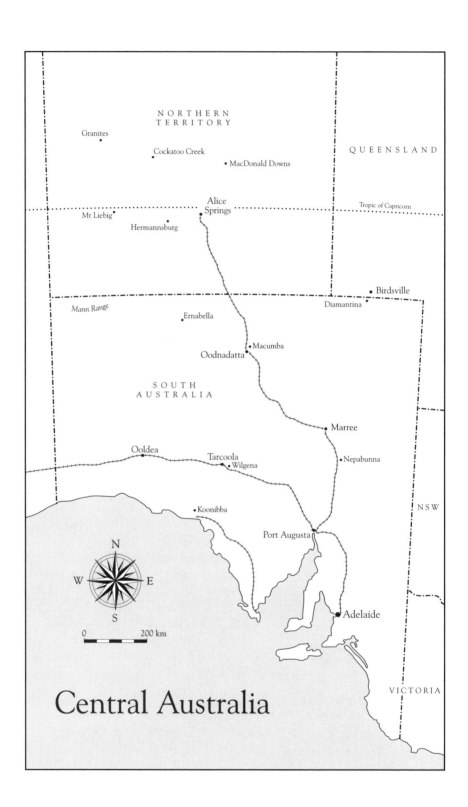

NORTHERN
TERRITORY

Granites

Cockatoo Creek

MacDonald Downs

QUEENSLAND

Alice
Springs

Tropic of Capricorn

Mt Liebig

Hermannsburg

Birdsville

Mann Range

Diamantina

Ernabella

Macumba

Oodnadatta

SOUTH
AUSTRALIA

Marree

Ooldea

Tarcoola
Wilgena

Nepabunna

Koonibba

Port Augusta

NSW

N
W   E
S

Adelaide

0   200 km

VICTORIA

Central Australia

CHAPTER 7

FROM DESERTS THE PROPHETS COME

FULL OF OPTIMISM AFTER World War I, E. J. Brady predicted that even the arid center of Australia would soon be covered with prosperous white settlements. Brady, who had imbibed literary nationalism with the poet Henry Lawson around the campfire at Mallacoota, in eastern Victoria, proclaimed that "instead of a 'Dead Heart of Australia' there exists in reality a Red Heart, destined one day to pulsate with life." He meant white life; Aboriginal Australians were missing from his vision of *Australia Unlimited*. "I must unreluctantly announce to those chronic pessimists who have clung for three generations to a belief in an ever-receding 'Australian Desert,' that this bogey is now definitely relegated for all time to the Limbo of Ancient Lies." Brady had never passed through the evaporating central deserts, but he heard from his bush mates that "the whole continent is good from its inmost core to its outmost rind."[1] Although Brady deplored popular allusions to a "Dead Heart of Australia," he readily found common cause with J. W. Gregory, the geologist who had coined the term. In *The Menace of Colour*, Gregory observed that "the proportion of desert land has been overstated," and he asserted that the center of the continent was destined to become a white pastoral region. Aboriginal Australians would continue to "wither away" with further European colonization.[2] Both Brady and Gregory reproved T. Griffith Taylor, Ellsworth Huntington, and any other effete geographer who regarded the arid center as a limitation to the implanting of white civilization across Australia.[3] Taylor and Huntington were calling for more sensitivity to the environmental limits to whiteness while Brady and Gregory were working to ensure that the allegedly hostile Australian desert disappeared as completely as had the allegedly hostile Australian tropics a decade or so earlier. All of it must become white man's country.

But as yet there was little "white blood" pulsing through the Red Heart. No more than a few hundred European sojourners clung to the land along the overland telegraph, strung from Adelaide to Darwin in 1872. Few white women had ventured into the center, and hardly any stayed more than a season or two. In the 1920s, as Brady, Gregory, and others promoted inland settlement, the region was enduring a prolonged drought, and even the toughest white residents thought of leaving. Aboriginal Australians, most of them "full-blood," still outnumbered whites by a ratio of at least ten-to-one. In 1927, Jens Lyng, the Melbourne statistician, calculated that 60,000 "full-bloods" remained in the country, with the "half-castes" numbering more than 15,000. Although he was still convinced that full-bloods were dying out, and the half-castes would be absorbed into the white community, Lyng warned that "the idea of the white Australia ideal being shattered from within cannot be dismissed as altogether absurd."[4] When the plucky reporter Ernestine Hill traveled across the Top End and into the center in the 1930s, she was wary of the "savages" who molested Europeans, but she was always prepared to have a yarn with the blokes—reassuringly white, of course—in outback pubs.[5] As white women were "as rare as roses" in the bush, Hill found that even the hard cases were friendly and attentive. But European numbers were few, and she too lamented that "the future of white Australia in the north looks very dark indeed."[6] A few years later, A. Grenfell Price was echoing her concerns: "Despite the 'white Australia' policy, a great part of the continent is black Australia still."[7]

One might imagine that a demographic abnormality of this kind would disconcert the scientists who had reported so recently on white triumph in tropical Australia. But it did not. Instead, the persistently black heart of Australia occasioned a readjustment of racial categories and a new calculation of the rate of full-blood decline. Most experts still believed that contact with whites had doomed full-bloods to extinction, but this inevitable biological process would take a little longer than previously predicted. More interestingly, the unforeseen delay allowed medical scientists and physical anthropologists to assay in novel ways the character of Aboriginality in Australia. Aborigines were subject to far more biological and medical scrutiny in the 1920s and 1930s than ever before. Previously viewed by amateur anthropologists as living exhibitions in a natural history museum, Aborigines were dragged into the biomedical present and accorded an ambiguous, unsettling status, more kin than stranger, but not quite either. Thus recognized belatedly in medicine, persistent Aboriginality irritated scientists into a recharting of racial boundaries and a reassessment of disease patterning in Australia between the wars.

A series of expeditions sent into central Australia from Adelaide and Sydney during the interwar years conducted physiological experiments and hematological studies on full-bloods and half-castes. In the outback, medical scientists found tribes of "tawny" natives and "white blood" in even the most deceptively dark of the blacks. It appeared that the University of Adelaide expeditions were confirming earlier, scattered speculation that Aborigines were in fact "archaic" or "dark" Caucasians.[8] As Grenfell Price reported, "Blood tests appear to show that the Aborigine is akin to the white man."[9] So even if, as he thought, large parts of the center were black Australia still, it was a spurious blackness, a Caucasian sort of blackness. Here is a striking local example of a more general effort to consolidate groups with a hitherto dubious status into a unitary "Caucasian" race. As Matthew Frye Jacobson points out, this project is pursued perhaps most thoroughly and definitively in the United States during the 1920s.[10] In Australia the process may have had less popular appeal, but uniquely the category of "Caucasian" was enlarged so as to take in even the indigenous inhabitants.

Brady was among the first to announce the new scientific findings. In his travels during the 1920s the poet encountered a doctor attached to the hookworm survey, examining blood specimens. "When Nipper's smear went under the microscope Mac came as near to excitement a fellow of the Rockefeller Institute ever permits himself to go," he wrote. "It was neither the hookworm— with which Nipper was at first glance obviously infected—nor the disease clamorously manifest . . . but a rare and precious discolouration which Mac thought he saw on the little glass slide below the lens." As Nipper had gone bush, it was nearly a week before Mac came back "with those further samples of Nipper's venous and arterial personality which his scientific soul coveted." The doctor looked again at the blood and "after a reflective pause he imparted the fact that this particular nigger's smear presented distinct European characteristics!"[11] If nothing else, Brady captures well the predilection for racial classification, and the perfunctory attention to disease diagnosis, found in much of the medical research conducted on Aborigines during this period.

The reframing of Aboriginal racial identity caused scientists to reflect again on the meanings of whiteness in Australia. In the nineteenth century, the character of antipodean Britishness had been defined primarily in opposition to the devitalizing soil and climate of the new country; in the early twentieth century, new understandings of a more mobile whiteness emerged from medical disparagement of foreign races. As these projections of European desire and fear gradually faded from the scene, medical scientists and others began to use novel understandings of Aboriginality in order to reimagine their own lives and destinies. In the past, science had etched more deeply the demarcation between whites and the land, as well as between whites and other races. Now scientists would instead attempt to shift the boundaries of "whiteness" and incorporate Aboriginal Australians into the category as distant relatives and object lessons. In the 1920s, medical doctors and physical anthropologists were able to discern an alternative Caucasian destiny, one that marked more clearly the peculiar features of their own development and allowed many of them to express ambivalence toward modernity. Scientists had discovered a whiteness of a truly different color and quality, associated with a different mentality and spirituality and distinguished by a close relationship with place and circumstance—in fact, it seemed to be a racial variant almost consumed by its environment, the blood soaking deeply into the soil. And yet this difference—even such significant and illuminating difference—was now subordinated to similarity, to a common physiology, and to common pathological processes. Scientific investigations of racial kinship would thus appear to validate, and often might even propose, later policies of Aboriginal absorption that especially targeted half-castes.[12]

In this chapter I will consider research on full-bloods, a people rarely regarded as absorbable in social practice (though probably so in biological theory) and yet a group whose extinction had been deferred indefinitely. These dark Caucasians in the heart of white Australia not only demonstrated an alternative racial destiny and another way of relating to the land; they also incited a continuing debate on the value of a colonial variant of white civilization. Most experts never doubted that Aborigines were the latest victims of white "civilization," at least in a metaphorical sense; a few scientists began to wonder whether this destructive civilization was not itself degenerate. In general, of course, the march of civilization had been viewed as little more than an inevitable biological process, not as a phenomenon that might be judged as good or bad. The opinions expressed by H. L. Wilkinson, a Melbourne political scientist, were typically distanced. Aborigines, he wrote in 1930, "were a primitive people who did not and could not absorb the newcomer's higher civilisation; and their ways of life were too different to permit of their being absorbed. They simply retired into the Australian wilderness as the new civilisation advanced; if they remained, they died as a result of their contact with it."[13] But some scientists expressed profound reservations about this civilizing process. Frederic Wood Jones, the professor of anatomy at Adelaide and an instigator of scientific expeditions into the center during the late 1920s, lamented that "blankets will not save the Australian race, flour will not provide the panacea that will render those who have singed their wings in the flame of degenerate civilisation whole again."[14]

There was more to this argument than a conventional structuring of contrasting typologies, in which tradition illuminates the modern, the primitive reveals the civilized—with these polarities embodied in the virile, but endangered, nomad and the increasingly effeminate city-dweller. Wood Jones and his colleagues were also recognizing the racial affinities of Aboriginal Australians and Europeans; they had demonstrated the deep identities of bodily function and malfunction that underlay minor structural variations; they were inserting Aboriginal bodies into a modern time frame. For them, Aboriginality was not anachronistic; it was functionally contemporaneous. It is almost as though they were issuing a sort of biological license to attend to Aboriginal expressiveness and spirituality in the modern world. In thus representing an alternative, if ultimately tragic, destiny for Caucasians in a contemporary setting, Aboriginality could even be taken up by literary nationalists in Adelaide in the 1930s and used to inform a vision of another way of being modern in Australia. In the beginning was science; then, as we shall see, came Jindyworobak.

THE DISCOVERY OF THE ARCHAIC CAUCASIAN

With the extension of white settlement in the nineteenth century, Europeans began to speculate on the place of Aboriginal man in nature. How did the Aboriginal type differ from a European type? Where did Aborigines fit in the racial hierarchy? What did it mean that providential design or evolutionary mechanism had placed blacks, not whites, in the Australian environment? In Britain, naturalists such as Charles Darwin and T. H. Huxley found it necessary to address these questions, and in so doing they drew often on unpleasant antipodean experience to fashion their theories. When Darwin, for example, visited Australia on HMS *Beagle* in the 1830s, he found that the Aborigines were not "utterly degraded beings," and he placed them "some few degrees higher on the scale of civilisation than the Fuegians." At the time, the naturalist wondered about "some more mysterious agency at work. Wherever the European has trod, death seems to pursue the Aboriginal."[15] When the science of race, or anthropology, emerged in Europe in the middle of the century, most of its practitioners were especially keen to classify and rank the disappearing Australian type, even if many of them still had to rely on odd reports from explorers and early settlers.

In Australia the immigrant interest in Aboriginal man was always more than theoretical. Few medical doctors regarded the country's original inhabitants as worthy clinical material, or even as pathological threat, but some of the more self-consciously cultivated of colonial savants, many of them physicians, did attempt to explain scientifically the obvious physical and mental differences between the races. Should Aborigines be considered one type or many? What was their origin? Had they degenerated in a vitiating environment, or was their development merely stalled? Would they become extinct as the result of a racial struggle for existence?[16] As they represented Aboriginal man, some of the more scientific of colonizers wondered if they were forecasting a dire white destiny in hostile circumstances. Later, as Darwinian doctrine—especially when viewed through the lens of hard heredity—helped to allay fears of European deterioration, medical doctors and academic scientists instead began to cast Aborigines as the rapidly dwindling precursors, or rather aged collateral relatives, of ascendant Europeans. Whether prognostic or genealogical, such typological framings of Aboriginality usually served better to express, or at least to project, white anxieties and hopes than to describe accurately the indigenous population of the continent.

Many early observers had asserted that Aborigines, though undoubtedly inferior, could yet advance and become civilized; but by the 1830s, with closer settlement, most commentators were more pessimistic, predicting the inevitable extinction of the race.[17] In 1846, William Westgarth, generally a sympathetic observer, reported from Melbourne that the local Aborigines had a low "aptitude for civilised life." Although an Aborigine may show "a facility of imitation of European manners and habits," he eventually would "suddenly throw aside the loose and cumbrous mantle of civilisation, and return with unabated zest to his native woods and his original barbarism." Westgarth noted that "they soon exhibit symptoms of impatience, and a sensation of irksomeness under the monotony of ordinary daily labour."[18] Westgarth, one of the Port Phillip District's leading intellectuals, believed, with most of his less sophisticated contemporaries, that body form and mentality manifested "such variations as the nature of the climate and other conditions of life might impress upon the human frame." With dark skin, "the forehead low, eyes large and far apart, nose broad and flat, mouth wide, with large white teeth and thick lips, the lower jaw unusually short and widely expanded anteriorly," and a disturbing facial angle between 75 and 85 degrees, Aborigines clearly had emerged as a distinct and degraded type.[19] Yet if this was a case where physical and mental faculties "exist in perfect accordance with the circumstances by which each [race] is surrounded," what then did such woeful transmutation presage for immigrant whites? Westgarth chose to insert a moral and behavioral paradox into the prevailing environmental determinism. "Barbarous, unreflecting, and superstitious," he wrote, "how strangely contrasted is an object so obnoxious and so useless with the brightness of a southern sky, and the pastoral beauty of an Australian landscape!"[20] Without dwelling on this conundrum, Westgarth predicted "the diminution of his number, and the final extinction of savage man, as he makes room for the civilised occupants of his territory." Contact with European society, and the effects of dispossession, would soon lead to the extinction of the race. It was best to leave them to themselves, though some temporary success might come from "the training of the Aboriginal children, particularly when they can be separated from their parents and tribes."[21] But even if pastoralist whites could thus displace Aborigines under southern skies, their own antipodean destiny was still clouded.

A later generation of settlers would continue to echo Westgarth's prediction of Aboriginal extinction, but they also began to assert more confidently the successful implantation of British bodies and civilization in the temperate parts of Australia. In 1876, R. Brough Smyth, a Melbourne meteorologist and geologist, agreed that "it was the kindness of the civilised immigrant that swept off the native population." Brough Smyth, the difficult, energetic secretary of mines and director of the geological survey, described a peculiar sickness that afflicted natives who mixed with whites: "They mope, they sit stupidly over a fire, and at length the lungs or some other parts of the body are attacked and they die."[22] Brough Smyth went on:

> In the artificial life which the whites have forced upon him, he is not always very strong nor very healthy. The process of selection which nature has employed in fitting him for the haunts he loves is one which renders him a ready victim to the diseases that are the results of the kind of civilisation now existing; diseases which would be unknown were civilisation based on natural laws, and not crippled by old superstitions nor held in bondage by vicious intentions.[23]

When "uncontaminated by contact with the whites," Aborigines were robust and remarkably healthy. Insanity was unknown among those who did not mix with Europeans. Now they were prone to consumption, other lung problems, rheumatism, skin diseases, and syphilis—and European methods of treatment rarely helped them.[24]

Like Westgarth, Brough Smyth expressed more interest in fate of the Aborigines than in their origins, though he did remark that they seemed to conform "to one pattern as regards features, colour, and mental character." He distinguished mainland Australians from the Tasmanians, who were "darker, shorter, more stoutly built and generally less pleasing in aspect than the people of the continent. Their hair was woolly and crisp, and some bore a likeness to the African Negro."[25] A few years earlier, T. H. Huxley had decided that the Tasmanian people were Negritos, "men with dark skins and woolly hair who constitute a special modification of the Negroid type."[26] Paul Topinard, his French counterpart, disputed this classification and suggested instead that the Tasmanians were a pure autochthonous race, separate from Melanesians and Australians and distinct from those around them.[27] After the publication of Darwin's *Descent of Man* in 1871, the fashion for classification and for speculation about the origins of the types of mankind soon caught on in Australia too. H. Ling Roth, basing his conclusions on linguistic and osteological affinities, confirmed that the Tasmanians were a Negrito stock who once had occupied the whole of the continent "until annihilated and partly assimilated by the invaders now known as Australians."[28] The recent formation of Bass Strait had turned Tasmania into their island citadel. But what the continental natives had begun, Europeans would complete. When George Augustus Robinson attempted to collect the remnants of the Tasmanian people in the 1830s, he could find no more than 200, who were then consigned to Flinders Island in Bass Strait.[29] There, Roth reported, "they sank into a life of listless inaction, in which they lost their natural vigour, and became an easy prey to any disease that attacked them. . . . In fact, the unhappy captives pined and died from 'home sickness.'" In particular, "the use of clothes had a most injurious effect on their health," destabilizing their constitutions and leading thus to pulmonary disorders. Roth believed that "the white man's civilisation proved scarcely less fatal than the white man's musket." As a result, the last full-blood Tasmanian died in 1877.[30] Edward B. Tylor, the professor of anthropology at Oxford and a correspondent of Roth, declared in 1890 that the Tasmanians "stand before us as a branch of the Negroid race illustrating the condition of man near his lowest known level of culture." But Tylor knew that in fact there were no Tasmanian "types" left alive to stand before him in Oxford or anywhere else. He admitted this and lamented the great loss to science.[31]

Scientists in Europe and in Australia had much to learn about white adaptation and evolution from further investigations of the remaining inhabitants of the Australian continent, but it often seemed to them that these objects of investigation would disappear before their natural history was fully understood. From the late nineteenth century onward, an army of medical doctors, scientists, anthropologists, and antiquarians set out expeditiously to cover the inland, documenting local customs and habits, collecting and examining Aboriginal artifacts and body parts.[32] The investigations of Aborigines were less orderly and contained than we might now expect. Disciplinary boundaries between the nascent sciences were indistinct; the collectors and analysts often occupied different social spaces, or then again, the same person might perform both activities; specimens might circulate locally, or they could gain value in global transactions; conclusions would take the form of simple descriptions or otherwise be elaborated into complex taxonomies.[33]

A few key elements in this ambitious racializing project were commonplace. A classificatory impulse drove most scholars; they generally felt a need to rank each definite type in a more or less fixed hierarchy of physical and mental attainment, with Aborigines inevitably at the bottom. No one doubted that culture, usually termed "customs and habits," derived from inherited racial capacities, not from historical circumstances—indeed, until the early twentieth century it was assumed that race, and in particular race struggle, shaped history. The relations of these types to their circumstances—and their capacity for transmutation when environments changed—were less obvious. For some the antipodes reiterated natural theology, with inflexible types perfectly placed by God in their proper environment; more commonly, scientists detected a

Lamarckian dynamic in the apparently rapid adaptation of Aboriginal man to local needs. In the 1870s, though, the latest Darwinian theories seemed to endorse a general sense of stability of racial type, white or black. According to the *Descent of Man*, the rise of civilization, even in its meager indigenous forms, meant that natural selection had virtually ceased to operate on the races, which therefore became fixed, or at least insignificantly variant—stuck at whatever stage their ecological niche had once permitted.[34] From careful scrutiny of contemporary types, one might therefore derive ancestral forms; and so by the end of the nineteenth century, genealogy had become, for the more romantic of scientists, the poetry of nature. Aborigines came to represent the past of advanced Europeans, and not their antipodean future, as the more pessimistic Lamarckians had suspected, or yet their current concern, as some, like Grenfell Price and Wood Jones, would later claim.

Among less sophisticated observers, pigment might obscure deeper affinities. As a squatter in the western district of Victoria, Edward Curr beheld a "remarkable homogeneousness" of type among Aboriginal Australians. They were a "rather dark copper colour," and "the forehead is low, and the brows largely overshadow the eyes, which are of medium size and far apart. . . . The eye lashes are often long, and the eyes soft, lustrous, quick and intelligent." Fascinated yet also somewhat repelled, Curr had found that their hair "is plentiful, long, wavy, and hangs in heavy curls," and the skin is "soft and velvety to the touch," but with a "disagreeable odour." He considered the half-castes "the reverse of an improvement" on this type.[35] Similarities of physical features, customs, and languages suggested to Curr that "the Australian is by descent a Negro, crossed by some other race," but "with hair and colour such as no Negro possesses," and he thought that Africans had advanced much further.[36] Still, Curr was convinced that Aborigines might yet become civilized. "The only success which our treatment of them has had is in the cultivation of their intellects; and if their education is preserved with for several generations, I see no reason to prevent their being brought in this particular level to ourselves." But this was unlikely to occur, as white diseases ravaged Aboriginal society and white medicines were not in harmony with the Aboriginal constitution. "The White race seems destined," Curr concluded, "not to absorb, but to exterminate the Blacks of Australia."[37]

Much as they might endorse his dire predictions, most experts chose to deride Curr's classification of mainland Aboriginal Australians. Brough Smyth had implied that the straight- or curly-haired continental type might be Caucasian; T. H. Huxley already had noted the similarities between Aborigines and Dravidians, a Caucasian branch living on the Deccan plateau in India.[38] In an extremely influential zoological account, W. H. Flower and R. Lyddeker described the original peopling of Australia by frizzy-haired Melanesians who had later been displaced, or absorbed, by "a low form of Caucasian melanochroi," a wavy-haired type from whom Dravidians also descended.[39] In 1893, the aged Alfred Russel Wallace, who alongside Darwin had once proposed a theory of natural selection, observed a resemblance between Aboriginal Australians and "the coarser and more sensual types of western Europeans." Wallace thus confirmed his colleagues' suggestions that "in all essential characters" the natives of the continent must be classed as Caucasian, even if they were the lowest and most primitive of this noble breed. As the primitive Caucasians occupied "undesirable" country, Wallace, more sentimental (or perhaps more naive) than many of the younger scientists, did not expect their rapid extinction.[40]

In the 1890s, then, the leading biological authorities regarded Aboriginal Australians as predominantly a form of archaic Caucasian. But John Mathew, a genial Presbyterian minister in Melbourne who had grown up among the Aborigines of the Burnett River in Queensland, disturbed the emerging accord, discounting the dominance of Caucasian characters and emphasizing instead the hybridity of Aboriginal type. In *Eaglehawk and Crow*, Mathew concluded from linguistic evidence that Papuans, a Negroid form, had initially occupied Australia, but a mixed Dravidian and Malay race later invaded the continent and amalgamated with them. The two biological races, he claimed, were represented socially by two primary classes, or phratries, whose names—eaglehawk and crow—indicated an ancestral color-consciousness.[41] As Mathew, a liberal and eloquent preacher and a close friend of Sir John MacFarland, the chancellor of the University of Melbourne, later put it, the social classes thus "stand for blood distinctions." Aborigines, it seemed, were as sensitive to color difference as any European colonizer: "The colour of the skin," he wrote, "is supposed to correspond to the colour of the blood."[42] Although primarily concerned with demonstrating Aboriginal racial heterogeneity, Mathew also expatiated on the mental attributes that the mixture had produced. He found that Aborigines lacked application and concentration, showing little determination; and yet they could also "exhibit powers of mind anything but despicable" and were capable of routine work.[43] From the manse at Coburg, in Melbourne, he recalled their gaiety, their sunny disposition, along with their vanity. But without "complete detachment" the Australians were "doomed to perish rapidly by contact with European civilisation and vice." "A black gin," the preacher warned, "lolling about the camp, clad in an ill-fitting, cast-off, tattered gown, begrimed with grease and ashes, is a sad picture of Aboriginal degeneracy and parasitism."[44]

But the trend of modern biological thought was away from Mathew. A. W. Howitt, one of Melbourne's leading naturalists, was most trenchant in his criticism. Conceding that invading Caucasians had "absorbed" an earlier Negroid element, Howitt chose to emphasize Caucasian dominance in the amalgamation; he denied altogether any Malay contribution.[45] Howitt was, in any case, more interested in documenting Aboriginal social structure, in describing the social organism, than in ascribing racial origins. An experienced bushman who had been involved in the attempt to rescue the explorers Burke and Wills in 1861, Howitt frequently mingled with Aborigines during his tours of Victoria as a magistrate. After reading Darwin in the 1860s, he began to record the customs and habits of the Kurnai; he acquired a collaborator, the Reverend Lorimer Fison, who introduced him to the evolutionary theories of Lewis Henry Morgan, an American anthropologist.[46] Morgan, an expert on ancient societies, valued the research of Howitt and Fison on a people who "now represent the condition of mankind in savagery better then it is elsewhere represented on the earth—a condition now rapidly passing away."[47] In order to understand the evolution of modern society, Howitt and his colleagues would have to hurry to document the kinship arrangements of such ancient survivals.

In taking up anthropological study, Baldwin Spencer, the professor of biology at the University of Melbourne, became, in general, an ally of Howitt. A staunch Darwinian evolutionist, Spencer, like Howitt, believed that Aborigines "represent the most backward race extant and, in many respects, reveal to us the conditions under which the early ancestors of the present human races evolved."[48] In his reflections on fieldwork in central Australia, Spencer recalled that

> we had been carried far back into the early history of mankind and . . . we had enjoyed an experience such as now falls to the lot of few white men. We had actually seen, living in their primitive state, entirely uncontaminated by contact with civilisation, men who had not yet passed beyond the palaeolithic stage of culture.[49]

Spencer concentrated on recording primitive kinship structures and culture forms, but he did also take issue with Howitt's theory that the higher race that had migrated from Asia to the continent might later have mixed with Negrito Tasmanians to produce the current Australian race. As Spencer could not imagine a majority of a higher race readily joining with those of lower status, he was convinced that Australians must be pure Caucasians.[50] Spencer's anthropological studies and his experience as protector of Aborigines in the Northern Territory led him to believe that these pure, archaic Caucasians would eventually succumb to the combined assaults of Asians and their superior brethren. In 1913, he reported from the settlement at Darwin that "one thing is certain, and that is that in all parts where they are in contact with outsiders, especially with Asiatics, they are dying out with great rapidity."[51] The process might be delayed by the white Australia policy and the creation of reservations, as well as through moral "uplifting" and medical care, but it was difficult to imagine it being circumvented entirely. As protector, Spencer recommended the expansion of reserves, or sanctuaries, for the true "nomads," segregation of Asians and full-bloods, and the removal of half-castes from reserves so that they might learn hygiene and receive a basic education.

The ethnographic concerns of Howitt and Spencer signaled a growing interest in recording Aboriginal social organization and cultural forms, with speculation on racial identity relegated to remarks in introductory or closing chapters, or to occasional addresses to learned societies. Physical investigation did not cease, but as the methods of race determination grew more sophisticated, medical supervision was more often required, and it was becoming difficult to replicate these increasingly complex procedures in the messy conditions of outback fieldwork. And yet if the laboratory was not easily delivered to the field, the field might be brought to the laboratory. From the late nineteenth century through to the 1920s, morphological studies generally took place in anatomy departments or in surgical institutes. In the 1870s, Paul Topinard and Armand de Quatrefages had measured Aboriginal skulls in Paris, and they found them homogeneously dolichocephalic, or long-headed, thus implying a distinct racial identity, even if its origins remained obscure.[52] In Edinburgh, William Turner reported on the metric characters of thirty-five skulls and confirmed their unitary classification.[53] Hermann Klaatsch, an anthropologist from Germany, examined a further eighty-seven skulls from a Queensland collection and again determined that Aboriginal Australians were a homogeneous group of dolicho-cephalics.[54] In 1910, R.J.A. Berry, the Melbourne anatomist, measured the bones and the calvaria of eighty-six Tasmanians, 100 Aboriginal Australians, and 191 Papuans, finding that all were dolichocephalic, especially the Australians. But then Berry, who had learned his anatomy from Turner, noticed a gradient of "purity," with the Tasmanians most homogeneous, the Australians intermediate, and the Papuans least so. He ventured the rather unorthodox opinion that the Australians might represent a "dual type."[55] But it was not until the Adelaide expeditions of the 1920s that these and other complex medical procedures could be taken back into the field and tested on living subjects.

At the end of World War I, Australia was a thoroughly Caucasian nation, even if much of the type was archaic, dark, and passing away—and thus forever, it seemed, deferred from modernity. It is striking to observe the extent to which Aborigines had been given precise, antique, typological anatomies, whereas their physiology and pathology, their bodily function and possible malfunction, were sketched only in very broad outline. Evidently archaic Caucasians would wither upon contact with their civilized brethren, but what was the pathophysiological mechanism of this antipathy? The doctors who were drawn to Aboriginal studies had generally been more interested in discerning racial type and tracing human genealogies than in conducting research on the normal and abnormal functioning of Aboriginal bodies. The epidemiology of Aboriginal "extinction" was hardly known. Instead, scientists and amateur naturalists had unintentionally produced a displaced, allegorical account of white racial history in Australia. The parallels are now obvious, but they went unremarked at the time. Caucasians had invaded the continent once before. They had eliminated the original inhabitants—or had they absorbed them? They were a pure race— or were they perhaps secretly hybrid? The anxieties of European Australians about their own racial purity and racial destiny were thus projected onto earlier Australians; Aborigines provided a background for scientific speculation on whether antipodean whiteness would remain unitary or become multiple and what the consequences might be. Just as European safety had demanded isolation from Asians, so too did Aboriginal survival appear to depend on the erection of barriers between indigenous people and the most recent invaders. It was the old logic of quarantine. Some scientists called for what was, in effect, a "dark Caucasian" policy within a white Australia policy; others simply accepted the tragic consequences of promiscuous and unregulated contact with a fatalism they would never countenance were European existence at stake.

Traveling through the continent's "Dead Heart" at the beginning of the twentieth century, J. W. Gregory was favorably impressed with the local Aborigines. "Instead of finding them degraded, lazy, selfish, savage, they were courteous and intelligent, generous even to the point of imprudence, and phenomenally honest; while in the field they proved to be born naturalists and superb bushmen." Gregory was thus convinced of their racial purity. "The Australian has some of the characteristics of the Negro; but he appears to me to be essentially Caucasian," he surmised. "He has the kind-heartedness of the Negro, with the capacity for dignity and self-respect of the Caucasian."[56] These Caucasian Aborigines were certainly more honest than "Negros and Asiatics," but they were lazy and not quite as truthful as "the Teutonic race." To the geologist's "trained eye," Aboriginal man resembled "an intelligent but untrained European." Even though his colleague Berry was demonstrating their small cranial capacity, Gregory believed that "given a fair chance, kind treatment, and a suitable education, the Australian Aborigine will develop into an intelligent, industrious and careful member of society."[57] But he conceded that this was idle speculation, as it was certain that the race would be extinct before such progress could take place. Contact with advanced Caucasians was proving terminal. The Dead Heart would soon be suffused with modern European blood. "The sight of white men engaged in severe manual labour, under the midday sun in the hot climate of the Lake Eyre depression, certainly suggested that a 'white Australia' is no impossible ideal even in the hottest regions of the Centre."[58]

A decade after Gregory's visit, Elsie Masson was keeping house for Baldwin Spencer in Darwin. Soon to elope with the anthropologist Bronislaw Malinowski, Masson began to ask "how may this vast land be civilised and settled, how may its wealth be exploited, keeping it at the same time a white man's country?" Like Spencer, Masson believed that the eventual extinction of the natives would, lamentably, greatly simplify the problem:

> White man's drink, white man's diseases, neither of which he has the stamina to withstand, have already begun their work of degeneration. It seems as if Nature were determined that the race, which has not toiled by slow ways to civilisation, made mistakes, given sacrifices, shall not be fit to accept its benefits and shall only perish by it.

Spencer was trying to use his knowledge of evolutionary anthropology to bridge primitivism and civilization, but Masson feared it might be too late. "At the best it can only be an imitation of civilisation, but, if the Aboriginal race can survive for two or three generations, its savage instincts may be replaced by those of a civilised community."[59]

NOMADIC CAUCASIANS AND WHITE CIVILIZATION

Into the 1920s, most scientists and general observers loosely followed an evolutionary logic that implied that Aboriginal Australians represented a Caucasian past that was withering away on contact with the civilized Caucasian future. Although a few experts still discerned some Negroid elements in the Aboriginal body, most physical anthropologists were more impressed with indigenous homogeneity and purity. Only the sentimentalists among them believed that the archaic Caucasians had a future. Before the full-blood Aborigines—the "uncontaminated tribes"—passed away, physical anthropologists would try to document their morphological and physiological features, and social anthropologists would seek out explanations of kinship structures and cultural patterns.

During the 1920s, medical scientists from Adelaide began regularly to visit the central deserts with measuring devices and physiological apparatus in an attempt to determine the structure and function of Aboriginal bodies in the wild. They were applying the medical techniques that Townsville scientists had used a decade or so earlier to test poor white subjects. Such modern practices tend eventually to create modern bodies. The Aborigines they studied functioned, or malfunctioned, contemporaneously, not in a distant racial past. Gradually, then, as evolutionary logic gave way to functionalist methods and assumptions, archaic Caucasians were refigured in medical texts as merely dark Caucasians, coexistent in all senses with white Caucasians. Of course, in entering the present, Aborigines did not necessarily gain a future, but their tragic destiny was more often (though not always) attributed to the predictable consequences of mundane contact with disease organisms, less often to some mystical antipathy of primitive and civilized or of archaic and modern. Scientists, such as W. Ramsay Smith and Wood Jones at Adelaide, might still refer to evolutionary terms and schema, but their assumptions were nuanced by a context quite different from any that Howitt or Spencer might recognize. In becoming contiguous, persistent, and functional, Aboriginality had become a modern problem, not just an antiquarian interest. Studies of Aboriginal Australians in the nineteenth century had produced a monitory antithesis—primitive against civilized—resolvable in racial struggle; but further scientific research was inadvertently regenerating Aboriginal identity as an antinomial motif within modernity, giving it a persistently ambivalent status that ultimately would prove unresolvable.[60]

Adelaide, the capital of South Australia, was the organizing center for the biological study of Aboriginal Australians for most of the twentieth century. Founded in 1836 by ambitious middle-class Nonconformists and Dissenters, apostles of enlightenment and progress, the colony boasted that it had avoided any convict stain. An advanced democratic society, it also valued respectability and good works. Revealing every summer its arid circumstances, Adelaide was nonetheless a carefully planned and well-built, solid city. The wealthier members of the small community generously supported worthy and improving institutions such as an art gallery, a museum, and a university.[61] By 1885 the university had established a small medical school, a rival to long-established Melbourne and to the recently opened Sydney school. The Adelaide medical school was located close to the museum, and the two institutions would work together on the investigation of Aboriginal people in South Australia and the Northern Territory, which was controlled from Adelaide until 1911.[62] The Adelaide investigators chose a subject that, with few exceptions, had elicited little interest from their medical colleagues in Melbourne and Sydney, and they brought to their project some unusual assumptions and methods.

Ramsay Smith, head of the health department for South Australia, was one of the Adelaide doctors and scientists who sought to test their theories of heredity and adaptation among the Aborigines of the nearby central deserts. Initially he was spurred on solely by evolutionary zeal. Nature had "side-tracked" a people in Australia, a group of research subjects that might supply anthropologists "with data regarding the bodily variations occurring in primitive races, and the place and the value of variations in estimating the zoological stratum or horizon to which races belong."[63] Later, in the 1920s, during his wanderings in central Australia, Smith insisted that "the more we know of the blackfellow, the more we are convinced that there are whole subterranean rivers of anthropology unmapped and untapped."[64] Some of these depths would continue to reveal evolutionary patterns. Which characters, for example, mark primitiveness?

Which features indicate a departure from primitive conditions? Smith accepted that "the Aboriginals are a homogeneous race, unmixed in descent, of Caucasian stock, not Negro or Negrito . . . a primitive race, a relic of the oldest human stock." But Smith had begun to recognize that Aborigines, even "tribal full-bloods," had to function, for a time, in a modern world. He was convinced that a change in the environment might change the ancestral type, perhaps to a degree unrecognizable. He found the indigenous inhabitants "observant, self-reliant and quick" in native conditions, but as yet "civilised man knows little regarding the possibilities of the mind of his uncivilised brother."[65] Here, then, was a being that was more than a mere evolutionary remnant.

In the early twentieth century, Edward C. Stirling, dean of the Adelaide medical school and director of the South Australian Museum, also had nurtured local interest in physical anthropology. Having absorbed evolutionary theory at Cambridge, Stirling traveled in 1892 as an ethnologist with Baldwin Spencer and Francis Gillen on the Horn Expedition and later documented the remains of the Swanport burials.[66] At the museum, he encouraged a rising generation of medical doctors and scientists to study the physical anthropology of the Aborigines; his associates and successors included John Burton Cleland, Robert Pulleine, Frederic Wood Jones, and Thomas Draper Campbell.[67] They committed themselves to an investigation of the racial origins of the Aborigines, using the methods of anatomy, physiology, and, later, hematology. In general, the medical scientists believed the race to be homogeneously Caucasian, though a later generation in Adelaide, including N. B. Tindale and F. J. Fenner, would rework theories of a hybrid constitution. Most members of this intellectual community shared a high estimate of the impact of the environment on the human organism; in the view of the Melbourne medical faculty, a few had even drifted into Lamarckism.[68] Conventionally, all of the early Adelaide anthropologists assumed that culture, or the capacity for civilization, followed race, but the hereditary categories that seemed so influential were for them quite soft and flexible.

In 1926, in his presidential address to the anthropology section of the Australasian Association for the Advancement of Science, Frederic Wood Jones accused white Australians of neglecting "the study of the Aborigine from the purely scientific point of view." "Although a great deal has been written concerning the ceremonials and tribal organization of the Australian native," the Adelaide anatomist continued, "we are still profoundly ignorant concerning him as a distinctive psychical and physical type." Masses of "superficial details" had thus obscured the fundamentals of biology and psychology. While at Adelaide between 1920 and 1926, Wood Jones led a group of medical scientists in their efforts to redress such "basal ignorance."[69] With T. D. Campbell from the dental school, he had conducted anthropometric investigations of South

Australian full-bloods, "the most rapidly vanishing section of a dying race," and determined, yet again, that they were dolichocephalic, platyrhinic (or broad-nosed), with long legs and forearms.[70] Every year the Adelaide teams went back to the deserts to record from other "tribes," concentrating on defining typical physical features but also making perfunctory attempts to document local customs, songs, and technologies. They had no trouble finding research subjects. In studies of the outback Aborigine, "a pure stock with well-defined and constant physical characteristics," Campbell and his colleagues reported that "judicious bribery will generally overcome any scruples about being examined."[71] At the end of the 1920s, physiologists began to accompany the anatomists, taking blood and conducting experiments to establish baselines of Aboriginal bodily activity.[72] In 1936, Campbell and his colleagues were able to summarize their anatomical findings. They had found no "intraracial differentiation": The typical Aborigine was dolichocephalic, broad-nosed, and "compared with European standards . . . his thigh and lower limb are thin, his trunk is short, and his shoulders and trunk are narrow." Hair was thick and wavy, covering the body; in females, hair was "more strictly confined to the external surface of the labia majora and only slight in amount over the mons pubis"; breasts were "pendulous"; and ear lobes were distinctive.[73] Obesity was rare, but they found no evidence of dietary deficiencies.[74]

It may seem paradoxical that Wood Jones's deep sympathy for the plight of Aborigines was predicated on his efforts to objectify their bodies. But anthropometry had demonstrated that the "uncontaminated" nomads were fine physical specimens, Caucasian in type and not degenerate. When settlers extended to these people "the crudities of living that in the circumstances have passed for the white man's civilisation," the results were deplorable.[75] The fragility of the Aboriginal bodies that modernity was giving form reproved their author. "We have taken his lands," Wood Jones declared, "we have used his hunting grounds as pastures for sheep and cattle, we have dispossessed him, we have doomed him to a lingering but certain death wherever we have come into any prolonged contact with him." Because "entry into white civilisation and continued existence are incompatible where the Aborigine is concerned," Wood Jones recommended an expansion of reservations and yet more scientific investigation. He condemned missionary and state efforts to civilize the natives:

> They wear the white man's clothes, but know not of his hygiene—even that terribly rudimentary form of it met with in outback life. They lose interest in their racial and tribal activities and become apathetic and idle. In the vast majority of cases they become degenerate hangers-on to the fringe of civilisation, neglecting the best of their own activities and adopting the worst of the defects of that mode of life frequent among men in out-stations.[76]

Wood Jones discerned that the nomads—as he thought of them—were following an alternative and, in some senses, superior Caucasian destiny in the deserts. Aboriginal embodiment had more than mere evolutionary significance. The persistence of full-blood independence, virility, and sensuality presented a telling contrast to the degeneracy of the colonial variant of white civilization.

In 1934, Wood Jones, by then an unhappy professor of anatomy at Melbourne, gave a series of passionate talks on the radio about Australia's vanishing race. While the majority of white inhabitants of the continent still seemed to regard "the Aborigine merely as some sort of lowly black man who happened to be in Australia when the conquering race came with its enlightened civilisation," science now suggested otherwise. Most importantly, the Aboriginal "is a pigmented member of the human family; but he is no Negro."[77] Indeed, blood tests implied a Mediterranean origin. Wood Jones pointed out that his skin is brown, with a velvety texture; his hair is wavy, and often quite light; his eyes are large and dark, with overhanging brows; his nose is broad; and his hands show "fine-shaping and beautiful proportions." Although Berry, his predecessor at Melbourne, had documented the small head of the Aboriginal, Wood Jones disputed any links between cranial capacity and intelligence. "Physically and physiologically he is of our family—an older branch it is true, and one that left the ancestral homeland long before we did."[78] White Australians had much to learn from their dark brethren. The uncontaminated Aboriginal, Wood Jones pointed out, "has elaborated an extraordinarily complicated, but highly efficient, social code for the regulation of the moral and physical welfare of his communities." Complicated kinship rules "safeguard the eugenic welfare of the race." It was imperative to preserve this paragon "from contamination by the establishment of inviolate reserves for his sole occupation."[79]

For Wood Jones, the romance of the dark Caucasian nomad suggested a lingering alternative racial destiny, one that would not only reveal the degeneracy of white civilization but might also provide an example of an ethical relationship with place. In the nineteenth century, Brough Smyth and others had taken Aboriginal decline as an opportunity to denounce the nastier features of colonial culture, but they resigned themselves to the evolutionary mechanism that determined this tragic fate, and they rarely, if ever, regarded Aboriginal patterns of existence as models for modern life. Wood Jones, however, hoped, rather forlornly, to preserve uncontaminated Aboriginal society, and he even implied that an injection of some elements of "primitive ethics" into modernity might do some good. The scientist wanted to isolate full-bloods in ethnic enclaves, not to consign them to an ethnological museum; he wanted to keep them available to the present, not seal them in the past.

But a younger generation of Adelaide scientists had mixed feelings about the feasibility of such separate development. For them, full-bloods remained valuable objects of investigation, but by the late 1930s the rising generation of Adelaide scientists were more inclined to recognize only two possible destinies: extinction, or a thorough biological and cultural absorption into white Australia. And if unscientific racial prejudice were to prevent full-blood assimilation, the path might yet be cleared for half-castes.

DARK CAUCASIANS IN THE MODERN NATION

During the 1930s, the Board of Anthropological Research of the University of Adelaide sponsored repeated scientific studies of the bodies of Aboriginal Australians. Adelaide medical scientists had established the board with the hope that it would attract some support for their research from the Rockefeller Foundation. In 1923, representatives of the Galton Society of New York had approached the foundation to suggest an intensive study of Aboriginal tribes in north and west Australia. It seemed that full-bloods, before they passed away, offered an unrivaled opportunity to study processes of natural selection among peoples in a primitive state.[80] C. B. Davenport, the head of Eugenics Record Office at Cold Spring Harbor, wrote urging a comparison of the anatomical structures of the primitive race with those of Europeans and anthropoid apes. He was interested also in comparative studies in physiology, hematology, and pathology; and he hoped for an answer to the question of "how far the lowest race is capable of intellectual development." Davenport had a grand vision. "Besides a surgeon, a pathologist and a serologist there would be needed for longer or shorter periods an anthropologist, an anatomist, an embryologist, an endocrinologist, a psychologist, a student of comparative culture and others."[81] The Rockefeller trustees decided to consult with Grafton Elliot Smith, an Australian physical anthropologist and a leading promoter of notions of cultural diffusion, who was based in London. Smith toured Australia to determine the best site for Rockefeller investment. He narrowed the choice to Sydney, with its access to the Pacific, and to Adelaide, where his former student, Wood Jones, had already built a program in physical anthropology. Smith eventually recommended the establishment of a chair in anthropology at Sydney.[82] Following the appointment in 1926 of A. R. Radcliffe-Brown, the new department focused its research on social anthropology, contrary to the initial request of the Galton Society for eugenic studies. But some Rockefeller money was reserved primarily for support of the Adelaide work in physical anthropology, and it is extraordinary just how closely the Adelaide medicos later would follow Davenport's advice.[83]

John Burton Cleland, the professor of pathology at the medical school, was the most committed advocate of assimilation at Adelaide. An industrious amateur botanist and ornithologist, Cleland had trained in medicine at Adelaide and Sydney. He then worked for a time as a bacteriologist in Western Australia and New South Wales, where he established that local outbreaks of dengue were spread by *Aedes aegypti*, before moving back to Adelaide in 1920.[84] Throughout his career, Cleland demonstrated an interest in physical anthropology and, more generally, a propensity to speculate on mechanisms of heredity and adaptation. While in Perth, he had challenged August Weissmann's claim that the individual "is merely a protecting and nourishing envelope for the continuity of the germ plasm for all time," suggesting instead that the environment might transmit characters to the germ cells through the influence of recently discovered hormones.[85] Cleland later came to believe that individuals possess hidden hereditary potential that awaited a means of expression, a capacity that a stimulating environment might yet call forth.[86] In his anthropological work, conducted with Wood Jones and Campbell, Cleland hoped to gauge the hidden potential of Aborigines, to investigate below the surface, exploring the physiological and genetic interior. While the anatomists still used bones and teeth to reveal patterns of heredity and adaptation, Cleland and other physiologists would study laboratory markers of descent and function. But there was little time left. "The pure-blooded Australian Aborigine is fast dying out," Cleland wrote. "Already over very large areas in the settled parts he has entirely disappeared. With the march of civilisation only a few years will see, in all probability, the complete disappearance of pure-blooded natives."[87]

Cleland became the chief blood grouper of the Board of Anthropological Research in Adelaide. In the late 1920s, he accompanied a number of expeditions to central Australia, bleeding full-bloods and botanizing along the way.[88] For almost twenty years it had been accepted that the patterns of agglutination determining the major human blood groups (A, B, and O) remained constant throughout life and were inherited according to Mendelian principles, that is, according to whether the factor giving rise to a character was dominant or recessive. During World War I, the Hirszfelds had made thousands of investigations on men of different races in Serbia, demonstrating that the A factor was more common in the inhabitants of northeastern Europe and diminished in the southeast; the B factor was more frequent among those from Asia. They called the distribution of the ratio of A to B the biochemical index and claimed that the wandering and intermingling of races accounted for its variation.[89] In 1923, A. H. Tebbutt reported that a survey of almost 200 Aborigines in southern Queensland showed an extremely low frequency of the B factor; a few years later, D.H.K. Lee, as a young doctor briefly attached to the Australian Institute of Tropical Medicine, found that few of the 377 Aborigines whom he bled on

Palm Island belonged to group B.[90] In 1926, Cleland took blood from 158 Aborigines in central Australia and discovered no B factor at all. Although he conceded that "blood-grouping fails to provide an infallible test of race," he remained convinced that "the ease with which it yields measurable results, the precision of its applications, the definite inheritance of the factors concerned, furnish it with advantages that no other anthropological method possesses."[91] When precautions were taken to exclude persons of mixed origin, blood grouping demonstrated that Aborigines contained no B factor. But Cleland, perhaps with some irony, warned that "because the rather pathetic sub-man of Australia has a high frequency of the A factor, we need not suppose that it implies a close affinity with the Nordic superman who also possesses a high frequency of A." Blood grouping was just one of the many anthropological features worth considering in defining race. Certainly it implied that Aborigines were descended from very few ancestors and had remained a homogeneous population. It might also suggest that Australians were unlikely to be descended from Asians and Africans, but it would never "automatically by itself mint out the races of man."[92]

Cleland never tired of bleeding Aborigines as he traveled, even though the agglutination results soon became predictable. In 1929, at Hermannsburg mission—three days by fast camel west of Alice Springs—he took blood from seventy-one "Arunta" and "Loritcha" men, accidentally including one "half-caste." The authorities made sure there was no difficulty in carrying out the tests, and Cleland remarked that "we have never met with any opposition or any suspicions as to our intentions, in striking contrast to the experiences of others with some primitive peoples." All the same, in puncturing the ear lobe to obtain blood, the anthropologists "soon gained the sobriquet of 'the butchers' from the surrounding Aborigines, and our mild form of operation was designated, in cattle terms, as 'ear-marking.'"[93] Not surprisingly, Cleland found that most of the ear-marked full-bloods at Hermannsburg belonged to group A, with some in group O and none in group B. In 1933, Cleland joined an expedition that the Board of Anthropological Research sent out to Ernabella in the northwest of South Australia. Work began as soon as the party arrived "as previous experience had taught that our Aborigines, while enjoying the novelty at first, soon tire of intensive work; difficulty is experienced in holding them, as is necessary for such investigations, for more than about ten days." The team performed routine anthropometric measurements, blood grouping, and photography; collected genealogical information; and made a series of films and records. When Cleland tested the blood of sixty-four "natives," he again found no Asian B.[94]

Despite his interest in stable hereditary markers, Cleland still believed that the harsh desert environment had directly shaped Aboriginal physiology. Whereas the more advanced Europeans "controlled their surroundings by clearing forest lands and planting crops, by growing fruit trees and vegetables and domesticating wild animals," Aborigines had relied on a physiological adaptation to their harsh surroundings. Cleland based his remarks on the physiological work of his colleague, Cedric Stanton Hicks, who had proven over many years that "the Aboriginal has an extremely active control over the blood circulation in his skin."[95] A New Zealander, Hicks had been appointed in physiology at the University of Adelaide in 1926, having completed a Ph.D. at Cambridge on the function of the thyroid gland. In England, Howard Florey had warned him that he was going to "an intellectual desert," but on his arrival in Adelaide Hicks soon came into the academic orbit of Wood Jones, "then 47 years of age, black haired, keen eyed, with a handsome face and a perceptive, philosophical mind."[96] At Cambridge, Hicks's studies had stimulated an interest in metabolism, and during the late 1920s and the 1930s the young scientist and his Adelaide colleagues traveled frequently into central Australia to investigate Aboriginal physiology. With the support of the Carnegie Corporation and Rockefeller Foundation, Hicks found a place in the expanding Adelaide research expeditions, performing elaborate experiments in the desert in order to ascertain racial differences in basal metabolism. He had found not an intellectual desert so much as a desert for intellectuals.

But on his first trip to Koonibba mission station, Hicks was dismayed to find that the remnants of the "Kokata tribe" were no more than "pathetic and unattractive imitations of Europeans." To obtain accurate recordings of the basal metabolic rate, Hicks required his experimental subjects to lie still and relaxed for hours, with their noses clamped, and breathing through a rubber mouthpiece attached to a large and complex apparatus. At Koonibba, the local people were "venal and evasive, and it was no simple matter to get cooperation."[97] The chief difficulty, Hicks reported, "lay in occluding the nostrils, which were not only large and widely spaced, but in many instances strengthened by extraordinarily firm cartilages. In these cases an assistant closed the airway by hand."[98] The flies were bad, and it was hard to get native subjects to lie still for long. A twenty-three-year-old woman was "very nervous"; another was "apprehensive"; a thirty-five-year-old man was "amiably stubborn"; a nine-year-old boy was a "troublesome subject . . . a peculiar ape-like type." Hicks's notes are revealing: "subject became disturbed"; "stoicism amazing"; "many attempts on this big powerful native." But on occasions all went well: Another nine-year-old boy, for example, proved a "very good subject—lay like a corpse."[99] The experiments provided enough information for a scientific paper, but Hicks later had to retract the conclusions.[100]

In 1931, when Hicks visited Cockatoo Creek, north of Alice Springs, with his Adelaide colleagues, he came to admire the "wild, nomad Aborigines," who were "so intelligent, so courteous and good natured, and so willing and interested in cooperating in our experiments despite all the associated discomfort and restraint."[101] They were different from the detribalized Kokata with whom he had contended a few years earlier. (All the same, he soon realized that it was prudent to restrict his studies to males and not to try to take rectal temperatures.) Initially Hicks had been unsure if they would be any more cooperative than the Kokata. On arrival, he explained that he was a medicine man and that the rituals he performed would "greatly improve their wind." The next morning, "we plodded, muttering forebodings, through the mulga to our unpredictable, paleolithic objective"; and they found, to their astonishment, that the "natives" were waiting for them. "These fellows were magnificent, and the Koonibba experience by comparison, was nightmare evidence of decadence of a noble race under the influence of western civilisation." Hicks and his assistants conducted thirty-three experiments on twenty Aborigines and established that the Aboriginal metabolic rate was the same as the rate determined by W. A. Osborne, Henry Priestley, and others for Europeans in Australia. Using a different methodology, Hicks thus confirmed the conclusions of Cleland's blood group studies, demonstrating that "the Aborigines are, in fact, archaic Europeans."[102] And yet, as Hicks observed, "no white subjects could, or would, have behaved as such perfect experimental animals."[103]

Hicks was puzzled that Aborigines lying unclothed on cold desert mornings could still give such normal European values. In the late 1930s at Ernabella waterhole, 250 miles from Oodnadatta, Hicks and his team of physiologists returned to the desert to study the reactions of whites and Aborigines to cooling the skin. (Hicks still found it "amazing that it is possible to place a mouthpiece in a subject's mouth and carry out a metabolism estimation with no other explanation than can be given by dumb-show.")[104] Two tents were pitched side by side, and in one of them a physiologist lay naked on the ground and in the other an Aboriginal male did the same. The investigators found that the nomads of the desert possessed far greater powers of peripheral vasoconstriction (the ability to reduce the blood supply to the skin to reduce heat loss). As conditions became cooler, the Aboriginal subjects limited their skin circulation long before whites did. Hicks believed that this ability was a "biological adaptation," one that whites living in the bush—even a physiologist if given enough time—might also learn.[105]

Although Adelaide scientists found repeatedly that nomadic Aborigines conformed to European norms, physiological expeditions sent out from Sydney were observing regular, and apparently genetically fixed, deficits. When Henry Priestley left the Australian Institute of Tropical Medicine and moved to the University of Sydney, he extended his research interests in white physiology in the tropics to encompass nutritional studies in southern Australia.[106] With the assistance of the Rockefeller Foundation, he built up the physiology department, recruiting staff with a strong research record, including H. Whitridge Davies and H. S. Halcro Wardlaw.[107] After investigating their students in order to establish white norms for basal metabolism, Wardlaw and his colleagues went bush in the 1920s to get comparable Aboriginal figures. The Sydney researchers assumed that metabolism was racially determined and inherited as a more or less fixed package. Like most of the Melbourne scientists, they believed in a harder heredity than their Adelaide counterparts, and they were more inclined to look for racial differences than for similarities. For Wardlaw, the study of "racial factors in determining the level of basal metabolism" was a broad enterprise, because even "diet and general conditions of life are themselves, to some extent, racial characteristics."

In 1928, at the Aboriginal reserve at Runnymede, Wardlaw investigated full-bloods "living under civilised conditions," a group of people who spent much of their time "lounging about or sleeping." He recorded their pulse rate, temperature, and respiratory rate, and he collected the air they breathed out. He found that their basal metabolism was only 80 percent of "normal" white values but observed that "admixture of approximately 50 per cent of white blood brings that basal metabolism up to that of full-blood whites examined locally."[108] White blood evidently was genetically more industrious, but black blood did seem to signal better adaptation to local conditions. In 1934, Wardlaw and his colleagues compared the metabolic rates of ten "Aranda" and "Aluritja" men with four local whites and reported that white metabolism varied little between the center and Sydney, but native metabolism again was only 80 percent of the white standard. Aborigines proved better adapted to desert conditions, for when they lay naked under the sun they were able to lose more heat through perspiration than the white subjects. But as soon as they put on clothes and became semicivilized, this natural advantage evaporated.[109] The next year, at Hermannsburg, the Sydney physiologists determined that, after exercise in hot conditions, Aboriginal haemoglobin concentrations had increased less than their own. They therefore concluded that Aboriginal blood was thinner, less energetic, but preadapted to desert life.[110]

Although Adelaide and Sydney scientists may have disagreed on the extent of Aboriginal physiological difference, and disputed the relative contributions of environment and genetics to producing difference, they still shared many assumptions. The full-blood Aboriginal body that emerged from medical research in Adelaide and Sydney was a Caucasian variant, sometimes hybrid but more commonly homogeneous; naturally a nomad but frequently a dweller on urban fringes and therefore degenerate; primitive and childlike but possessing an indefinite capacity for advancement or assimilation. The question that exercised the minds of many of medical scientists between the wars was how biosocial processes of Aboriginal absorption might be managed scientifically. For

Wood Jones, it was necessary to delay or to circumvent Aboriginal "contamination"; but Ramsay Smith and Cleland usually recommended that the government hasten absorption and begin the "civilizing" even of full-bloods. Although most scientists agreed that Aborigines could be civilized, some doubted whether they should be forced to endure the process. Even Cleland could be equivocal. As a member of the Aborigines' Protection Board, he frequently visited "native institutions." In 1940, he reported that "natives cannot be expected to become good citizens if their upbringing is bad (e.g. camp natives, vicious or immoral parents)." Making no distinction between full-bloods and half-castes, he demanded that "children must be removed from their parents under such circumstances" and placed with white foster parents or in a home.[111] But on other occasions Cleland urged the establishment of reservations to delay "detribalization." In 1946, he reported from Woomera that:

> My Board is of the opinion that the intermixing of tribalised natives with white people inevitably leads to de-tribalisation. With de-tribalisation loss of interest in life occurs and the natives just cease to exist. Half-castes arise. As many of these are difficult to fit into the general community a number of them become a burden on the state.[112]

More often, Cleland argued that Aborigines were a people "we could absorb by marriage without fear of introducing a low type of mentality." Therefore, it was important to allow all white children and all Aboriginal children to mix and receive the same education; whenever possible, Aboriginal children should have white foster parents or guardians. "Brought up like this in a pure white community from a very young age," he wrote in the late 1950s, "all that nature can do will be done."[113] He looked forward to the day when "in generations far distant nearly every inhabitant of Australia will have had an Aboriginal ancestor." In order that this might occur, "it is the duty of the white population as a whole . . . to improve these living conditions, to teach proper sanitary measures, to provide washing facilities and encourage their use, and gradually lead these at heart nice people into the ways of European civilisation."[114] This was not a destiny that Wood Jones would have recommended for his cherished nomads.

From Ancestral Forms to Dark Caucasian Children

The transition, incomplete as it was, from notions of the savage mind to assessments of Aboriginal mental age indicates perhaps most clearly the ambivalent incorporation of full-bloods into modern Australia. The evolutionary significance of "primitive" became muted in the 1930s, and the term was applied more often to contemporary social and psychological development than to racial history. As Ernestine Hill admitted in 1937, "The worst that might be said of [the Aboriginal] is that he is a child of his environment, but a normal child, not a backward one."[115]

R.J.A. Berry had been among the first scientists to try to provide an objective measure of Aboriginal intelligence. It was a manifestation of the last part of his serial conversion from an anatomist to a physical anthropologist to a mental specialist. Reflecting back on when he began measuring skulls before World War I, he recalled that "even in these early days it was the brain within the skull for which we were groping."[116] According to Berry, Aborigines were simply another group of small-headed people and therefore might be classed, along with white delinquents and criminals, among the feeble-minded. Berry had measured more than 9,000 heads in Victoria, Tasmania, and South Australia, including the heads of university students, schoolchildren, the poor, and some Aborigines. He employed a young teacher, Stanley Porteus, to perform psychological tests on 100 who were below the 10th percentile of head circumference and another 100 who were above the 90th percentile. Those with larger heads on average did better on the Stanford-Binet intelligence test and on the new maze test that Porteus had designed. The average Aboriginal head was the same size as the head of the average thirteen-year-old white schoolboy, an average exceeded by 90 percent of adult whites.[117] But for Berry the racial element was insignificant. "The truth is," he lamented, "that about one in every ten of the population whom you meet in your daily pursuits has the physical and sexual passions of the adult with the brain control of an underdeveloped child." Berry dedicated the rest of his life to combating the generic "menace of the feeble-minded."[118]

Stanley Porteus, Berry's earnest young collaborator, had grown up in rural Victoria and trained as a teacher. As a keen bushwalker and enthusiastic football player—in his youth he frequently played against the Aboriginal team at Coranderrk and found "their running, kicking and handling of the ball were remarkably good"—Porteus was well prepared for his later fieldwork. In the Victorian education department, Porteus had met Harvey Sutton, the school medical officer, who directed his attention to the problem of the feeble-minded. It seemed to Porteus that the new Stanford-Binet intelligence test depended too much on verbal skills, and a more basic test of initiative was required. While teaching retarded children in Melbourne, he developed a series of maze tests that he claimed would gauge planning capacity in a way that was not culturally biased. Berry, "who had become greatly interested—perhaps over-interested—in the possible relation between the size of the brain and intelligence," soon became equally interested in this "psychologist of sorts" and offered Porteus a job in his laboratory of educational anthropology.[119] Although Porteus, who had an embarrassingly small head, later tried to distance himself from Berry's obsessions with head size and the problem of the feeble-minded, there are few signs of disaffection before the late 1920s. It was only after Porteus, who had been appointed professor of psychology at the University of Hawaii, met Wood Jones, who was briefly professor of physical anthropology at the same institution, that the psychologist's rapport with Berry began to dissolve.[120]

In 1929, Porteus and Wood Jones worked together on a synthetic account of neuroanatomy and psychology, *The Matrix of the Mind*. In it they argued that "education or environment writes on each slate the lessons of social inheritance, but some slates are much better as writing materials than others." But Wood Jones, in particular, wanted to make it clear that "extravagant claims have been made concerning the importance of heredity." He also took the opportunity to challenge conventional views of primitive mentality. "Though primitive man possesses many . . . childish or moronic characteristics he acquires in addition other abilities quite beyond the range of capacity of any race." Recalling his experiences in the central deserts, Wood Jones wrote that the so-called primitive in his own environment "exhibits an acuity of judgement which is the wonder and envy of the civilised white man."[121] The anatomist was thus able to excite the psychologist's interest in these children of nature. Porteus decided to return to Australia and investigate the remaining uncontaminated full-bloods. "Given a racially homogeneous people with a whole continent to range over, and segregation from all other human contacts for an untold period of time, what, psychologically speaking, will they make of themselves?"[122]

Porteus set up his "laboratory" among the "Arunta" people, not far from where Géza Róheim was gathering psychoanalytic data and adjacent to T. D. Campbell and the Adelaide medicos who were performing physiological tests.[123] He wanted to discard entirely the old evolutionary hierarchies of Spencer and Gillen and instead focus on Aboriginal psychological adaptation to a harsh environment. The psychologist now denounced Berry for using his essays on Aboriginal skulls merely as occasions for racial disparagement. In the deserts, Porteus decided that the Aboriginals he met were good-humored, scrupulous, patient, and generous to the point of improvidence. Convinced that his maze tests revealed "the fundamental traits underlying social adaptability," he applied them as often as possible. In whites the maze tests had shown "a distinct correlation with industrial trainability"; among Aborigines they would indicate "planning capacity and prudence."[124] Porteus found that in general the maze performance of full-bloods was low—equivalent to twelve white years—but not markedly inferior to many other racial groups, and some individuals could achieve white adult levels of proficiency. The results demonstrated "the selective influence of environment and the apparent malleability of human nature." Aborigines were perfectly adapted to the Australian environment, but they would find civilization a challenge. Still, Porteus did wonder if further schooling or the "admixture of white blood" might yet assimilate them.[125]

In the late 1920s and early 1930s, Adelaide investigators also were demonstrating the equivalence of "primitive" mentality and modern child mentality. R. H. Pulleine, the professor of medicine at Adelaide, wanted "a just estimate of the ability of the Aborigine"—with his colleagues, he could not see the point of the term "primitive" and denied any correlation between head size and intelligence.[126] In 1930, they gave the full-bloods at Koonibba a complete physiological and psychological overhaul. The mean blood pressure and basal metabolic rate were slightly lower than white norms; but visual, auditory, and tactile acuities were at least equal to white standards. After further observations, Pulleine and his coworkers concluded that, though "the physiological levels of the Aborigine are much better or much like our own," their mental function seemed to lag behind European achievements. But Aborigines could cope with basic work, such as stock-riding, and they were "keen, skilful, and often successful" footballers, showing excellent team spirit.[127] At Hermannsburg mission, H. K. Fry, a lecturer in clinical medicine at the Adelaide medical school, tried to perform more sophisticated psychological tests, carefully modeling his work on the reports of W.H.R. Rivers and A. C. Haddon from the 1898 Torres Strait expedition.[128] But Fry found it difficult to get the "natives" to understand many of the tests, and they were quickly bored; the task of estimating intelligence bristled with difficulties. None of them understood the Stanford-Binet test; few persisted with the puzzles; and the maze-testing was marred by the experimenter's mistake in copying the maze test at the fourteen-year-old level. Fry suspected that the average adult Aborigine was as intelligent as a white schoolchild but could not prove it.[129]

In or around 1931, Aborigines, having gained childish ways, also became sensitive to pain, according to psychological testing. When Aborigines were regarded as nothing more than dwindling evolutionary remnants—true primitives—they appeared notoriously indifferent to suffering. Natalie Robarts had closely observed the natives at Coranderrk and knew that these "savage" people "do not suffer pain as acutely as do the higher races, their skin seems not so sensitive."[130] In 1914, Herbert Pitts, a missionary who had "taken up the white man's burden" in northwestern Australia, reported that Aborigines, having "a much less developed nervous system, feel pain to a much less extent than we do."[131] Scientists like Ronald Hamlyn-Harris, the director of the Queensland Museum, confirmed this useful Christian knowledge. In an address dedicated mostly to eugenic measures that might prevent the deterioration of the white race, Hamlyn-Harris observed in passing that full-blood Aborigines "express no symptoms of pain" but may become more tender according to the proportion of white blood.[132] In 1931, Fry and Pulleine, having heard repeatedly that Aborigines do not feel pain, tested the response to pressure on the nailbeds of rather surprised research subjects at Macdonald Downs. Their victims did seem a little less sensitive to pain than whites, but the deficiency was "not as marked as is commonly assumed."[133] At Hermannsburg, Fry set up an "algesimeter," a spring balance with a drawing pin placed point up on the pan of the scales. Although the Adelaide investigators, testing their own sensitivity, generally stopped pushing before sixteen ounces, when penetration of the skin occurred, the obliging native subjects often kept on going to twenty-eight ounces or more.[134] In 1931, Porteus suggested that the correct interpretation of such tests was not that Aborigines are relatively insensitive to pain but that they have developed a habitual indifference to discomfort. This was no racial characteristic but a pattern of behavior set "by the common reaction of his group."[135] Aborigines felt pain like whites; they burned like whites; they were just like whites in so many ways, only isolated in a harsh, unstimulating environment that demanded stoicism. Whites might even learn from them.

White Pathology and Culture Contact

Whatever their quibbles about race origins, all of the experts on Aboriginal Australians in the nineteenth century had deplored the ravages of disease and degeneration among the "poor creatures" they were studying. On making contact with white civilization—more specifically, with a low colonial variant of it—Aboriginal society appeared to wither, to become demoralized, and to pass away. James Barnard, the vice president of the Royal Society of Tasmania, observed in 1890 that "following the law of evolution and the survival of the fittest, the inferior races of mankind must give place to the highest type of man, and . . . this law is adequate to account for the gradual decline in numbers of the Aboriginal inhabitants of a country before the march of civilisation."[136] Until World War I, a tragic outcome was commonly attributed to the mystic discord of civilization and primitivism and thus elevated to the realm of the teleological. Once contact had occurred, primitives either died off or they attempted to conform to the civilizing process. Like all transitions in life, the passage from primitive to civilized was perilous, especially so if racial capabilities provided only a limited repertoire of adaptive functions. Among Europeans, the growth of a child into an adult represented a threat to constitutional order that, according to nineteenth-century medical theory, might shade into illness or at least render one more susceptible to disease. Similarly, the civilizing process might meet a biological impediment and stall, leaving erstwhile primitives into a state of constitutional disequilibrium and decline. It is true that even before the general acceptance of germ theories in the late nineteenth century, bodily contact had been implicated in the spread of a few diseases, particularly smallpox and venereal disease. But on the whole, Aboriginal sickness, like most sickness, had appeared more often to derive from a reactive constitutional frailty, a failure of a dynamic bodily system to cope with new demands. Thus we find before us the indigenous sufferer of diseases of civilization and semicivilization; this is the lamentable figure of the "dressed native."[137]

But after the 1890s, the mechanism of Aboriginal decline is more precisely, more technically, traced to the transmission of germs, often from one person to another, sometimes through food and water, occasionally involving insects and other unpleasant vectors. Gradually the diseases of civilization become diseases of contemporary culture contact, and then they are further normalized as diseases of mundane personal contact. A once-grand evolutionary schema thus turns into a rather banal calculus of individual risk. As usual, Baldwin Spencer is a revealing transitional figure; he is equivocal on the causes of degeneration, apparently unsure whether disease among Aborigines has arisen from contact with civilization or just from bodily contact. At one point he muses: "The rapidity with which a tribe undergoes degradation, as soon as it comes into contact with civilisation, is astonishing."[138] On another, earlier occasion, he has a more technical explanation: "No sooner do the natives come into contact with white men, than phthisis and other diseases soon make their appearance."[139] Although scientists come to favor a modern bacteriological exegesis of Aboriginal decline, vague gestures toward "civilization" do persist, partly out of habit and partly because it provided a default etiology that conveniently diffused human agency. Better that a natural or mystical process than a technical problem for which specific economic or social arrangements might be held responsible.

It is not surprising that the Adelaide scientists who had constructed modern anatomies, physiologies, and even psychologies for the full-bloods of the central deserts also managed to insert them into modern pathological processes. J. B. Cleland opened his major survey of diseases of Aboriginal Australia with a conventional gesture toward evolutionary exculpation. "With the march of civilisation," he wrote in 1928, "only a few years will see, in all probability, the complete disappearance of pure-blooded natives."[140] But in the rest of his paper, which stuttered over fifteen installments in the *Journal of Tropical Medicine and Hygiene*, mundane personal contact was gradually substituted for civilization in his description of disease causation. Admittedly, "the adoption of cast-off European clothing, often filthy, and worn perhaps day and night, not dried when wet, must handicap the native"; and "access to alcohol, contraction of venereal disease, and the indolence induced by the doles of European rations must also lead to an undermining of the constitution." But for Cleland, as for most contemporary medical doctors, transmission of the seeds of disease had become far more significant than any general receptivity of the soil. Specific immunities did matter, but the broad constitutional robustness of the race was a relatively minor influence on disease transmission and expression. Cleland explicitly discounted the importance of "reactions inherent upon some racial peculiarity."[141] Of course, contact with civilization was demoralizing for these people, but more telling and more tragic was their contact with disease-dealing poor white males.

To the new diseases they encountered, Aborigines reacted in much the same way as anyone else born of a previously isolated population. As many of them had not yet had the opportunity to develop a specific immunity to infections like tuberculosis and syphilis, the germs of these conditions propagated widely and made their victims sicker. Tuberculosis, smallpox, influenza, measles, and whooping cough were all widespread and devastating. But they represented the predictable biological consequences of personal contact between the immunologically competent and the immunologically naive and were thus potentially separable from white civilization.[142] (Indeed, the dangers to Aborigines from contact with whites had come to resemble the threat that Asians allegedly presented to whites, and no one thought the latter predicament arose from the superiority, or the sophistication, of Asian civilization.) Studies of Aboriginal bodies and societies might still provide an opportunity for Wood Jones and others to express their ambivalence toward white civilization, without necessarily according civilization anything more than a metaphoric, or incidental, role in disease causation. The only possible exceptions to this medical deflation of teleological explanation were cancer and metabolic diseases, which, according to Cleland, occurred mostly among those in a civilized or semicivilized condition. Even so, civilization was not directly to blame; it merely signified exposure "to sources of irritation similar to those to which Europeans are subjected."[143]

Cleland thought that Aboriginal Australians displayed a rather ordinary and boring pathology. "There were very few diseases which seem to be peculiar to the natives. . . . It seems probable that the native suffers from the same diseases as the white man and in general in much the same way." He was not surprised that "pathological reactions do not seem to be of much value in differentiating human races from each other."[144] Previous geographical isolation was the best explanation of the prevalence and severity of affliction. But even if Aboriginal decline could now be construed in mundane and modern terms, it remained devastating. Most experts still predicted a tragic outcome. What, then, was to be done? As we have seen, a few experts, often those who were more sentimental, or perhaps more disgruntled with colonial modernity, emphasized above all the creation of special reserves for full-bloods. Given a reprieve, possibly no more than a brief one, these isolated Aboriginal Australians would have an ambivalent status within modern Australia. More commonly, scientists urged policymakers to hasten the absorption of dark Caucasians into a standard white modernity; if whites still refused to merge with full-bloods, some of them might consider blending with half-castes. It seemed that further racial absorption, with attendant cultural assimilation, might eventually solve the public health problem. Of course, a combination of full-blood isolation and half-caste absorption, as Cleland suggested, would prove very attractive. But in practice, as Cleland's own career demonstrates, one policy was generally favored over the other. By the end of the 1930s, it was half-caste absorption that most concentrated the minds of medical scientists.[145]

Considering the relentless pathologizing of Asians, it is perhaps surprising just how little pathogenicity was attributed to Aborigines. Cleland stated that Aborigines were definitely not a reservoir of infectious diseases for whites. The nastier tropical infections, such as malaria, were rare, probably because Aboriginal populations were mostly dispersed. Tuberculosis and syphilis prevailed, but any whites close enough to be at risk were either inured to these diseases, or suffered from them already, or would contract them only if they were mixing far too promiscuously with fringe-dwellers. Leprosy was becoming more common, but most Aboriginal suspects were isolated in the new leprosaria cropping up across the north. Conventionally, Aborigines appeared as natural, pathetic, and ignorant victims of the diseases they contracted through mixing with whites; they were not typically a disease threat to Europeans.[146]

But not every medical scientist was so ready to disarm Aborigines. Raphael Cilento, the country's leading tropical health specialist, continued to hope that they might represent the dangerous "native reservoir of disease" that he so longed to find. Hookworm was rife among the Aborigines clustered in the Queensland reserves, and Cilento, as we have seen, suspected that the germs of laziness were spilling out into surrounding white communities.[147] In 1931, Cilento asserted that Aboriginal populations in the tropics "represent foci for the dissemination of hookworm, malaria and other diseases"; in 1934, he reported that leprosy follows "very roughly with the degree of prevalence of coloured persons in the population."[148] Cilento thus recommended the segregation and medical policing of Aboriginal communities, more as a strategy to protect vulnerable whites than as a means of promoting indigenous health. A few other medicos concurred with Cilento's views on the pathological potential of Aboriginal communities but recommended, in place of segregation and policing, a cleansing assimilation into white communities. Thus C. E. Cook, the protector of Aborigines in the Northern Territory and later commissioner of public health in Western Australia, warned that:

The pernicious influences which the coloured races exercise upon the hygienic, social and economic development of areas where white settlement is sparse, and upon the public health where hybrid remnants concentrate in the poorer quarters of cities or on the fringes of country towns, continue for the most part unsuspected.[149]

In the 1920s, under the influence of Cilento at the Australian Institute of Tropical Medicine, Cook had agreed that "the lack of any disposition towards interracial intercourse which is a feature of Australian national character, has been a potent factor in protecting the whites in areas from which many coloured lepers have been reported."[150] But in later years Cook came to promote "education of the native in citizenship" and other efforts to "adapt him to white civilisation." Otherwise, "uneducated, bewildered, without any tangible point of contact with white citizenship and with no stable foothold in the social structure, psychologically unequipped for community life and outcast from white society, the native hybrid must remain a ready prey to agitators and a receptive field for subversive ideologies."[151]

The Return of the Native

Even as some medical scientists were reimagining Aboriginal difference as an odd stain that might be dissolved with careful population management or, like Cilento, were thinking of Aborigines as a threat requiring isolation and medical policing, a few literary nationalists in the 1930s were still reading Wood Jones, convincing themselves that the desert nomads offered an example of an alternative Caucasian destiny in Australia. No longer consigned to the primordial, the "primitive" had come to signify a people who were structurally and functionally adapted to the land, a people who had become part of the land, not alienated from it. The combination of images of virility, purity, blood, and soil made an exceptionally attractive brew in Australia in the 1930s. The primitive was licensed as a site for the expression, by some European Australians, of alternative modern possibilities.[152] Stan Larnach, traveling with a Sydney expedition to Haast's Bluff in the early 1930s, rode his camel alongside the Pintubi, a few of them with "quite blonde hair." "Walking along with an easy swing, erect, placing each foot on the ground, with toes pointing forwards, or sometimes slightly in-turned, they would make a wonderful demonstration to an adult European of how to walk."[153] R. H. Croll, a conservative Melbourne bookman and bushwalker who accompanied Porteus on his expedition, recollected that "central Australia, where I have now been five times, was long a place of desire." Each time Croll encountered the true nomads, his reaction was "one of disgust with my own kind."[154] In Katharine Susannah Prichard's powerful novel, the full-blood woman Coonardoo becomes "a sort of fantasy" for Hugh, an outback white man whose "repressions have rotted in him."[155] Modernized in science, the nomads triumphed—for a time—in literature.

These white fantasies and desires were expressed most fervently and most persistently by a group of Adelaide writers, the Jindyworobaks. Clustered around Rex Ingamells and Ian Mudie, they learned Aboriginal mythology and vocabulary from the books of Baldwin Spencer and Wood Jones, as well as from talking with Ted Strehlow, a contemporary who had grown up at Hermannsburg and become an associate of the Adelaide physical anthropologists.[156] They admired the nationalist tracts of P. R. Stephensen, and many of them became fellow travelers in his native version of fascism.[157] According to Ingamells, "Jindyworobak" meant to annex or to join, in this case to graft an idealized version of the primitive nomad onto modern literature and thereby to allow "the expression of environmental values." "Jindyworobak has, from the first," wrote Ingamells, "essayed the scientific method for helping to induce the needful cultural maturity of Australia in the modern world."[158] An epitome of Aboriginality might provide a distinctive modern Australian idiom. "Nature, the Aborigine, primitivism—these concepts do not of themselves make an Australian literature; but they cannot be ignored as components."[159] Ingamells deplored the pseudo-Europeanism that clogged the minds of most white Australians and alienated them from the land:

> *Australia is a land that has no people,*
> *for those that were hers we have torn away,*
> *we who are not hers nor can be till love*
> *shall make us so and fill our hearts with her.*[160]

Unable to abandon the convention of lyric poetry—even in one of its more dubious forms—the Jindyworobaks still longed for a reunion with the land, a primitive engagement of blood and soil that was, somehow, very modern.

Through biological investigation, strangers became kin, and the romance of the nomad became a family romance. In physical anthropology, as in social research, a psychophysiological functionalism was flattening evolutionary differences; similarities in contemporary biological function became more significant than minor differences in racial history.[161] The scientists who migrated to the central deserts every August, year after year, recognized that Aboriginal bodies shared with them a common location and temporality: they were coexistent, not antecedent. In thus entering the biomedical present, the "primitive" was given a mediated voice in modernity, and at the same time, white modernity was offered an opportunity to absorb it.

CHAPTER 8

THE REPRODUCTIVE FRONTIER

AFTER THE GREAT DEPRESSION of the 1930s, some writers on the edges of science described in vivid terms their journeys to the inland; in these popular narratives they extolled the "uncontaminated desert nomads," just as an earlier generation of city authors had praised the itinerant white bushman.[1] When H. H. Finlayson, the curator of mammals at the South Australian Museum, stayed at Ernabella, he found himself among skilled hunters adapted to desert conditions—an affectionate, generous people whose "normal state is an ambulant one." But he also observed with distaste "the miserable wreckage of the race which is strewn about the margins of settlement." It almost seemed that when the myall "dons the cast-offs of his white master he becomes a pitiful scarecrow." Accordingly, it would be best to reduce to a minimum white interference with traditional life.[2] A few years later, Charles P. Mountford also visited Ernabella, accompanying the Adelaide scientists, and there, among the spinifex and mulga, he encountered "one of the most lovable of the races of mankind, our Australian Aboriginal." A telephone mechanic from Adelaide, Mountford was acquiring a reputation as an ethnographer and photographer of the last of the nomads. Convinced that clothing and education would ruin their health, Mountford sought to collect as many myths and legends as possible before they disappeared. He believed that the desert full-bloods were "following a life rich in philosophical thought, in cultural expression and communal living." Pioneer environmentalists and natural communists, the remaining uncontaminated Aboriginal Australians appeared "free from the avarice, bitterness and strife that characterise the more complex civilisations."[3]

Not all popular writers endorsed the romance of the nomad. On his inland travels, Finlayson had stayed with old Charles Chewings, a geologist who founded Tempe Downs cattle station in the 1880s, not long after the completion of the overland telegraph line. Many years of observation had convinced Dr. Chewings that the Aborigines on his land "possess very remarkable faculties

225

of observation, and good reasoning powers" as well as the inevitable "nomadic instincts." But if the "natives are naturally indisposed to labour or physical exertion, and lack mental activity," it was also true that "under proper, kindly supervision the Australian natives are capable of very useful work."[4] As Chewings was fond of telling anyone who stopped to listen, as a station owner he preferred missionaries to scientists. He described his scientific visitors from the University of Adelaide and South Australian Museum as "insatiable." The scientist "wants the uncontaminated natives kept in their primitive state mentally, morally, and in every other way, so that they can be further studied. He has pleaded successfully for large reserves and would keep them there as zoological curiosities." In contrast, missionaries hope "of bringing about in them a complete transformation from barbarism to civilisation, from totemism to Christianity." The drift from the reserves to the towns and missions was continuing apace, so it was quixotic to imagine that one might shut off the full-bloods entirely from the allegedly contaminating touch of "wicked whites."[5] Chewings conceded that welfare and rations meant that the fringe-dweller "degenerates into a lazy, useless being, and soon dies of ennui." But the author of *Back in the Stone Age*—a paradoxical title—had found a secular answer: the transformative power not of the gospel but of employment. "No better examples can be found of the civilising effect of personal contact with the whites than the working native boys and women; and no other equally successful method has yet been devised to improve that natives as properly regulated personal contact with the respectable white man." The solution to Aboriginal ill health and degeneration was to civilize full-blood and half-caste alike and absorb them into the white economy, not to isolate them and study them. "By adopting the white man's ways they may overcome the tendency to 'die out,' for those in work are healthy enough."[6]

More and more, it was Chewings's vision of Aboriginal destiny that came to dominate the research agenda and policy debate in the 1930s. The ground had already been prepared for a scientific justification of policies of attraction and absorption. Medical scientists at Adelaide seemed to have confirmed that Aboriginal Australians were dark Caucasians, and they repeatedly demonstrated affinities of function and malfunction between pure whites and full-blood natives. By the 1930s, scientists had mostly discarded the notion that Aboriginal Australians were simply object lessons of evolutionary theory, and they had begun to locate indigenous bodies unambiguously in the biomedical present. Full-blood desert nomads were functioning efficiently and wisely in central Australia; their physiological adaptation to harsh conditions was exemplary. It still seemed likely that they were doomed, but the end had been deferred indefinitely, and the causes of their diminution were now the commonplace ones of immunological incompetence—a consequence of isolation—and "race-crossing," producing mixed offspring. Their eventual "extinction" was no longer attributed to a clash of races, to a mystic antipathy between civilized and primitive. With the decline of such teleological explanation, some basic, mundane interventions now seemed possible. One might, like Finlayson, Mountford, and Frederic Wood Jones, recommend continued isolation of vulnerable traditional populations, thus preserving them as paragons of environmental and communitarian virtue in a fallen modern world. Or like Chewings and J. B. Cleland, one might seize on their capacity to perform basic tasks in the white economy and urge that they become absorbed into the white nation as rapidly and as completely as possible.[7] With an acceleration of the trajectory from nomad to proletarian, the problems of Aboriginal ill health and degeneration would become simply the problems of poor white ill health and degeneration.

Inevitably, research and policy settings shifted to focus on the destiny of half-castes, who were becoming more numerous and who seemed more readily assimilated.[8] Chewings had criticized scientists for failing to recognize the successful incorporation of full-bloods and half-castes as stockmen and maids in the central Australian economy. But science had moved on, and by the end of the 1930s research on the management of half-caste assimilation had largely replaced investigations of full-blood physiology and racial identity. Half-castes, more than full-bloods, seemed tantalizingly absorbable. Not only were they fundamentally, and homogeneously, Caucasian; they were (in general) already part white, and so they could pass more easily in prejudiced white communities. Unlike "Negroes," it seemed that a Caucasian genetic identity would permit a gradual and indiscernible diffusion of genes throughout the white population, a "breeding out" of color without "throwbacks" to a dark type. (Of course, those who were part Asian appeared to present a serious biological impediment to this schema.) Cleland and his younger Adelaide colleagues predicted that dark Caucasian genes would eventually be submerged in the larger white Caucasian gene pool, and then proper training and instruction in hygiene—the same discipline as inculcated in poor whites—would do the rest. Unlike Wood Jones, the scientists of the late 1930s were modernizers and interventionists; they promoted the rational, biological management of populations. Their leader, Cleland, could thus predict a day when, as the result of a scientific breeding and education program, all Australians claimed some Aboriginal ancestry—and it would not matter. All of the continent, even its once-black heart, would at last be covered by a carefully supervised working white race—if not purely white, then white enough.[9]

The scientific rationalization of the "breeding out of color" was a project taken up most enthusiastically at Adelaide, which had long boasted a special expertise in studying the biology and physical anthropology of the Aboriginal inhabitants of the central deserts. Researchers in the medical schools at Melbourne, Sydney, and, later, Brisbane remained fascinated with white bodies, whether in the tropics or, more often, in the urban slums. During the 1930s, medical scientists and national hygienists in Melbourne and Sydney, such as Harvey Sutton, were focusing again on specifically British character, or else, like W. A. Osborne and Jens Lyng, they were subdividing whiteness into Nordic, Alpine, and Mediterranean types. But throughout this period, Adelaide scientists maintained a commitment to a broader, less differentiated concept of whiteness, sometimes even calling it Caucasian and suggesting that it might ingest and consume, without damage, anything on its margins. Many of the South Australians would, if pressed, default to a residual Lamarckism to explain how whiteness might come to encompass such a wide range of types and groups. One could, of course, justify absorption of Aboriginal people into whiteness, or a less color-conscious modern Caucasian identity, by pointing to the weight of European gene numbers, the disproportion of an Aboriginal gene droplet in a European ocean. But some of the Adelaide investigators also assumed that ultimately a common adaptation to the environment, heavily mediated though it was by advanced technology, would also contribute to ensuring a biological homogeneity, that persistent national goal. Thus a breeding out of color might still be complemented by a genetic convergence in a common hygienic environment, so that half-castes would indeed sink and show no trace.

Because Adelaide scientists were dealing specifically with Aboriginal bodies, whose eligibility for normalization and citizenship in white Australia remained marginal, they were allowed a greater range of interventionist strategies than their eastern counterparts. Although R.J.A. Berry and Wilfred Agar, among others, had advocated state-sponsored breeding programs to eliminate unfit whites, most national hygienists had deemed impractical any such reproductive intervention. Instead, retraining in hygiene became the preferred strategy for improvement of white Australian stock, a means of enhancing development during an individual's life span. But Adelaide modernizers in the 1930s, led by Cleland, felt they could go further, moving beyond the supposedly necessary reform of customs and habits. They had license to promote a breeding policy in order to remove the half-caste, an irritating and expanding group that was between "authentic" whiteness and "authentic" (and disappearing) Aboriginality.[10] In effect, they were able to urge the state to intervene, on scientific grounds, to replace, or at least to supplement, errant white males on the reproductive frontier. They were free to advocate, and to justify, a breeding program for half-castes—though not strictly "eugenic" in the sense of being directed toward the improvement of a race, it was nonetheless a scale of reproductive intervention that would not usually be countenanced in even poor white Australian communities.[11]

The elevation of the half-caste—a person with some Aboriginal ancestry who did not pass as a white—onto the scientific agenda and into public consciousness was a dramatic one. Few writers in the nineteenth century had passed judgment on the rare Aboriginal-European "hybrid." R. Brough Smyth was more interested in the new breed than most. The half-castes whom he observed in Victoria in the 1870s "partake in their form, features and colour more of the character of the male parent than that of the Aboriginal female." Indeed, they resembled southern Europeans, but they deteriorated after fourteen years of age.[12] Natalie Robarts, in describing the Aborigines of Coranderrk in 1913, echoed Smyth's faint praise. "The half-castes," she claimed, "are intelligent and capable of working, but the mother being the black parent, the moral tendencies lean towards the native on account of pre-natal influences. Also, the child, being brought up among an indolent, lazy people, contracts these habits." Physically "the white race strongly asserts itself. The white colour overpowers the black."[13] The few who cared to comment on "the half-caste" repeated the truism: physically almost white, but mentally and morally almost black. But it was not until the 1920s, when half-castes numbered in the tens of thousands and seemed destined to proliferate still more, that there were any scientific studies of the biological and social capacities of such novel "hybrids."[14] In defining a new problem for white Australia and suggesting a biological solution, these studies would reframe—and ultimately challenge—both Aboriginality and whiteness.

SCIENCE DISCOVERS THE HALF-CASTE

When Ernestine Hill, that intrepid reporter, ventured into the far north in the 1930s, she soon realized that "the steady increase of coloured and half-breed populations threatens an empty country with the begetting of one of the most illogical and inbred races in the world." She found the prospect most unsettling. Half-castes were "pitiable in that they are cursed with a dark skin in a white man's country, and all astray in life, menacing in that they alone are numerous where children of the white race are few."[15] But a chat in Darwin with Cecil Cook—"anthropologist, biologist, bacteriologist, Chief Medical Officer and Chief Protector of the Aborigines"—reassured her somewhat. Apparently the latest scientific theories suggested that one could breed out the black, and unlike crosses with "Negroes" or Asians, there was no danger of atavism, or throwbacks. Cook was directing "a vitally interesting ethnological experiment, teaching these children to live white and think white." Hill was taken to visit a special home in Alice Springs where "under the best conditions, these unfortunate little ones will be given every opportunity to outgrow their heredity—if they can."[16] She tried to be hopeful, but she remained skeptical at heart.

Hill's views stand in contrast to those of Xavier Herbert. In the 1930s, the novelist was working as a pharmacist (and in a variety of other jobs) in Darwin, and writing *Capricornia*, his Dickensian tropical epic. Herbert had fallen out with Cook because he thought the medical officer was not doing enough to civilize the half-castes. In the novel, Dr. Aintee—Herbert's version of Cook—regarded Aborigines "merely as marsupials being routed by a pack of dingoes; and he understood that his duty was merely to protect them from undue violence during the rout."[17] Herbert believed that the government did not really want blacks to flourish because this would lead to further miscegenation, to the proliferation of half-castes; the authorities would prefer to preside over the race's extinction. The novelist had the more sensitive, alcoholic characters give voice to his own thoughts. Sitting around a campfire, the grazier Andy McRandy reflected on the capacity of the Aboriginal:

> Gettin' to know him will lead to gettin' to honour him, givin' him the citizenship that it's to the everlastin' disgrace of the country he's been denied so long, and education, rights as a human bein', and the chance to learn this new system of society that's been dumped down in his country and so far done nuthen but wipe him out. The blackfeller aint a Negroid type. His colour's only skin-deep. Three cross-breedin's and you'll get the colour right out, with never the risk of a throw-back.[18]

McRandy pointed to Norman, the hero of the novel, as an example of an intelligent, capable half-caste. Elsewhere, Herbert declared that there was a pressing need to teach whites that half-castes are "intelligent human creatures like themselves." He could not countenance "wasting money on useless Commissions to investigate the problems of settling the land, which the blacks and half-castes would have settled in no time if trained to do it."[19]

Despite their different evaluation of the likely outcomes, Hill and Herbert both had based their stories on the latest scientific reasoning about the breeding of Aborigines with Europeans. In the 1920s, the proliferation of "hybrids" had occasioned a flurry of scientific speculation on the effects of mixing the races. Most experts argued that, given the accepted ethnological affinities, the offspring of white and dark Caucasians would present the government with decent material to work with. Absorption would virtually be complete; half-castes would sink and show no trace. Herbert Basedow, a medical doctor, anthropologist, and South Australian politician, was one of many who asserted that "our" half-castes soon lose color: "There is never any risk in a subsequent generation of having a black fellow born of a white woman."[20] But where were the studies to support this claim? And even if absorption were feasible, was it desirable for whites? In the 1920s, a few scientists had begun to outline a research program to investigate the destiny of the half-castes. In 1924, W. Ramsay Smith, the director of the South Australian Health Department, expressed his regret that no one had yet applied the principles of Mendelism to the study of the crossing of our Aboriginal with the white, so as to find out what characters are dominant and what are recessive. Speaking generally, we had noted that when white mates with black characters of the black disappear with the first generation, particularly the overhanging forehead and the deep notch at the root of the nose. Further, when half-caste mates with half-caste, the children are whiter than either parent, and the third or fourth generation is perhaps indistinguishable from the white. This goes to support the view that the Aboriginal and the Maori are both Caucasian in origin.[21]

But would Aborigines be Caucasian enough, or adaptable enough, to pass in white Australia? "I am not sure whether football is a recognised test of civilisation," Smith wrote, "but if cricket is any criterion the blackfellow has a strong claim to be civilisable."[22]

There were many self-styled experts, like Stan Larnach, who were prepared to endorse such a claim. Attaching himself to scientific expeditions to the central deserts, Larnach had come to believe that there was no reason to fear crossings of Aboriginal Australians and Europeans. "If wholesale miscegenation occurred their blood would be ultimately diluted to an insignificant amount." But Larnach was unusual: He could not see the point of abstract racial classifications and questioned the assumption that "it should be impossible for a white man to love an Aboriginal woman." "It would be much better," he wrote, "if we legislated for the Aborigines as if they were human beings, with human thoughts and feelings, instead of as if they were practically dingoes."[23] But where was the scientific support for the benefits of absorption? When A. Grenfell Price recommended the intermarrying of half-caste women and white men as a far-sighted policy, he was still lamenting the lack of clear scientific data. The policy, according to the Adelaide geographer, "looks towards breeding the Aborigine white, instead of letting the half-castes become black. Blood tests appear to show that the Aborigine is akin to the white man. There are no records of throwbacks. The black strain breeds out comparatively quickly, and the slight evidence available indicates that the octaroon is of good type."[24] When would further scientific investigation bolster this meager evidence?

Scientists hoped that this natural experiment in race-crossing might illuminate biological processes of global significance. In the 1920s, Griffith Taylor suggested that the successful amalgamation of Aboriginal Australians and Europeans implied that some other race-crosses might be beneficial, providing that the differences were not so great as to produce disharmony in the offspring. Uniquely, he recommended "Anglo-Mongolian marriages" and suggested that "a small influx of Chinese . . . would greatly stimulate our tropical settlement." But even he drew the line at miscegenation with "the Negro peoples." "On every count," he assured his readers, "they stand on a lower plane than white and Mongolian. Racial mixture with them may be a deterioration for the other races."[25] This reservation was not enough for J. W. Gregory, who condemned even such limited proposals for race-crossing. The professor of geology, who was also a race enthusiast, pointed out that most international experts—especially those from the United States and South Africa—believed that hybrids were inferior to both parents, more so if the breeding stocks were from widely distinct races. Accordingly, "if miscegenation between the primary races is undesirable, the co-residence of different races should be avoided in the interest of the future of mankind."[26] But were not Aborigines and Europeans branches of the same primary race? H. L. Wilkinson, the Melbourne political scientist, endorsed Gregory's general concerns. He was convinced that hybrids would always be inferior to their parents. "From what I have seen of the results of interbreeding between Europeans and Chinese, Indians, or native Africans," he wrote, "I can only come to the conclusion that it is bad from a physical, mental and moral point of view." At best, breeding between closely related human stocks would result in an increase of physical and mental strength in the first generation—hybrid vigor— but these gains always proved evanescent. At worst, "miscegenation between peoples far apart gives bad results which are not eliminated, but rather are accentuated, in successive generations."[27] If the white and dark Caucasians of the continent were as closely related as some scientists had claimed, then the results of interbreeding might at best be neutral—if not, then the policy of biological assimilation would prove misguided, imperiling the nation.

Framed as a modern experiment in race-crossing, the generation of mixed Aboriginal and European Australians attracted international attention. As early as 1914, after attending the British Association for the Advancement of Science meeting in Melbourne, Charles B. Davenport had traveled to Brewarrina in western New South Wales to investigate properly the physical and mental character of the new black-white hybrids. Davenport, the chief American promoter of Mendelism, wanted to take some simple anthropometric observations of the last of the full-bloods and what he called the "Australian mongrels." He did not get around to publishing the results until 1925, when the need for scientific data on half-castes was more widely recognized. The focus of his study was the first generation—the F_1 generation—examples of which could be found more commonly in Australia than in other parts of the world, where race-crossing had occurred for longer. Davenport found that members of the first hybrid generation had relatively short legs and a less dolichocephalic skull than their Aboriginal mothers; but hair and eye color were still dark, "showing the dominance of the Australian pigmentation." Based on measurements from only seven F_1 subjects, and undercut by ambivalence about the racial status of Aborigines, it was not a convincing paper.[28]

Later, with Morris Steggerda, a zoologist, Davenport made more extensive investigations of race-crossing in Jamaica and claimed that the results obtained there indicated that "mulatos" could not sustain white man's civilization. The brown hybrids seemed far more "muddled and wuzzle-headed" than either of the parent stocks.[29] Davenport was dismayed that disharmonious combinations such as the long legs of the black and the short arms of the white would mean that some hybrids could not pick things up off the ground. He condemned such dangerous race experiments.

Most of the other international authorities in the new science of genetics disagreed with Davenport on this matter and expressed some tolerance of race-crossing. W. E. Castle, a professor of zoology at Harvard, believed that if mixed races were physically feeble it was not simply a result of the mixture but because those individuals who were mixing were already feeble. "Mating out of the race, when mates in the race are available," he wrote in 1916, "is *prima facie* evidence that the individual mating is an outcast." But in principle, even when the breeding pair were robust, "human racial crossing in general is a risky experiment, because it interferes with social inheritance, which after all is the chief asset of civilization."[30] Ten years later, Castle had developed a more favorable opinion. Deploring fashionable race prejudice, he observed that much race science was no more than "assumption backed up by loud voiced assertion." He wondered if the poor achievements of half-breeds derived from heredity or from the environment in which they were forced to function. "Attainments imply opportunities as well as abilities." Although Castle still was worried that race-crossing might disrupt social inheritance, he had come to believe that it might also give rise to a population "more adaptable to a new or changing environment either physical or social." Any disharmonious combinations would eventually disappear with natural selection. He felt that Davenport's concerns were overstated: In the United States, when black-white hybrids were repeatedly back-crossed with whites, the "result is an approximation to the skin color and level of intelligence of whites in a few generations."[31]

In the 1920s, other geneticists in the United States and Britain joined Castle in attempting to distance themselves from eugenic enthusiasms, and in the process their concerns about race mixture also became somewhat more muted. Herbert Spencer Jennings, a professor of zoology at the Johns Hopkins University, frequently protested that hard-line race purists like Davenport were making all geneticists look like cranks. In 1930, Jennings reflected on the "eagerness to apply biological science to human affairs" and wondered if the science was equal to the burden placed upon it.[32] He criticized many of his colleagues for their recourse to a facile genetic determinism. Even so, Jennings could not resist using biological theory as a rough guide to human mating. He still felt that if gene sets were very different, the results might be disastrous, in that mixed individuals might be "less efficient physiological machines than the purer ones." But in other cases the combinations might be harmonious. "The mating of two slightly diverse races often gives offspring that are superior to either race"; the children might "excel the parent in vigor and efficiency." By mixing races, recessive defective genes were less likely to be combined in the offspring. Natural selection should in any case eliminate the more severe genetic disharmonies—but "while the poorer combinations are still present and in the process of elimination, the mixed race may expect a lively and varied history."[33]

Race-crossing continued to excite speculation among biologists, but their views on the effects of hybridization were becoming ever more equivocal and uncertain. Gregory and Wilkinson joined Davenport in condemning "mongrelization"; Griffith Taylor associated himself with the more "advanced" uncertainties of Castle and Jennings. But what status would these scientists finally assign to the offspring of Aboriginal Australian and European liaisons? It was unclear at the time just what sort of biological experiment was taking place in Australia. Were the gene sets of the parents sufficiently different to produce disharmony in their children? Or would racial affinities give rise to a more vigorous breed that would, after back-crossing of later generations, eventually become indistinguishable from pure whites? Was it, indeed, an example of race-crossing at all? Perhaps the very similarity of race that made interbreeding possible to contemplate would lessen its value as a racial experiment?

Having structured sex in the outback as yet another great experiment in human biology, the scientists predictably demanded more research into the matter. Davenport's perfunctory study of the Brewarrina "mongrels" had been inconclusive. In 1924, Griffith Taylor, hoping to extend knowledge of Aboriginal reproduction, went among the Kamilaroi in the valley of the Namoi, measuring more half-castes. By then, half-castes in New South Wales outnumbered full-bloods by 6,000 to 1,000, a reversal of the numbers forty years earlier. Taylor found his half-castes mostly on the reserves, the men working as shearers and drovers, the women employed as domestic help or nursemaids. He measured only seven "three-quarter castes" and eight half-castes, and his results too were dubious. The teachers told him that boys lost their "mental initiative" at the age of thirteen or fourteen, and the less black blood they had the more intelligent they appeared. The full-blood men had red-brown skin, and the half-castes were ochre; in skull shape there was "a slight change from the dolichopse towards the euryopse form with increase in proportion of the white blood"; and with a greater volume of white blood, the nose was more narrow.[34] But what could this mean to white Australia? Evidently there would need to be far more research.

In a remarkably influential essay on the effects of "culture contact," G. Pitt Rivers, the Oxford anthropologist, suggested in 1927 that the failure of native peoples to adapt to sudden changes in "culture forms" led to their gradual extinction. "A condition of culture disequilibrium is engendered," he wrote, "followed by the extinction or modification of the weaker culture and a variable degree of re-adaptation accompanied by a greater or lesser change in ethnos." He had heard that this was happening in Australia, but miscegenation was greatly complicating the process. "The gradual infiltration of European blood into a declining native population must favour a re-adaptation of the increasingly miscegenated stock."[35] But if white blood benefited native peoples, did native blood confer any advantage on whites in a settler society? Or was it still possible that such admixture would only hasten white deterioration?

The Harvard-Adelaide Half-Caste Survey

Norman B. "Tinny" Tindale, an entomologist, was drawn into Adelaide anthropology circles in the 1920s, assisting Thomas D. Campbell and others on archaeological digs and working at the South Australian Museum. Like most of his expedition mates, he was especially entranced by the natural history of the "authentic" full-blooded nomads, but during the 1930s his attention increasingly was drawn to the scientific aspects of "the half-caste problem."[36] Visiting Harvard University in 1936, he called on E. A. Hooton, a professor of physical anthropology, and met one of his graduate students, Joseph B. Birdsell. Tindale talked with them at length about "the desirability of having an anthropometrist to measure the mixed blood Tasmanians and Australians."[37] Eager to find a dissertation topic, Birdsell seized on the possibility of studying race-crossing in Australia.[38] In 1938, with Hooton's encouragement, Birdsell proposed a joint Harvard-Adelaide study of hybrids of mixed Aboriginal and European ancestry, an investigation in which the Harvard graduate student would concentrate on the anthropometric aspects and Tindale would help with ethnological and genealogical issues. The numbers of half-castes in Australia were rising at a great rate—from 9,000 in 1911 to 23,000 in 1936, according to Birdsell—and given their recent origin most of them would be first-generation, with easily traced maternal parentage (standard figures could be used to represent putative white paternity). Birdsell regarded this project as an example of applied physical anthropology and promised to focus on "the capacity of the hybrids for adapting themselves to European civilization, since this group of the population constitutes a government problem."[39] Hooton was delighted, assuring James B. Conant, the president of Harvard, that the collaborating anthropologists at Adelaide "are extremely competent workers—the best among the Australian universities."[40] Hooton's support ensured that Birdsell and Tindale received financial assistance from the Carnegie Institution for their 1938–1939 expedition across Australia. (Ever helpful, Hooton also supplied his student with an impressive letter of introduction, using the format that worked so well for the department in South America and known at Harvard as the "dago dazzler.")[41] When Charles Davenport heard about the plan, he immediately invited Birdsell down to Cold Spring Harbor to discuss new measuring techniques. "My sole interest," Davenport told Hooton, "is to get the best possible set of data concerning these living representatives of Neanderthal man before they are all hybridized. If I were ten years younger I would go myself."[42] But it would seem that the aging eugenicist had sadly missed the point of the expedition.

Arriving in Adelaide in 1938, Birdsell introduced himself to Cleland, who was the local sponsor of the research project. Both Tindale and Birdsell found Cleland rather stiff and officious, and they resented his repeated warnings to confine their investigations to South Australia. Cleland frequently chided them for the ambitious scope of their plans, but they would do their best to ignore him. Tindale and Birdsell had already decided to start at Swan Reach and then travel along the Murray River before going north to Cairns and returning along the coast to Victoria; in December 1938 they would visit Tasmania; January and February of 1939 would be spent in South Australia; and they intended to go later to Western Australia. Strangely, they chose to avoid central Australia, the usual hunting ground of Adelaide investigators, even though no studies of race-crossing or half-caste absorption had yet occurred there. In view of Tindale's and Birdsell's later fascination with Aboriginal origins, it is hard not to suspect that they were from the beginning also interested in completing a full-blood survey in areas where none of the Adelaide group had yet ventured—just as Davenport had suggested.

Tindale and Birdsell departed from Adelaide in May 1938, full of enthusiasm and relieved that Cleland was by then in Europe.[43] Within a few days they were in Swan Reach, where "in the evening many children gathered around us and we had great fun with them." "The 3/4 black children seem to be of two types which we classified as Veddish and Dravidish at once."[44] Later in May, Tindale reported from Coomeragunja, north of the Murray River, where they had studied ninety-eight people and tested forty schoolchildren "whose genetic placing is satisfactory."[45] There Tindale observed a distinct "Tasmanian strain" among the Briggs family, who had darker skin and curly hair. "Even when present to the extent of 1/16th part it seems to stand out clearly from the Australian Aboriginal cross. . . . Birdsell is quite excited about it and I confess I am also."[46]

The ostensible research interest in white-black crosses did not really become evident until they reached Brewarrina in June, where the young investigators measured 250 adults—thirty of them full-bloods and twenty-five of them "the important and elusive F_1." Birdsell concentrated on measuring those of known ancestry and determining their blood groups while Tindale obtained genealogies—to determine their "effage"—and information about the local way of life and tested the intelligence of the children. Using standard tests, Tindale found that "scale scores usually show a year or more retardation on white children, but some of mixed parentage are outstanding in performance." The anthropologists reassured Cleland that the "costs of rewards to natives have been kept very low, so far we have used only boiled lollies and cigarettes."[47] At Goondiwindi, Tindale found himself chatting with "a 3/8th" who was "so white that he would pass anywhere as a European; his children are fair, one is blue-eyed and blond; none have much indication of abo blood."[48] In October, at Yarrabah in Queensland, Birdsell measured more than 900 adults, many of them F_1, and Tindale tested more than 300 children. "We have seen numbers of practical examples of what can be done by natives, even on their own, to adjust themselves to a full life in the white community," Tindale told Cleland. "Whole groups of quarter castes have passed over into the white community and are even climbing the social scale."[49]

At the end of November 1938, Tindale and Birdsell had measured more than 1,200 Aboriginal bodies, grouped their blood, and recorded their genealogies—175 of these were adult F_1. Among the "exotic crosses" were twenty-six F_1 Aboriginal-Chinese and seven F_1 Aboriginal-"Hindus."[50] At Menindee, Birdsell had also acquired some recent human remains, the bone fragments of about twenty people, which he decided to send back to the Peabody Museum at Harvard. "I intend to bring home the human stuff for study, regardless of the fuss Tindale and the local people kick up," he wrote to Hooton.[51] For the Harvard graduate student, the whole enterprise had exceeded his expectations. He was especially impressed with the abilities of the Australian hybrids. They are "rather pleasing in feature, and although showing Aboriginal morphology markedly, somehow the product of crossing here seems to show less disharmony than among American mulattos, to give more the impression of a dark, aberrant white type, than reveal any true Negro strain in the background."[52] It looked almost as if "*two* kinds of *whites*" had mixed."[53] At Brewarrina—which Birdsell referred to as "a dream," so prolific were the F_1 hybrids—the scientists observed that the faces of the mixed offspring "tan rather markedly, but their unexposed skin is very light, probably less swarthy than southern Europeans" (see Figure 8.1). The prospects of the white and dark Caucasian amalgam seemed bright. But Birdsell noted those few hybrids with some "Negro blood" reacted "entirely differently to the ordeal of measuring, verging on hysteria, as compared to the stolid white-black crosses, and the former also seem to inherit the Negro body odor, at least in some individuals."[54] (Aboriginal-white crosses, however, "smell like dirty whites, not offensive in kind only in degree.")[55] As the team moved south into Victoria, Birdsell found that the "daily catch" decreased appreciably.[56] Yet he was still able to report to Hooton that "the material to be obtained here in Australia is so rich as to leave the field worker gasping with astonishment that it has never been adequately touched before."[57] Hooton believed that the expedition had performed "the most comprehensive work on race mixture which . . . has ever been accomplished."[58] It was, he wrote to Cleland, "epoch making."[59]

Opposition to the investigations was rarely reported. Early on, Birdsell had found that the "difficult points are direct limb measurements and most subjects sensitive about extent of oral examination. Offer of cigarettes seems to be cheapest bribe."[60] In Cairns, Tindale had encountered "a slight element of distrust of our work," partly deriving from memories of Hermann Klaatsch's rude and intrusive investigations.[61] On Palm Island, "the people were a little suspicious at first but when rumour had passed around that we were out to help them we were well-received."[62] But later, on Cape Barren Island, in Bass Strait, "nine of the islanders refuse to come and be examined; a few are stubborn, a few shy and one is in active opposition to us."[63] At Mt. Barker in Western Australia, Tindale and Birdsell by the end of the first day had "settled the racial constitution of the majority of the 22 children in the school." Most of them were "1/4s" with some F_2 and "3/4"—"one of the whitest groups we have seen." But Tindale detected some hesitancy in "the confession of the white parentage of children of school age for owing to [A.O.] Neville's policy of seizing all 1/4 children the mothers fear to tell us."[64] In general, though, with the help of the local missionaries and police, the investigators had no trouble eliciting the information they sought.

Surprisingly, Cape Barren Island, occupied by descendants of the un-Caucasian "Negrito" Tasmanians, provided Tindale with perhaps the best example of half-caste absorption. "Our first impression," he wrote in his journal early in 1939, "is that we are not dealing with a group of half-castes, but with an isolated island group of white people."[65] Many of the Islanders had married white folk and "'disappeared' into the general white populace. Most of those who have made the break with the old life are still on the lesser rungs of life but a few have attained the lower ranks of middle-class life." They were just like any white community that intermarried too much. Despite a degree of indifference, or resistance, the investigators had measured some 135 Islanders, about 80 percent of the population, and they were gratified by the results. "Their modes of life and methods of thinking are essentially white and relatively few traces survive of their native ancestry. Considering their cramped surroundings and isolation, their code of morality is surprisingly high." Tindale felt that their problems should therefore be regarded as those "of a white people who have a dark strain running through them, rather than as Aborigines."[66]

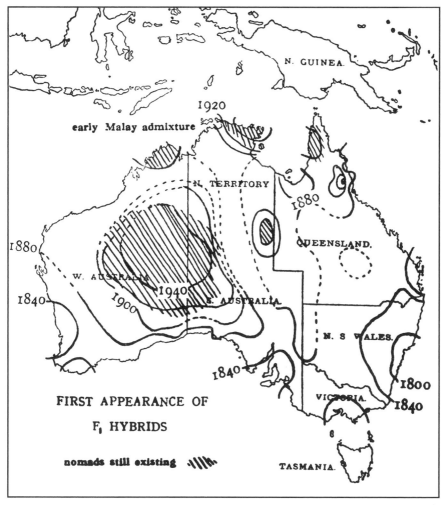

Figure 8.1: The reproductive frontier: the first appearance of F_1 hybrids in Australia. (*Proceedings Royal Geographical Society of Australasia, South Australian Branch,* vol. 42, 1940–41)

In an extensive report on the whole expedition, Tindale described race-crossing in Australia as a unique experiment, the results of which were unusually illuminating because genealogical determination was more certain in Australia than elsewhere. Some white Australians might be tempted to urge the segregation of half-castes (as in the United States and South Africa), but Tindale concluded that the racial experiment supported hybrid absorption. Aboriginal Australians "should not be treated as if they were a highly developed species of animal," he wrote, "to be viewed only as though they were inhabitants of a zoological gardens. They should not be shut away in segregated (almost caged) communities."[67] The measurements and the tests performed by Tindale and Birdsell had not revealed any half-caste degeneration. Absorption, not isolation, was therefore the best scientific solution of the half-caste problem:

> Complete mergence of the half-castes in the general community is possible without detriment to the white race. Their Aboriginal blood is remotely the same as that of the majority of the white inhabitants of Australia, for the Australian Aboriginal is recognised as being a forerunner of the Caucasian race. . . . Two successive accessions of white blood lead to the mergence of the Aboriginal in the white community. There are no biological reasons for the rejection of people with a dilute strain of Australian Aboriginal blood. A low percentage of Australian Aboriginal blood will not introduce any aberrant characteristics and there need be no fear of reversions to the dark Aboriginal type.[68]

The proper scientific management of the Aboriginal population would require a dispersal of mixed-bloods into the general white community. "Dispersal," Tindale assured his readers, "will mean rapid dilution of these dark ethnic pockets." He had devised a genealogical table of "absorbability," with "octaroons" the most readily absorbed and those with 7/8th Aboriginal ancestry requiring further crossing with whites.[69]

Increasing the index of absorbability through mating with whites was not necessarily a flouting of the white Australia policy. "'White Australia' requires there should be as little possible disturbance of the present biological balance. The absorption of ethnic strains of any widely different type is, therefore, discouraged." But Tindale took this to mean that any mixture with Asian types would not be countenanced, whereas Aboriginal miscegenation should be acceptable. The most important policy consideration was how absorption might be expedited. Tindale condemned Queensland and Western Australian "herding" arrangements, where large numbers of mixed-bloods and full-bloods had been concentrated in small areas. He praised Victorian policy, which since the 1880s had "enabled many mixed bloods to become dispersed and culturally and otherwise absorbed into the general population." In Tasmania, he had identified "a rather fair admixture between white and Aborigine, the white blood so predominating that, on the whole, they can be regarded as 'dark-whites' rather than as Aborigines."[70] Thus with careful breeding, improved nutrition, and proper education (in English only), those who were part Aborigine might become swarthy whites. Indeed, "the introduction of a low percentage of a primitive Australian strain may provide just that extra range of variation necessary for the ultimate selection and development of a white stock adjusted to the tropical parts of Australia."[71]

Tindale signaled that Birdsell would soon publish a study of the physical results of racial admixture, supplementing the sociological reports. But Birdsell's war service delayed his analysis of the measurements of hybrids, and by the time he returned to his Australian data in the late 1940s, he had come to distrust racial typologies. In 1950, Birdsell warned Hooton that the project was no longer "a conventional racial analysis so much as the exploration of the evolutionary processes of selection, mutation, hybridization and drift." Influenced by new work in population genetics, Birdsell was trying to write about "population characteristics," not racial types, but it proved difficult to fit his old data to his changed frame of reference.[72] In the late 1930s, he had aggregated physical characters into abstract types, but now he wanted to trace the geographical distribution of variations among populations. The information he had collected with Tindale proved incompatible with his new analytic framework, and he was compelled to undertake more fieldwork in the early 1950s in Western Australia before he could write on contemporary evolutionary processes.

Before genetic nominalism corroded his confidence in racial type, and dissolved the categories that had structured the race-crossing data, Birdsell did publish some studies of the racial origins of Aboriginal Australians. From the beginning of their expedition, Tindale and Birdsell had obviously been interested in identifying traces of a number of original types in the Aboriginal population—they were already skeptical of the claims made by Cleland and others in the previous Adelaide generation for Aboriginal homogeneity. At the time, Birdsell in particular held a belief in hard heredity, in the preservation of ancestral elements or factors more or less unchanged—only recombined—in contemporary populations. His regression analysis of physical characters and blood group data seemed to confirm that Aborigines were not a pure, homogeneous race but consisted of three ethnic elements, variously blended. According to his trihybrid theory, the continental Australians were an amalgam of early Oceanic Negritos ("Barrineans"), a large element of primitive Caucasians ("Murrayians"), and a previously unidentified racial group ("Carpentarians"). Residual features of the Oceanic Negritos could be identified among the Tasmanians and a few rainforest tribes in the hinterland of Cairns, around Lake Barrine. Birdsell's measurements traced their origin to a people of short stature and dark skin, with woolly hair, a round head, and a narrow face.[73] Tindale's genealogical studies confirmed that "the Barrineans owe their unique traits to an ancient Negritic substratum, not to late prehistoric Papuan or historic Melanesian hybridisation."[74] A second wave of immigrants, "an archaic white or Caucasian group," the "Murrayians," had driven the primitive Negritos into the rainforests and to Tasmania or amalgamated with them elsewhere. Birdsell described them as short in stature, with light skin and wavy hair, a long head, large brows, and a wide nose. A third racial type, clustered around the shores of the Gulf of Carpentaria, had arrived still later. They were tall and dark, with wavy hair, a narrow head, and a very broad nose. According to Birdsell, their general appearance was "extremely primitive, generalised and non-white." They seemed to represent a fourth major racial division, equivalent in status to "the white, Mongoloid and Negroid groups." The last surviving representatives of this group were "the much-mixed dark-skinned peoples of India and the less-mixed Aborigines of northern Australia."[75]

Where Tindale—perhaps opportunistically—had discerned some advantage in the hybridization of European and Aboriginal Australians, Birdsell went further and claimed that the parental stocks were already thoroughly hybridized. Since the 1920s, the fragmentation of Europeans into Nordic, Alpine, and Mediterranean types had become a commonplace of racial thought—Jens Lyng, for example, had devised an elaborate calculation of the contributions of each type to the white population of Australia.[76] At the beginning of the century, John Mathew and others had suggested that the Aboriginal population was a biocultural hybrid, but Ramsay Smith, Wood Jones, and the rest of the Adelaide investigators had derided his views and claimed repeatedly that the continental type was purely, homogeneously Caucasian. Toward the end of the 1930s, the Adelaide consensus had begun to break down. In particular, Tindale began to doubt his colleagues' assertions of Aboriginal racial purity, and he conveyed his uneasiness to Birdsell and to Frank Fenner, a young craniologist at the South Australian Museum. Fenner, using craniological materials and techniques, had suggested that appreciable physical differences separated the Aborigines of southern Australia from those in the Northern Territory.[77] Birdsell's analysis of the anthropometric data that he collected during the 1938–1939 expedition implied an even greater diversity and dynamism in Aboriginal populations. Most of the earlier authors had viewed Aboriginal populations in static terms, as entities that remained intact through a series of migrations. Birdsell, by contrast, felt it was more profitable "to consider existing populations as merely transient by-products of the complicated processes of racial dynamics, a field in which hybridisation seems nearly always to have played an important role."[78] Thus in the 1940s Birdsell and Tindale were discussing the hybridization of already hybridized parent stocks: The mensurational and statistical complications were staggering, and the manifestations of such complex antecedent factors in hybrid offspring were unpredictable. The analysis of ever-proliferating hybrids of hybrids seemed to be leading to a hopeless disintegration of racial categories, perhaps to a raceless chaos.

For Birdsell, races—whether colored or white—were disappearing during the 1940s in a seemingly infinite regress of hard heredity, a process that ineluctably preserved antecedent factors. Although he remained a biological determinist, he was unable, on further reflection, to delimit any clear racial boundaries. Hybridity came to appear biologically persistent, even ineradicable; and as it proliferated through reproduction it rendered everyone heterogeneous and ultimately deracinated—there were no pure types, and perhaps there never had been. How, then, could one conduct an analysis of race-crossing? It proved impossible. The issue had not, in theory, presented many difficulties to an earlier generation of scientists at Adelaide: For Cleland and those others who assumed a softer heredity, absorption and biological homogeneity would eventually be determined by a genetic submergence and by adaptation to a common environment. But Birdsell and others, who at the time were more rigidly Mendelian and believed in a harder, more persistent heredity, found that the racial types that supposedly were crossing had become fragmented, so a framing of reproduction in terms of race-crossing would make little sense. Race-crossing was not so much a bad thing as meaningless. But if race was proving so difficult to define, then what was left as an organizing principle in human heredity? Birdsell and others during the 1940s increasingly turned to the analysis of families and tribes or clans and abandoned the search for any ideal type—and to a large extent their genealogical methods must have influenced their recognition of families as a useful unit of genetic analysis. Indeed, one of the great ironies of Tindale's genealogical research is that the information he collected would become the basis of the Aboriginal family history project, an effort to reconstruct the families whose destruction his science had initially promised to rationalize in the service of racial homogeneity.

The internal contradictions and confusions of racial analysis in Australia, the breakdown of the classificatory grid, had prepared the ground for Birdsell's abandonment of racial categories. There is no doubt that after World War II he became appalled by the revelations of Nazi racial policies. Furthermore, he was inspired by the work presented at the Cold Spring Harbor conference on quantitative biology, organized by Theodosius Dobzhansky in 1950, which emphasized population dynamics rather than racial typologies. But the origins of his conversion can be traced back to Australia a decade earlier, to his failed effort to explain its heterogeneous and disorderly reproductive frontier in terms of race-crossing.[79] Unfortunately, though, he did not publish his recantations of race theory until much later, long after his further fieldwork in Western Australia in the early 1950s—and he did so in North America, not Australia.

As a professor of biological anthropology at the University of California–Los Angeles, Birdsell would become a leading opponent of racial analysis and an advocate of microevolutionary studies. In the 1970s, he observed that no one has ever "produced a scientifically successful, closed taxonomy system" for humans. It was more realistic to think about interbreeding populations and the "continuous variation of biological characters in space," a complex process of blending and hybridization that might be analyzed quantitatively.[80] In particular, the biologist ought to consider evidence for the operation of gene flow and drift, as well as for evolutionary change in small local breeding populations, such as those found in the western deserts of Australia. "The game of classification," he wrote, perhaps reflecting on his work in the 1940s, "cannot be conducted scientifically because of the biological complexities inherent in subspecification." Birdsell recalled "a brilliant American physical anthropologist"—probably E. A. Hooton—who was "unfortunately not knowledgeable in biology" and resorted to a discussion of racial types. "Needless to say," Birdsell continued, "this typological approach was totally in biological error."[81] Thus in his textbook of the new physical anthropology, Birdsell warned that "the use of the term 'race' has been discontinued because it is scientifically undefinable and carries social implications that are harmful and disruptive." Moreover, "in the modern world it is not enough for an educated person to know that modern human variation is a product of micro-evolution; it is necessary to be able to grapple with and disarm racist dogma and argument."[82] At the end of his career, Birdsell admitted that working with Aboriginal people had "left the investigator with a profound feeling of the injustices suffered by native peoples under colonial regimes."[83] By then he and Tindale, who had retired as curator of ethnology at the South Australian Museum, had become supporters of Aboriginal self-determination and the land-rights movement that emerged in the 1970s.[84]

The Policy of Absorption

Cecil E. Cook, the chief medical officer, chief quarantine officer, and chief protector of Aborigines in the Northern Territory between 1927 and 1939, was among those who dreamed of giving the half-caste an "opportunity to evolve into a white man."[85] As far as he was concerned, science offered nothing but support for this project. The son of a general practitioner in west-central Queensland, Cook had studied medicine at Sydney and later specialized in tropical hygiene at the London School of Hygiene and Tropical Medicine. In the 1920s, he investigated leprosy in Aboriginal communities in the Northern Territory and Western Australia and looked for hookworm in Queensland. His studies of leprosy, and his quarantine duties, led him to advocate the segregation of Aborigines already suffering from contagious diseases.[86] But he thought that others, especially half-caste women, should be absorbed as much as possible into white society, partly to make sure they did not later become a "native reservoir" of disease.[87] In 1933, Cook declared that "experience shows that the half-caste girl can, if properly brought up, easily be elevated to a standard where the fact of her marriage to a white will not contribute to his deterioration."[88] Training and discipline might improve the prospects of all half-castes, turning the women into more skilled and dedicated homemakers and fitting the men for work as stockmen and drovers. Accordingly, the more absorbable children, especially the half-caste girls, should be removed from allegedly baleful influence of the native camp and brought up in a sanitary home, where they would receive appropriate instruction.

Cook had absorbed the absorptionist arguments of contemporary science:

> It is not to be supposed that such marriages are likely to produce an inferior generation. On the contrary, a large proportion of the half-caste female population is derived from the best white stock in the country, whilst Aboriginal inheritance brings to the hybrid definite qualities of value—intelligence, stamina, resources, high resistance to the influence of the tropical environment and the character of pigmentation which will serve to reduce the at present high incidence of skin cancer in the blond European.[89]

The protector of Aborigines assumed that half-caste girls would be acceptable as partners of white men, whereas half-caste men were unlikely swains of white women. Thus Cook's scientific breeding program would focus on Aboriginal women: Instead of ad hoc, unsupervised couplings of white men and Aboriginal girls, the state would take control of Aboriginal reproduction. In this way, state intervention substituted for frontier white men, rendering them reproductively invisible. Cook and others viewed such state involvement as a racial salvage operation, saving half-caste girls from returning to perversely masculine full-bloods or disreputable white bushmen. In Germany during the 1930s, these girls might have been regarded as undesirables and therefore sterilized; in Australia, however, they were to be absorbed in order to produce a biologically consolidated nation.

In his later reflections on the "native problem," Cook lamented the earlier failures of Aboriginal absorption. At first, "the fundamental incongruities of the native life-pattern prevented its harmonious assimilation intact into the fabric of the white social order." In particular, the indifference to wealth of the true nomads seemed incompatible with adaptation to white commercialism. Some anthropologists had proposed the establishment of inviolable reserves to protect the remaining traditional full-bloods. But in so doing, they had ignored "the fate of the bedraggled and pauperised remnant of broken tribes," the destiny of the fringe-dwellers. Moreover, such a policy would have promoted "the unchecked dissemination of communicable disease and inviolable sanctuary for the law-breaker."[90] The alternative policy of training Aborigines in the ways of civilization seemed more promising, but Cook believed that a reluctance to invest generously in assimilation had also led to disappointing results. The result of mission training and government supervision "was too often a youth unqualified for comfortable existence either in a native or a white society, a prey to a multitude of newly acquired wants which his limited abilities and impaired efficiency would not permit him to satisfy in the environment into which he was discharged." Cook argued instead for an education in self-reliance in the white community. "If the native is successfully to achieve integration into the general community he must evolve under environmental stresses from which he has hitherto been sheltered."[91]

In 1937, Cook and his state colleagues had gathered together in Canberra to discuss Aboriginal destiny in Australia. They generally agreed that the best hope "of the natives of Aboriginal origin, but not of the full-blood, lies in their ultimate absorption by the people of the Commonwealth."[92] Cook expressed his fears that segregation, the alternative to assimilation, would lead to black dominance in the north and the eventual subversion of white Australia. J. B. Cleland expatiated on the scientific justification for miscegenation, pointing out that the mixing of such closely related types would certainly produce "increased virility." But the leading advocate of assimilation at the conference was A. O. Neville, the chief protector of Aborigines in Western Australia. He could find no scientific reason not to absorb the dark Caucasians into the white race. What was the alternative? "Are we to have one million blacks in the Commonwealth," he asked the delegates, "or are we going to merge them into our white community and eventually forget that there were any Aborigines in Australia?."[93]

In Western Australia, Neville had abandoned efforts at segregation, convinced that the native's "emergence into civilisation or acceptance of a fuller civilisation is being forced upon him whether he likes it or not."[94] The Adelaide scientists assured the protector that there was no risk from intermarriage, as Aborigines are "people already allied to us by association, consanguinity and ancestry"—because they "predate us in some vague Caucasian direction," the mingling of blood presented "no marked antagonistic features."[95] Nonetheless, Neville predicted "a period of transition, a hiatus so to speak, between the present incongruity and a future of complete assimilation, a period of intense training in every sense of the word."[96] He supported the establishment of institutions for the further education of half-castes in white ways, but like Cook, Neville criticized the contemporary failure to invest properly in such retraining. The current half-caste camps fostered "dreadful conditions under which human life spawns and increases like an unhealthy fungal growth." The inmates "crowd together in mutual misery or transient enjoyment upon the flea-ridden, germ-impregnated soil of their reserves." Neville believed that the answer was to replace this site for the welding of Aborigines into "an ethnic coloured whole" with a total institution for the production of hygienic, self-possessed citizens.[97] He proposed an institution that focused on technical training, hard work, and compulsory sport, a place where "matters of hygiene should be an essential part of an inmate's training." Above all, and everywhere, "the unseen sympathetic hand of Authority should be there to support and guide."[98]

And though some adults might live at the training institution, the most important, and most susceptible, inmates were young half-caste children. From infancy, these special candidates for absorption would "sleep in their own exclusive dormitories, have their own classrooms, cooking, dining arrangements and playgrounds." According to Neville, Aboriginal families were invariably incompetent, and only "Authority can teach their children the right way to live."[99] All colored children should therefore be treated as orphans. But the protector remained frustrated by "our easy-going, oft-times sentimental attitude towards the semi-civilised natives." There was a naive mind-set that caused some to hesitate to take children from their parents. But if these potential partners for whites were not removed as infants, "they develop into weedy, undernourished semi-morons with the grave sexual appetites which characterise them." In contrast, "quadroons and nearer whites" who received white training soon "learn to forget their antecedents" and seldom reverted.[100] Within a few generations, Neville claimed, his plan for institutional assimilation would have "raised the social and moral outlook of the coloured people generally—instilled into them a sense of usefulness and a desire to create homes in accordance with white standards. . . . In short, it will complete their emancipation."[101] Residual blackness was the only thing preventing their recognition as citizens in the modern nation. Authority would train this out of them and allow them to merge into hygienic whiteness.

Not all authorities shared the "egalitarian" enthusiasms of Cook and Neville, though most were similarly interventionist. In Queensland, J. W. Bleakley, the chief protector of Aborigines between 1914 and 1942, was an advocate of the "benevolent supervision" of reserves for full-bloods and half-castes, but he opposed policies that would produce a race of "poor imitation whites." He sought to make Aborigines more socially acceptable, but he was not so committed to their biological absorption.[102] With Bleakley's departure, Queensland fell into line; by the 1950s all states and territories were vigorously pursuing policies of attraction and assimilation. It is likely that, from 1910 until 1970, between one in three and one in ten Aboriginal children were forcibly removed from their families, thus becoming stolen generations.[103]

THE CULTURES OF "HYBRIDITY"

In his introduction to Neville's *Australia's Coloured Minority*, A.P. Elkin, the professor of anthropology at the University of Sydney, observed that 30,000 or more half-castes "are in our midst, and partly of our blood, but they are not yet 'of us.'" Elkin, the leading social anthropologist in Australia, believed that "all human beings, irrespective of skin-pigmentation and ancestry, are born with like potentialities for living worthily, intelligently and happily." He called on his fellow whites to forget their "antipathy to darkish skin colour and broad noses" so that the egalitarian ideal of biological and social assimilation might be realized within two or three generations.[104]

The Sydney department of anthropology since its establishment in 1926 had been dedicated to guiding the management of native populations. From the beginning it had trained administrative cadets for the Australian territories of Papua and New Guinea; and the senior anthropologists at Sydney had frequently advised commonwealth and state governments on the appropriate treatment of Aboriginal communities. "Special attention," wrote Raymond Firth, "has been given to the discussion of the application of anthropological methods to colonial administration and the effects of the contact of Europeans with native peoples."[105] And where Elkin's predecessor at Sydney, A. R. Radcliffe-Brown, and most of his colleagues had reported mainly on traditional groups in Australia and the Pacific, Elkin came to realize in the 1930s that the half-caste problem was calling out for further anthropological analysis—but not for more physical studies. As a social anthropologist, Elkin showed little interest in the sort of biomedical investigations conducted by the Adelaide researchers. In 1935, reviewing the discipline in Australia, Elkin pointed out that "mere superficial measurements of the length and breadth and height of this, that, and the other, and of the colour and form of various external parts, no longer form the prevailing interest, though they are by no means overlooked, being of value for purposes of classification." Neither was Elkin advocating further academic studies of kinship and social structure. He had moved away from the rather arid and formulaic structuralism of Radcliffe-Brown; instead, he emphasized the importance of viewing Aborigines, whether full-blood or half-caste, as human personalities in challenging contemporary settings. "We anthropologists," he warned, "must take care lest, as a result of our scientific urge to systematise whatever we study, we abet the dehumanisation of a living people."[106] Elkin and his colleagues still felt that the biological capacities of Aboriginal Australians might limit their advancement, but they believed even more strongly that social anthropology and social psychology should smooth, as much as possible, the path of full-bloods and half-castes to adjustment. Just as it was necessary for whites to understand the traditional native in order to govern internal and external colonies, so too was knowledge of half-caste social life and psychology needed for whites to ensure that their charges fulfilled biological potential.

In 1934, Elkin made it clear that the Sydney social anthropologists "have no desire to preserve any of the Aboriginal tribes of Australia or of the islands in their pristine condition as 'museum specimens' for the purposes of investigation." Rather, they, "like all members of a 'higher' and trustee race, are concerned with the task of raising primitive races in the cultural scale"—as practical social analysts, they just wanted to make sure that such major change occurred smoothly.[107] Recent anthropological research had indicated the sources of social cohesion in Aboriginal life, the meaning of native customs, the close association with place, and the effects of European interference. Using this knowledge, government policies might be framed more effectively and more sensitively. Elkin argued for the preservation of totemic sanctuaries, or sacred sites, and the reservation of traditional land, with good hunting, for the remnant tribes. He called on the government to adopt a "sane native educational policy," which would help tribal and detribalized Aborigines to understand white customs and the market economy. "Wise teaching on religion and in the rudiments of science," he wrote, "should do much to enable the natives to pass through the difficult transition period for which we are responsible." The natives to whom he referred on this occasion were full-blood—half-castes were not yet major figures in his calculations. In the early 1930s, it was primarily to full-bloods that he wanted to guarantee "in the future a livelihood, justice, the opportunity to maintain and develop their social life, and a real share in the land which is their spiritual home as well as the source of their economic necessities."[108]

Even as Elkin was trying to promote the psychosocial adjustment of Aborigines to white civilization, a few psychologists were still expressing a low estimate of Aboriginal capacity to thrive in the new conditions. In *The Psychology of a Primitive People*, Stanley D. Porteus had praised the social intelligence of Aboriginal Australians while suggesting that other indices of mental ability placed the race at the level of the young white adolescent. Thus he reasoned that Aborigines might find employment at low levels in the white economy, but, like white adolescents, they would not engage in abstract thought at the higher levels of civilization. Aborigines, Porteus claimed, were so completely adapted biologically and mentally to their own environment that they could not adapt fully to a culture of a different type—unfortunately, they probably lacked the ethnic capacity for civilization.[109] Some other psychologists, Ralph Piddington most prominent among them, challenged Porteus, arguing that their own research demonstrated the capacity of individual Aborigines to adapt readily to the dominant culture pattern. Piddington urged more effort to ensure "a harmonisation of the native's scheme of values with our own." His studies in the Kimberley had implied that "just as we approach the neurotic, and try to persuade him to face his conflicts squarely instead of attempting to evade them, so we may attempt a cultural 're-education' by which our social neuroses shall resolve themselves."[110] Elkin attacked Porteus for basing his conclusions on small sample sizes, for the cultural bias of his tests, and for his unfamiliarity with native social life and habits. There had been few attempts to understand scientifically how the native might be helped to adapt to change. "Until this has been done," Elkin wrote, "we cannot say that it is impossible for the Aborigines to advance along the road of civilisation and be of positive value in the exploitation of Australia."[111]

During the 1930s, Elkin began to incorporate "mixed-blood" Aborigines in his plans for the great transition to civilization.[112] He criticized the lack of European-Australian vision, which condemned the Aborigines "to be but hangers-on to our civilisation, having no real part in it and yet more and more drawn or forced away from their own culture." Elkin wanted to know what effect this "catching" of civilization might have on the outlook of Aborigines—a class of people that included half-caste as much as full-blood. It seemed to him that Aboriginal custom was remarkably flexible and persistent, that those Aborigines who were adjusting to civilization were also retaining and adapting elements of traditional culture—they were not utterly detached and alienated. For example, during his fieldwork with the "Wailpi" in South Australia, Elkin had met "a half-caste who had been most of his twenty odd or thirty years amongst whites, and yet he was fully possessed by all the emotions attached to this symbol of the secret life [the bullroarer]; and this was just as true of the other half-castes."[113] For Elkin, the attachment seemed to derive from an education in traditional ways, not from any blood drive. Provided they were raised in the native camp as children, full-blood and half-caste alike continued to show interest in the totemic ancestors. Elkin could provide many other examples. "In spite of the evangelistic efforts and of the part played by the natives in our economic activities, their own culture was still functioning remarkably efficiently." Moreover, these persistent functions were aiding, not impeding, the civilizing process. The task of "civilising agents" was therefore "to preserve and modify or supplant the Aboriginal view of life and the rites and practices arising from it, that primitive man may still feel at home in the universe."[114] The Aboriginal might be civilizable, but only if social anthropologists could carefully guide and define the process.

Elkin had signaled the development of new hybrid cultures in Australia, a hybrid complexity linked only incidentally to the concurrent proliferation of biological hybridity that Birdsell was describing.[115] The social anthropologist recognized that half-castes, in particular, were not merely convertible figures in between cultures—not simply stranded in states of no culture or tracing cultural trajectories; rather, they were putting together functional cultures of their own, forms that might prove lasting and acceptable. Birdsell was pointing to an unpredictable generation of hybrid bodies; Elkin was suggesting a separable and stable multiplication of hybrid cultures within white Australia. In the 1940s and 1950s, many of Elkin's students—Marie Reay and Ronald and Catherine Berndt among them—would study the mixed native/proletarian cultures of emergent half-caste communities.[116] Whereas Cook and Neville, inspired in part by Adelaide arguments for biological absorption, hoped to assimilate and engulf the remnants of Aboriginal Australia—they would sink and show no trace—Elkin and other social anthropologists in Sydney and Melbourne documented the persistence, and recombination or readaptation, of half-caste cultural traits. A devout Anglican and humanitarian, Elkin promoted the recognition and acceptance of such hybrid difference in "white" Australia. His policy advice in the 1940s was "based on the hypothesis that the Aborigines (even of full-blood) could eventually become worthy citizens of the Commonwealth." Cleland and other medical scientists had proposed biological absorption; Elkin was more committed to cultural amalgamation and adjustment, with or without miscegenation. The acceptance of some physical and cultural hybridity, defined and managed by anthropologists, implied a notion of citizenship that pushed at the physical boundaries of whiteness, though it still was organized around conventions of whitelike behavior. "We must not be afraid to try new ways," Elkin wrote in 1944, "and trust to human nature—even if it be clothed in a dark skin."[117] It was a more generous notion of citizenship.[118]

By the 1940s, the biological substrate of population management in Australia had begun to fall apart. For a brief moment in the previous decade a sort of consensus had emerged. A combination of biological and educational measures, including selective immigration, institutional segregation of the unfit, and proper training, offered to solve the problem of the degeneration of the urban white child. Similarly, a combination of further racial mixing and natural selection, together with institutional segregation, drill, and discipline, might remedy the equally pressing problem of the half-caste child. Scientific management thus offered to preserve, or even improve, "white" Australia. But in the 1940s, elements of social and physical inheritance independently began to appear more persistent than ever before. Corporeal and cultural units might be recombined and readjusted, but they would not sink and disappear. Whiteness was fragmenting, both within the urban fortresses and out on the reproductive frontier. And as whiteness disintegrated into Nordic and other types, into ethnic groups, into the fit and unfit, into persistent nationalities, into durable half-castes, or into hybrids of any of these imagined types, not even an enlarged category such as Caucasian could consolidate it again. Scientists began to scoff at fictions of racial and cultural purity or homogeneity, and they predicted that Australia, biologically and socially, would come to take on a more variegated whiteness—if it remained white at all. Before the encouragement of immigration from the Mediterranean, far in advance of immigration from Asia and Africa, the intellectual foundations of Aboriginal self-determination and European multiculturalism were laid by fieldworkers on the fringes of outback towns and in the slums of the eastern cities. But elsewhere, in the broader European-Australian community and among many policymakers, an utterly absorbing white dreaming—manifested still in goals of racial exclusion or absoprtion—would continue for some time yet.

Conclusion:
Biology and Nation

DURING THE NINETEENTH CENTURY, biology had come to represent destiny, and ideas of nature would continue to give form to ideas of sociality and civility well into the next century. Nature's interlocutors, mostly scientists and medical doctors, seemed generally to speak a language of racial type and circumstance, blood and soil, heredity and adaptation, purity and danger, fit and stress. Their arguments resonated through the national public sphere. Accordingly, a writer in the first issue of the *Lone Hand*, a Sydney literary journal, praised the early white settlers who had "found that an absolutely virgin country was theirs to exploit"; they had displayed "that roving instinct which bespeaks the unconquerable Norse element in the British blood." Such "strenuous blood" now covered, and was apparently seeping deep into the soil of, "a country eminently suited for the founding of another home for our race in the Antipodes."[1] In science and literature, it thus appeared that race, nation, and citizenship were inextricably entwined. A few years later, in 1912, when Walter Murdoch, a literary critic and popular essayist, was putting together an account of civic rights and duties in Australia, it seemed natural for him to include a warning against the mixing of races in the new nation, "for such mingling always leads to the creation of a mongrel people," a contaminated stock that would never develop into a "true community." After all, he wrote, as citizens "we believe in 'racial purity.'"[2] The very word "Australia" had come to presuppose the biological qualifier "white"—the nation was, by then, the apparently predestined place of the working white man.

But Australia was not unique: The assumption that settlement and nationality would have a biological foundation was common to other settler societies, though perhaps it was rarely as pervasive as in the antipodes. Reading Charles Pearson's warning to the white races, *National Life and Character*, in 1894, Theodore Roosevelt, for example, reflected on what might cause "new nations of an old stock to spring up in new countries," such as Australia and the United States. In his opinion, "the peopling of the great island-continent with men of the English stock is a thousand-fold more important than the holding of Hindoostan for a few centuries." It was the "ethnic conquest" of a territory, a place that must henceforth be kept entirely white. The presence of the "Chinaman," whether in Australia or the United States, would be "ruinous to the white race," but these democracies, "with the clear instinct of race self-ishness, saw the race foe, and kept out the dangerous alien."[3] In 1910, Roosevelt, still a careful observer of race struggle in Australia, claimed to see "strange analogies in the phenomena of life and death, of birth, growth and change, between those physical groups of animal life which we designate as species, forms and races, and the highly complex and composite entities which arise before our minds when we speak of nations and civilizations." Moreover, it appeared that some races were better at building such highly complex entities than others. "For the last three centuries," the former president of the United States mused, "the great phenomenon of mankind has been the growth of the English-speaking peoples and their spread over the world's waste spaces." Like so many others, Roosevelt rejoiced to "see our blood live young and vital in men and women fit to take up the task as we lay it down; for so shall our seed inherit the earth."[4]

To understand the nation, one had to know the race. The clinic, the laboratory, and the public health office might be engaged in disease diagnosis, treatment, and prevention—but they were also sites where the national body was checked, registered, and restored. Doctors, medical scientists, public health officers, and, later, physical anthropologists, were experts in bodily reform and hygiene; therefore they also could represent themselves as experts in white citizenship and national destiny. Such biosocial expertise assumed various forms. In the nineteenth century, doctors had studied specifically British bodies in the antipodes, looking for any disease or degeneration that might have arisen from racial dislocation, from the potential mismatch of heredity and environment, of blood and soil. Later, medical scientists and national hygienists would attempt to survey and to regulate white bodies in the tropics and in the urban slums, searching for sources of disease and degeneration on the national frontier and deep within the national fortress. As the strange Australian environment, even in the north, was gradually exonerated, attention shifted to the bad seeds that must be excluded from the white nation or the bad seeds that must be sifted out from its urban beds. Eventually, other doctors and scientists, many of them now calling themselves "physical anthropologists," would try also to erase the "black spots"—the half-caste bodies—at the heart of white—or Caucasian—Australia. Although these projects might seek different targets, they all shared the goal of stabilizing a white national body.

And yet the whiteness that all these experts craved was changing over time; it varied according to disciplinary commitment; it responded flexibly to clinical demands and to political needs. This is not to say it was an empty category, but it does suggest that "whiteness" was a remarkably reactive subject position, a variable signifier of difference, not an assertion of fixed qualities.[5] In other words, medicalized whiteness in Australia did have content, but its content was generally heterogeneous and contingent, even if misrecognized and marked, at any one time and place, as homogeneous and stable. Whiteness thus was both a sovereign category and a flexible one. Whether framed as British, white, or Caucasian, there was always a desirable racial substance that might be investigated, registered, and disciplined—it was just that each white ideal was regularly transformed into another, requiring more research, more monitoring. Inevitably there was always an opposing, and defining, entity or type—sometimes an environment or climate, sometimes another race—but there was nonetheless something about whiteness itself that could be marked physiologically and behaviorally and imagined as an ideal of citizenship. In thus marking whiteness, even within such broad parameters, doctors and scientists gave the nation a type of body and mentality to which it might aspire, as well as a range of variants that could be included in the category, or excluded from it, as the need arose. In practice, of course, the white body was marked most obviously only at the margins of the nation—in the tropics and in the slums. For most other citizens—those deemed to have internalized the rules of bourgeois civility—their sense of whiteness simply became normal. That is, they eventually came to be recognized, and to recognize themselves, as unremarkably Australian, not white Australian.

Medicine had provided a vocabulary for talking about a territory and a means of taking imaginative possession of it; later still, it created a syntax for social citizenship and a means of living up to it. Once a resource for knowing and mastering the land, medicine focused in ever more narrowly on civility and responsible behavior, the guidance of proper living, discarding most— though not all—of its antecedent geographical concerns. Early settlers had tried to cultivate the land in order to establish a natural harmony of race and circumstance, to feel comfortably at home and thus healthy; later, national hygienists proposed instead a cultivation of the white social body in order to maintain or restore national vigor and efficiency. Whiteness still required cultivation, but in a significantly different way. Medical modernizers were attempting to break the old nexus of race and proper place and to mobilize carefully cultivated white bodies that would not need to feel "at home."

An association of civilization with the autonomous racial capacity for self-cultivation was gradually supplanting, except in geography, an older understanding of the environmental determinants of civilization. Degeneration, the specter that haunted civilized communities, had in the past seemed to derive from a depleting, degraded environment or climate; increasingly it appeared to sprout up from bad seeds within the autonomous race.[6] By the end of the nineteenth century, it was the social terrain, organized primarily by race and then by class and gender, that really mattered, not the physical topography and climate. Once a means to describe, or reinvent, "home," to resettle a race after the trauma of migration, medicine became more often a way to calculate modern kinship and civic responsibility, to articulate and negotiate biological qualifications for citizenship. The more "advanced" members of the profession, like W. A. Osborne, regarded the alienation and mobility of stable white bodies as sure signs of modernity, as examples of modern possibilities. With good breeding and meticulous hygiene, white bodies might reside anywhere and work efficiently; there would be no cause for nostalgia, for homesickness, in the modern nation.[7] After World War I, the state could harness science to identify, register, and simplify the population—it could try to get standardized white bodies to behave in standard, civilized white ways, whether at "home" or not.[8]

Scientific visions of white Australia commonly conjured up an ideal of biological homogeneity, a fantasy of organic integrity and stability. There were, as we have seen, many paths to the common destination, to this imagined community. Some experts postulated a Lamarckian alteration and convergence of national type; others pointed to a continuity of the white germ plasm, regardless of surroundings; still others proposed the submergence into the white gene pool of related Aboriginal elements. For some the ideal type was British; for others it was old white; for many it was new white; and for a few, after the 1920s, it might be Caucasian. In any case, the result would be a biologically homogeneous national body and mentality. Until the 1880s, many doctors and scientists, and probably the majority of their patients, had believed that a combination of novel environmental influences and absorption of other stocks would eventually produce a unique white Australian type, a new amalgam of blood and soil. But in the south, especially around Melbourne, the circumstances came so much to resemble British conditions that at the end of the nineteenth century few medicos could imagine much change in type. The tropics, however, still seemed so different from the ancestral environment that it was commonly expected, until well into the twentieth century, that whites residing there would degenerate, or at least alter their character. But by the end of the 1930s, even in the north, a sense of harder heredity, or at least an assumption of a more insulated and protected heredity—implying a happily alienated mobility of type—would prevail, though it was never undisputed. Raphael Cilento was one of the medical doctors still predicting change, and he confidently forecast an improvement of type, a virilization of tropical whites. Meanwhile, scientists in Adelaide were arguing for the absorption of dark Caucasians into a purely white Australia, a mergence that would hardly alter the predominant Eurotype—half-castes would supposedly sink and show no trace.

But then, just as a purely white Australia, populated by an old or a new type of white, seemed to take shape, to become flesh, it was beginning to pass away and dissolve. Increasingly confident assertions of white triumph in the tropics or the slums—the declarations of the successful establishment of a working white race—in fact disguised an underlying anxiety about white possession, both of self and territory. Making a national body was inevitably a process of loss and denial, and it involved uncertainty and ambivalence. Whiteness in Australia kept exciting more commentaries, more definitions, more proposals, but no matter how prolific they became, they never quite satisfied; no matter how apparently redundant the claims, there was always something that they could not cover. Whiteness in Australia, like its accompanying modernity, was "on endless trial."[9] The attempt to register and simplify and normalize whiteness in Australia would ultimately prove both excessive and inadequate. For every Cilento there was a Griffith Taylor; for every J. B. Cleland there would be a Joe Birdsell. Harsh landscapes and persistent Aboriginality—each substituting at times for the other—repeatedly returned to unsettle the modern white nation, making it feel strange and uncanny again.[10] Some geographers were undermining white territorial possession; a few anthropologists, sociologists, and biologists were challenging white self-possession. The geographers, such as Taylor, continued to disagree with assertions of white triumph in arid and tropical environments, devaluing the white carrying capacity of the continent.[11] Physical anthropologists, like Birdsell, began to question the biological reality of race and to deny the possibility of delimiting whiteness or seeking racial purity.[12] And so, by the 1940s, E. J. Brady's brittle construct of an unlimited white Australia was, in scientific circles at least, coming to appear ever more insubstantial and vacant.

In 1947, A. P. Elkin wondered if white Australia was doomed. According to geographers, it was still possible that "regions like Burketown and Cape York are not suitable for continuous habitation by Caucasians," and only selected persons would tolerate Cairns.[13] The anthropologist asked if "it may be necessary to open our doors to an ethnic group more adapted to the conditions. If it come to this point, shall we turn to southern Europe or to the Orient?" But Elkin preferred to make Aboriginal Australians into tropical settlers and citizens. "The result may not be a one hundred percent white skin colour; but Australia is not all-white now." In any case, he thought that far too much had been made of color and racial type—scientists had shown that color was no index of intelligence or cultural worth, and standards of living were related to social conditions, not some biological essence. For Elkin, in the late 1940s, "the slogan 'white Australia' seems like an echo, as from a parrot shut in a cage back in the 1880s—and it doesn't make sense."[14]

By the early 1970s, a white Australia policy could not be said to exist: The programs of racial exclusion and half-caste absorption were formally abandoned; few, if any, scientists and doctors were prepared to defend the old order. But even as multiculturalism was promoted, many Australians still yearned for a comfortable biological and cultural homogeneity and felt that much of the newly valorized diversity was "un-Australian." Indeed, ideas and categories from the medical past continue to shape contemporary discussions of cultural aspirations, national character, immigration barriers, and population policy. Organic models and biological analogies, by now well-disguised, still inflect arguments for and against Aboriginal assimilation or self-determination. It is perhaps too simple to listen to a contemporary politician, or a leader of some social movement, and claim to detect an echo of Cilento or Griffith Taylor, for times have changed, and the meaning of words and phrases has often altered considerably. But then again, one does not have to try very hard to discern some of the deeper contours of old biological thought under all the recent recultivation of Australia.[15] Race science may not inform research and practice in the clinic and the laboratory, but it remains the partly hidden bedrock underlying much public debate. Perhaps we should ask how one might imagine otherwise a nation that has from the beginning been predicated on biological homogeneity, on an organic unity that seemed to demand alienated exclusiveness. If these residues of race science—the legacies of pioneering medical research—were finally to erode away, what sort of nation would Australians find themselves in?

ABBREVIATIONS

Author's Note: The following abbreviations are used in the Notes and the Bibliography.

AAAS	Australasian Association for the Advancement of Science
ADB	*Australian Dictionary of Biography*
AITM	Australian Institute of Tropical Medicine
AMG	*Australasian Medical Gazette*
AMJ	*Australian Medical Journal*
BMA	British Medical Association
BMJ	*British Medical Journal*
MJA	*Medical Journal of Australia*
NAA	National Archives of Australia
PJS	*Philippine Journal of Science*
RAC	Rockefeller Archive Center

NOTES

1. Examples of the recent scholarly discovery of whiteness include bell hooks, "Representing whiteness: Seeing *Wings of Desire*"; David Roediger, *The Wages of Whiteness: Race and the Making of the American Working Class*; Theodore Allen, *The Invention of the White Race, Volume 1: Racial Oppression and Social Control*; and Richard Dyer, *White*. The intimate framing of colonial whiteness is revealed in Ann L. Stoler, *Race and the Education of Desire: Foucault's History of Sexuality and the Colonial Order of Things*; and Vicente L. Rafael, *White Love and Other Events in Filipino History*. One of the few historical accounts of whiteness to engage with medicine and science is Matthew Frye Jacobson, *Whiteness of a Different Color: European Immigrants and the Alchemy of Race*.

2. On the framing of disease, see Charles E. Rosenberg and Janet Golden, *Framing Disease: Studies in Cultural History*; and Robert Aronowitz, *Making Sense of Illness: Science, Society and Disease*. For a vivid account of some aspects of the experience of illness in Australia, see Janet McCalman, *Sex and Suffering: Women's Health and a Women's Hospital: The Royal Women's Hospital, 1856–1996*.

3. The models are Richard Hofstadter, *Social Darwinism in American Thought*; Greta Jones, *Social Darwinism and English Thought: The Interaction between Biological and Social Theory*; and Nancy Stepan, *"The Hour of Eugenics": Race, Gender and Nation in Latin America*. See also Bernard Smith, *European Vision and the South Pacific, 1768–1850*.

4. On the construction of the nation, see Benedict Anderson, *Imagined Communities: Reflections on the Origin and Spread of Nationalism*; and Richard White, *Inventing Australia: Images and Identity, 1688–1980*.

5. I should point out here, at the beginning, that "Irishness" is not addressed as a category separate from "Britishness" or from "whiteness"—simply because the doctors and scientists writing about race in Australia did not distinguish it in this manner. While the Irish were often the victims of popular prejudice, they did not figure in medical and scientific texts produced during this period, perhaps because

the "experts" regarded them as British enough or white enough in a sparsely populated continent.

6. Henry Reynolds, *Frontier: Aborigines, Settler and Land*; Patrick Wolfe, *Settler
Colonialism and the Transformation of Anthropology: The Politics and Poetics of an
Ethnographic Event*. Racial thought in Australia is also addressed in Tom Griffiths,
Hunters and Collectors: The Antiquarian Imagination in Australia. On the Aus-
tralian racialization of Asians, see David Walker, *Anxious Nation: Australia and the
Rise of Asia, 1850–1939*.

7. For the general history of race science, see Nancy Stepan, *The Idea of Race in
Science: Great Britain, 1800–1960*; and George W. Fredrickson, *The Black Image in
the White Mind: The Debate on Afro-American Character and Destiny, 1817–1914*.

8. Indeed, it is virtually impossible to identify any true polygenists in Australia
in the nineteenth century, even though Australian material was sometimes used by
North American and British polygenists to support their theories.

9. On "situated knowledges," see Donna Haraway, *Simians, Cyborgs and
Women: The Reinvention of Nature*. On the production of subject positions, see
Michel Foucault, *Discipline and Punish: The Birth of the Prison* and *History of Sex-
uality*.

10. Warwick Anderson, "Disease, race and empire," "Immunities of empire:
Race, disease and the new tropical medicine," and "Race, geography and nation:
Remapping 'tropical' Australia, 1890–1920."

11. A more detailed account can be found in Russell McGregor, *Imagined Destinies: Aboriginal Australians and the Doomed Race Theory, 1880–1939*.

12. On the discrediting of typological thinking in biology, see Elazar Barkan,
*The Retreat of Scientific Racism: Changing Concepts of Race in Britain and the
United States between the World Wars*; and Richard Lewontin, Steven Rose, and
Leon J. Kamin, *Not in Our Genes: Biology, Ideology and Human Nature*. The de-
ployment of biosocial notions of race in contemporary Australian debates is re-
viewed in Ghassan Hage, *White Nation: Fantasies of White Supremacy in a
Multicultural Society*; and John Docker and Gerhard Fischer, eds., *Race, Culture
and Identity in Australia and New Zealand*.

Chapter 1

1. George Wakefield to father, 30 November 1853, Wakefield papers, ms.
6331, State Library of Victoria. Wakefield had practiced as an apothecary in Reading, England, for ten years before heading to the Victorian diggings in search of
gold.

2. To mother, 23 November 1862, ibid. On human acclimatization (in particular, ideas about the adaptation of Europeans to tropical climates), see Philip D.
Curtin, *The Image of Africa: British Ideas in Action 1780–1950*; David N. Livingstone, "Human acclimatisation: Perspectives in a contested field of inquiry in science, medicine and geography," and "Climate's moral economy: Science, race and

place in post-Darwinian British and American geography"; Warwick Anderson, "Immunities of empire: Race, disease and the new tropical medicine, 1900–20"; Michael A. Osborne, "Resurrecting Hippocrates: Hygienic sciences and the French scientific expeditions to Egypt, Morea and Algeria"; Dane Kennedy, "The perils of the midday sun: Climatic anxieties in the colonial tropics"; and Mark Harrison, "'The tender frame of man': Disease, climate and racial difference in India and the West Indies 1760–1860," and *Climates and Constitutions: Health, Race, Environment and British Imperialism in India 1600–1850*. Although the colonial tropics became, in the nineteenth century, the locus classicus of acclimatization, the process might occur wherever the atmosphere or soil differed from the itinerant's home.

3. J. William McKenna, *Mortality of Children in Victoria*, pp. 4, 5.

4. R. E. Scoresby-Jackson, *Medical Climatology*, pp. viii, 3.

5. For the background to this environmental understanding of health and disease—known as medical geography, see Mirko Grmek, "Géographie médicale et histoire des civilisations"; Erwin Ackerknecht, *History and Geography of the Most Important Diseases*; L. J. Jordanova, "Earth science and environmental medicine: The synthesis of the late Enlightenment"; Warwick Anderson, "Disease, race and empire"; Caroline Hannaway, "Environment and miasmata"; and Conevery Bolton, The "Health of the Country": Body and Environment in the Making of the American West, 1800–60.

6. Charles E. Rosenberg, "The therapeutic revolution: Medicine, meaning and social change in nineteenth-century America." Of course, predisposition was influenced as much by recent intemperance and immorality as by heredity.

7. Ibid., p. 5.

8. John Harley Warner, *The Therapeutic Perspective: Medical Practice, Knowledge and Identity in America, 1820–85*, chapter 3.

9. In this chapter I will focus on southern mainland Australian perceptions and experiences. Unfortunately, there is very little medical material available from the island colony of Tasmania and the Swan River settlement, later Western Australia, during this period. This largely reflects the smaller scale of medical work in these communities, the lack of opportunity to publish, and the narrowly practical orientation of the local doctors.

10. On the uses of Hippocrates' tract, see Genevieve Miller, "*Airs, Waters and Places* in history"; Osborne, "Resurrecting Hippocrates"; and Hannaway, "Environment and miasmata."

11. L. Cowlishaw, "The first fifty years of medicine in Australia"; Edward Ford, "Medical practice in early Sydney, with special reference to the work and influence of John White, William Redfern and William Bland"; Bryan Gandevia, "The medico-historical significance of young and developing countries, illustrated by Australian experience"; and W. Nichol, "The medical profession in New South Wales, 1788–1850."

12. John White, *Journal of a Voyage to New South Wales*.

13. Arthur Phillip to Lord Sydney, 12 February 1790, *Historical Records of Australia*, ser. 1, vol. 1, p. 144. On variation in the perception of the new country, see

Alan Frost, "What created, what perceived? Early responses to New South Wales"; and Ross Gibson, *The Diminishing Paradise: Changing Literary Perceptions of Australia.*

14. David Collins, *An Account of the English Colony in New South Wales*, vol. 1, p. 40.

15. Watkin Tench, *Sydney's First Four Years*, p. 69. Tench stayed in the colony from 1788 until 1793.

16. John Hunter, *An Historical Journal of Events at Sydney and at Sea 1787–92*, p. 138. Hunter had been Phillip's deputy in the first years at Sydney.

17. Collins, *Account of the English Colony*, vol. 1, p. 127.

18. Tench, *Sydney's First Four Years*, pp. 266, 265.

19. Collins, *Account of the English Colony*, vol. 1, pp. 157, 229.

20. Peter Cunningham, *Two Years in New South Wales*, p. 94. Cunningham, who studied surgery at Edinburgh (1806–1810), took up land on the Hunter River, north of Sydney. He traveled widely in the colony in 1821–1822 and 1825–1826. In the 1830s, based in South America, he studied the effects of tropical climates on European constitutions. Barron Field, a judge of the Supreme Court of New South Wales, pointed out in 1825 that "no miasmata come from the marshes or fallen leaves of Australian forests. Intermittent fevers are unknown here" (*Geographical Memoirs of New South Wales*, p. 425).

21. Cunningham, *Two Years in New South Wales*, p. 94. Phthisis, or consumption, was what we might now call tuberculosis, the great scourge of the nineteenth century.

22. Ibid., pp. 94, 12.

23. John Dunmore Lang, *Emigration; Considered Chiefly in Reference to the Practicability and Expediency of Importing and of Settling Throughout the Territory of New South Wales, a Numerous, Industrious and Virtuous Agricultural Population*, p. 2.

24. John Dunmore Lang, *Cooksland in North-Eastern Australia; the Future Cotton Field of Great Britain: Its Characteristics and Capabilities for European Colonisation*, p. 218.

25. Samuel Butler, *Handbook for Australian Emigrants*, p. 4.

26. Ibid., p. 6.

27. Ibid., pp. 5, 6. Accordingly, Butler notes that "colonial disease in general, when it attacks the frame, is more acute and arrives more speedily at the crisis" (p. 6).

28. George Bennett, *Wanderings in New South Wales, Batavia, Pedir Coast, Singapore and China*, vol. 1, pp. 50–1. Bennett later settled at Sydney where he taught medicine and supervised the introduction of foreign plants and animals.

29. Ibid., pp. 340, 341.

30. Sir James Clark, *The Sanative Influence of Climate*, pp. 354, 348–9, 349. Scoresby-Jackson, in *Medical Climatology*, echoed Clark's opinions, confirming that "diseases are said to assume a milder form in New South Wales than in European countries" (p. 149). On the recurrent interest in Australia as a *temporary* sanatorium for British troops worn down by service in India, see Tasmanian Parliament, *Military Sanitarium: Report of the Board of Commissioners*; J. Stirling, *Ob-*

servations on the Climate and Geographical Position of Western Australia, and on Its Adaptation to the Purposes of a Sanatorium for the Indian Army; and Western Australian Parliament, *Dispatches on the Subject of the Establishment of a Sanitarium in Western Australia for British Troops Serving in India.*

31. Thomas Bartlett, *New Holland: Its Colonisation, Productions and Resources*, pp. 190, 194, 195.

32. Ibid., pp. 197, 198.

33. To Mary Wilsone, 6 April 1839, Wilsone papers, ms. 9825, box 267, State Library of Victoria.

34. To George Wilsone, 9 Sept 1839, 13 March 1840, ibid.

35. Ibid., 18 June and 30 August 1840. In his last letter to his brother, Wilsone (1791–1841) reflected that "I have been very successful in my medical profession and would have done well were I spared" (26 February 1841, ibid.). In one of the earlier exploring parties in the Port Phillip District, Joseph Tice Gellibrand "found the gleams of heat extremely oppressive and which brought on violent palpitations and a termination of blood to the head" (25 January 1836). Around Melbourne, he frequently had to lie down in the shade and take some calomel pills. See his "Memorandum of a trip to Port Phillip" in Thomas Francis Bride, ed., *Letters from Victorian Pioneers, Being a Series of Papers on the Early Occupation of the Colony*, esp. p. 8. Gellibrand died the following year, 1837.

36. P. Divorty, "The influence of an Australian climate on the constitution of the western European," pp. 85, 86.

37. Ibid., p. 86.

38. Ibid., pp. 87, 88, 90.

39. On the disputes between "moral enlightenment" and "conservatism" during the 1840s, see Michael Roe, *The Quest for Authority in Eastern Australia*. George Nadel provides the intellectual context for a slightly later period in *Australia's Colonial Culture: Ideas, Men and Institutions in Mid-Nineteenth-Century Australia.*

40. E. Alan Mackay, "Medical practice during the goldfields era in Victoria"; and Bryan Gandevia, "Land, labour and gold: The medical problems of Australia in the nineteenth century." More generally, see Centenary Celebrations Council, *Victoria, the First Century: An Historical Survey*; and Geoffrey Serle, *The Golden Age: A History of the Colony of Victoria, 1851–61.*

41. Gandevia, "Land, labour and gold." Mackay ("Medical practice") points out that in 1857 there were 487 registered medical practitioners active in Victoria, including seventy members of the elite medical society. On the strong Scottish contingent, especially in Victoria, see Laurence M. Geary, "The Scottish-Australian connection, 1850–1900."

42. Diary, 22 December and 9 December 1852, Selby papers, ms. 9866, State Library of Victoria.

43. To father, 1 May 1856, 10 October 1857, Wakefield papers, ms. 6331, State Library of Victoria.

44. Diary, 11 January 1854, McMillan papers, ms. 11634, box 1882, State Library of Victoria. McMillan (1825–1892) had come to Victoria through California

and practiced in Melbourne and near Geelong, visiting the diggings intermittently during the 1850s.

45. Ibid., 11 June 1855.

46. James Robertson, "On the nature or essence of disease in Victoria," p. 252.

47. Edward Hunt, "On colonial fever and on some recent cases of remittent fever," pp. 167, 170, 172. See also P. H. MacGillivray, "Notes of dissections of colonial fever."

48. Letter to editor, *Australian Medical Journal* 12 (1867), p. 96. In this letter, Thomas also speculated on the nature of "colonial pock" and "colonial itch." Thomas graduated in medicine from St Andrew's and became a leading surgeon at the Melbourne Hospital. See D. M. O'Sullivan, "David J. Thomas: A founder of Victorian medicine." "Garryowen" [Edmund Finn] describes Thomas as "in some measure addicted to stimulants [and] the most skilful surgeon and queerest fellow of his time" (*The Chronicles of Early Melbourne 1835–52: Historical, Anecdotal and Personal*, vol. 2, p. 882).

49. Thomas, quoted in Hunt, "Colonial fever," pp. 180, 181.

50. For the early work and organization of the "disciples of Aesculapius" in Melbourne, see "Garryowen," *Chronicles of Early Melbourne*, vol. 2, pp. 878–90; J. E. Neild, "The medical profession"; T. S. Pensabene, *The Rise of the Medical Practitioner in Victoria;* and Diana Dyason, "The medical profession in colonial Victoria 1834–1901." On the development of learned societies in colonial Australia more generally, see Michael Hoare, "Learned societies in Australia: The foundation years in Victoria 1850–60," and Science and Scientific Associations in Eastern Australia 1820–90; and Ann Moyal, *A Bright and Savage Land: Scientists in Colonial Australia.*

51. On the importance of the local and the regional in nineteenth-century medicine, see John Harley Warner, "The idea of Southern medical distinctiveness: Medical knowledge and practice in the Old South." For an overview of the nineteenth-century medical world, see W. F. Bynum, *Science and the Practice of Medicine in the Nineteenth Century;* and Christopher Lawrence, *Medicine in the Making of Modern Britain, 1700–1920.*

52. James Kilgour, *Effect of the Climate of Australia upon the European Constitution in Health and Disease*, pp. 3, 5, 9. David Wilsone knew Kilgour well, regarding him as "an active, pushing fellow" (letter to George Wilsone, 30 August 1840, Wilsone papers).

53. Ibid., pp. 26, 23.

54. C. B. Mingay Syder, *The Voice of Truth in Defence of Nature; and Opinions Antagonistic to Those of Dr. Kilgour*, pp. 3, 53. Syder, whose medical degree was from London, arrived in Geelong in 1850. A radical, he was a good friend of many Chartists and bequeathed his skeleton to the University of Melbourne. See Anon., "Obituary," *Australian Medical Journal (AMJ)* 16 (1871): 312–13.

55. W. J. Sterland, "Hints on the climate of Australia," pp. 671, 672.

56. Andrew Ross, "The climate of Australia viewed in relation to health," pp. 195, 196. Ross points out that previously "the unsettled disposition of the inhab-

itants and their migratory life" had hopelessly complicated the issue (p. 131). Moreover, the military and the convicts had been "too much under routine and discipline to be considered either a true or safe guide for us in speaking honestly of the effects of climate on health, or its influence on the constitution of the European immigrant" (p. 131). For more on Ross and Divorty, see Susan Hardy, "Ferments, zymes and the west wind: Adapting disease theories and therapies in New South Wales, 1860–80."

57. Kilgour, *Effect of the Climate of Australia*, pp. 8, 27.

58. James B. Clutterbuck, *An Essay in the Nature and Treatment of Australian Diseases, Including More Especially Dysentery and Fever*, p. 35. Clutterbuck, who had received his medical degree from Erlangen and practiced in Kilmore, north of Melbourne, persisted with depletive therapeutics long after his colleagues had adjusted their practices. "Garryowen" remarked of Clutterbuck that "his manner was as out of the way as his name" and joked that after he had moved to Kilmore it would more accurately be known as "Kill-more" (*Chronicles of Early Melbourne*, vol. 2, p. 884). In the first years of settlement other doctors had resorted more enthusiastically to the lancet. "I bled largely and never regretted it," the Paris-trained Dr. James W. Agnew wrote to Dr. Edmund Hobson on 20 April 1842. "I have often had the patient propped up in bed when he could not sit and bled to fainting" (Hobson papers, ms. 8457, box 865, State Library of Victoria). Agnew was practicing along the Saltwater River, now the Maribyrnong, near Melbourne.

59. Divorty, "Influence of an Australian climate," pp. 83, 84, 90.

60. Kilgour, *Effect of the Climate of Australia*, pp. 28, 25.

61. S. J. Magarey, "Our climate and infant mortality," pp. 4, 8. Magarey was a member of the South Australian Legislative Council and honorary physician to the Adelaide Hospital from 1850 until 1901.

62. Ross, "Climate of Australia," pp. 197, 196, 197. For more on gold fever, see Serle, *The Golden Age*; and David Goodman, *Gold Seeking: Victoria and California in the 1850s*, chapter 6.

63. Anon., "Local topics," p. 193. I am grateful to Cathy Coleborne for this reference. The eccentricity and insanity of shepherds was a commonplace of colonial Australia; see, for example, Edward M. Curr, *Recollections of Squatting in Victoria, then Called the Port Phillip District, from 1841 to 1851*, pp. 442–44.

64. C. Travers Mackin, "Sunstroke, or *coup de soleil*: Its causes, consequences and pathology," p. 6. See also Graham A. Edwards, "Sunstroke and insanity in nineteenth-century Australia."

65. Mackin, "Sunstroke," pp. 7, 9.

66. Ibid., pp. 10, 12.

67. Ibid., p. 85.

68. Kilgour, *Effect of the Climate of Australia*, p. 27; and Ross, "Climate of Australia," pp. 132, 230.

69. On colonial masculinity, see David Walker, "The getting of manhood"; and Marilyn Lake, "The politics of respectability: Identifying the masculinist context." For the development of ideas of manhood in the United States during this period,

see E. Anthony Rotundo, *American Manhood: Transformations in Masculinity from the Revolution to the Modern Era*. Australian anxieties about masculinity may be related to the subsequent assertiveness of the "Australian legend"; see Lake, "Politics of respectability," p. 117.

70. Divorty, "Influence of an Australian climate," p. 87.

71. Kilgour, *Effect of the Climate of Australia*, pp. 32, 33.

72. Mackin, "Sunstroke," p. 6n (emphasis in original).

73. Ross, "Climate of Australia," p. 134.

74. Syder, *Voice of Truth in Defence of Nature*, pp. 23, 19, 29, 30.

75. Hardy, in "Ferments, zymes," points out the neglect of indigenous therapies—they may have suited the climate, but they would have been inappropriate for the British physiological system.

76. Desmond Manderson indicates that until the end of the century opposition to the Chinese was rationalized largely on economic and aesthetic grounds. The Chinese may themselves have been described as "diseased," and their "filthy" or "loathsome" camps and quarters may have been regarded as dangerous, but they were not themselves given a major role in the transmission of disease to whites. See "'Disease, defilement, depravity': Towards an aesthetic analysis of health. The case of the Chinese in Australia." More generally, see Andrew Markus, *Fear and Hatred: Purifying Australia and California, 1850–1901*; and Kathryn Cronin, *Colonial Casualties: The Chinese in Early Victoria*.

77. For more detailed accounts, see J. B. Cleland, "Some early references to tuberculosis in Australia"; B. Thomas and B. Gandevia, "Dr Francis Workman, emigrant, and the history of taking the cure for consumption in the Australian colonies"; and J. M. Powell, "Medical promotion and the consumptive immigrant in Australia." Michael Roe surveys the Tasmanian scene in *Life over Death: Tasmanians and Tuberculosis*.

78. Sterland, "Hints on the climate of Australia," p. 672.

79. "Medicus," "Correspondence," pp. 156, 157.

80. S. D. Bird, "On chest complaints in Australia," p. 33. See also his "On consumption in Australia." Bird was a physician to the Benevolent Asylum and the Immigrants' Aid Society's hospital. "Medicus" would have read Bird's *On Australasian Climates and Their Influence on the Prevention and Arrest of Pulmonary Consumption*. For similar arguments, but with more emphasis on the benefits of sea voyages and change, see Isaac Baker Brown Jr., *Australia for the Consumptive Invalid: The Voyage, Climates and Prospects for Residence*. These theories derived largely from Ebenezer Gilchrist, *The Use of Sea-Voyages in Medicine, and Particularly in Consumption, with Observations on That Disease*.

81. Bird, "Chest complaints," pp. 43, 44–5.

82. I discuss the bacteriological critique of Bird's theories in Chapter 2.

83. S. D. Bird, "Climate and consumption," pp. 112, 117, 118. At the end of Bird's address to the Medical Society of Victoria, Dr. W. J. Thomas commented that the Melbourne climate in summer was notorious for "its depressing influence upon the human frame, and its baneful effects upon the digestive organs" (p. 20),

but he was prepared to endorse Bird's view that it was the best climate in the world for consumption. Even Isaac Baker Brown Jr. criticized Bird for his exoneration of the hot winds: In Sydney, Brown observed that the consequent "feverish heat and determination of blood to the head, with a difficulty of breathing, are symptoms confined to the white race alone" (*Australia for the Consumptive Invalid*, p. 40).

84. For a description of health-seeking on the U.S. frontier, see Sheila M. Rothman, *Living in the Shadow of Death: Tuberculosis and the Social Experience of Illness in American History.*

85. C. Faber, "Australasia and South Africa as health resorts, especially for consumptive immigrants," p. 30. See also his "Australasia, South Africa and South America as health resorts, comprising a medical climatology of the southern hemisphere." Faber was the medical officer at the German Hospital in London.

86. Warwick Anderson, "The natures of culture: Environment and race in the colonial tropics"; and Bolton, The "Health of the Country."

87. On the vast accumulation of detail that characterizes Humboldtian science, see Susan Faye Cannon, "Humboldtian science"; Michael Dettelbach, "Humboldtian science"; and Nicolaas Rupke, "Humboldtian medicine."

88. Sterland, "Climate of Australia," p. 671.

89. John Dickson Loch, Information in Regard to Adelaide and South Australia (c. 1838), ms. A2755, Mitchell Library, NSW.

90. To mother, 24 February 1864, Wakefield papers.

91. Divorty, "Influence of an Australian climate," p. 85. R. Brough Smyth thought that the Victorian hot winds were dangerous because they lacked ozone. He recommended a colonial ozone survey in "Ozone."

92. Ross, "Climate of Australia," pp. 164, 231.

93. R. G. Jameson, *Australia and Her Gold Regions*, pp. 6, 37.

94. William Kelly, *Life in Victoria, or Victoria in 1853, and Victoria in 1858*, vol. 1, pp. 300, 43. Kelly had arrived from California in 1853 in search of gold.

95. Ibid., pp. 300, 292. Kelly did concede that it was "not yet a climate for developing mellow beauties of the 'fat, fair and forty' category—at least, I have not seen any of them amidst a chaos of 'new ruins'" (p. 294).

96. Sterland, "Climate of Australia," p. 672.

97. Diary, 26 May 1855, McMillan papers.

98. Ross, "Climate of Australia," p. 260.

99. James E. Neild, "Some remarks on the diarrhoea and dysentery of this colony," p. 9. Neild, a trenchant and dogmatic physician and theater critic, was the editor of the *Australian Medical Journal* (1862–1879), a lecturer in forensic medicine at the University of Melbourne, and a leader of the profession in the 1860s and 1870s. See Harold Love, *James Edward Neild: Victorian Virtuoso.*

100. J. Gentilli, "A history of meteorological and climatological studies in Australia."

101. Bolton observes a similar concern in her wonderful study of perceptions of the healthfulness of Arkansas and Missouri (The "Health of the Country"). For other features in common with U.S. medical geographies (especially Southern

examples), see also Michael Owen Jones, "Climate and disease: The traveler describes America"; Karen Ordahl Kupperman, "Fears of hot climates in the Anglo-American colonial experience"; James H. Cassedy, "Medical men and the ecology of the Old South"; and Mart A. Stewart, "'Let us begin with the weather?': Climate, race and cultural distinctiveness in the American South."

102. On the colonial interest in improvement, physical culture, cultivation, gardening, and farming, see Roe, *Quest for Authority*.

103. William Howitt, *Land, Labour and Gold, or Two Years in Victoria with Visits to Sydney and Van Diemen's Land*, pp. 8, 9. Howitt (1792–1879), a Quaker writer, visited Australia between 1852 and 1854; his son Alfred stayed in Victoria and became a pioneer anthropologist (see Chapter 7). William Howitt spent his last years in Rome and was responsible for introducing eucalypts to the Campagna in the 1870s.

104. Howitt, *Land, Labour and Gold*, pp. 95, 70. F. Lancelott, in *Australia as It Is: Its Settlements, Farms and Goldfields*, urged gold-seekers to acclimatize in Sydney before heading inland, in order to prepare themselves for the chaotic diggings.

105. Howitt, *Land, Labour and Gold*, pp. 127, 84. C. R. Read, in *What I Heard, Saw and Did at the Australian Goldfields*, warns that the exposure to damp on the diggings would cause rheumatism and colds.

106. Howitt, *Land, Labour and Gold*, pp. 128, 129.

107. J. W. Mackenna, "On the comparative effect of climate on certain diseases," p. 16.

108. Christopher Rolleston, "The sanitary condition of Sydney," p. 38.

109. Ross, "Climate of Australia," p. 166.

110. See Warner, *Therapeutic Perspective*. In "The idea of Southern medical distinctiveness," Warner discusses a regional therapeutics that more closely resembles Australian precepts.

111. Divorty, "Influence of an Australian climate," p. 88.

112. Ross, "Climate of Australia," p. 200.

113. Clutterbuck, *Nature and Treatment of Australian Diseases*, pp. 1, 50.

114. George Bennett, *Gatherings of a Naturalist in Australia: Being Observations Principally on the Animal and Vegetable Productions of New South Wales, New Zealand and Some of the Austral Islands*, pp. 92, 94.

115. James Ballantyne, *Homes and Homesteads in the Land of Plenty: A Handbook of Victoria as a Field of Emigration*, p. 22. "Rolf Boldrewood" [T. H. Browne] also found another England in southern Victoria, according to his *Old Melbourne Memories*, pp. 43, 229.

116. J. Cecil Le Souef, "Acclimatisation in Victoria"; Linden Gillbank, "The Acclimatisation Society of Victoria," and "The origins of the Acclimatisation Society of Victoria: Practical science in the wake of the goldrush"; Michael A. Osborne, "A collaborative dimension of the European empires: Australian and French acclimatisation societies and intercolonial scientific cooperation"; Warwick Anderson, "Climates of opinion: Acclimatisation in nineteenth-century France and England"; and Thomas R. Dunlap, "The acclimatisation movement and Anglo ideas of nature."

117. "The Vagabond" [John Stanley James], *Vagabond Country: Australian Bush and Town Life in the Victorian Age*, p. 81. (This dispatch appeared in the *Argus*, 24 January 1885.)

118. Syder, *Voice of Truth*, p. 6. As early as 1825, Barron Field had suggested that "the climate of New South Wales is becoming generally cooler, as the colony gets cleared of timber" (*Geographical Memoirs*, p. 425). Similar speculation is found forty years later, in Brown, *Australia for the Consumptive Invalid*, p. 36. On the long-standing interest in the effects of human intervention on climate, see Clarence J. Glacken, *Traces on the Rhodian Shore: Nature and Culture in Western Thought from Ancient Times to the End of the Eighteenth Century*. More specifically, on the impact of civilization on the terrain, see Gilbert Chinard, "Eighteenth-century theories on America as a human habitat."

119. Kelly, *Life in Victoria*, p. 293. Evelyn P. S. Sturt, a brother of Charles Sturt, the explorer, had settled near Mt. Gambier, before "the march of civilisation." Even in 1853 he looked back to early days "as to some joyous scene of school-boy holidays." He too believed that the seasons appeared to "have undergone a considerable change, and to have become both colder and more moist, for, although a fire was fully appreciated, the weather generally was mild and dry." See his letter to C. J. La-Trobe (29 October 1853) in Bride, ed., *Letters from Victorian Pioneers*, p. 365.

120. "Garryowen," *Chronicles of Early Melbourne*, vol. 1, p. 35. See also vol. 1, p. 415.

121. James Bonwick, *Climate and Health in Australasia: New South Wales*, p. 2.

122. On the "innocence" of the observing bourgeois European in colonial circumstances, see Mary Louise Pratt, *Imperial Eyes: Travel Writing and Transculturation*.

123. To father, 25 January 1861, Wakefield papers.

124. Ibid., 21 March 1861.

125. Ibid., 25 November 1861. Wakefield died in Kerang in 1888 after being knocked over by a cab; he was alone and had been trying to raise some money for the passage home.

126. Curr, *Recollections of Squatting*, pp. 418, 182.

127. Howitt, *Land, Labour and Gold*, p. 447.

128. Ballantyne, *Homes and Homesteads*, pp. 97, 6.

129. Ibid., pp. 100, 102.

130. Bonwick, *Climate and Health in Australasia: New South Wales*, pp. 53, 54. Roe describes Bonwick as speaking "the unalloyed language of moral enlightenment" (*Quest for Authority*, p. 155).

131. James Bonwick, *Climate and Health in Australasia: Victoria*, pp. 41, 42.

132. "A Resident" [John Hunter Kerr], *Glimpses of Life in Victoria*, p. 81.

133. For a brilliant account of similar (but nonmedical) representations of the Australian landscapes, see Paul Carter, *The Road to Botany Bay: An Exploration of Landscape and History*. Carter's own phenomenology, his understanding that "biological constitution is itself a spatial configuration" (p. 82), echoes nineteenth-century medical theory.

134. For a more thoroughly psychoanalytic perspective, see Gillian Rose, *Feminism and Geography: The Limits of Geographical Knowledge*.

CHAPTER 2

1. "Henry Handel Richardson" [Ethel Florence Robertson], *The Fortunes of Richard Mahony*. The central figure of the trilogy, Richard Mahony, represents her father. See also "Henry Handel Richardson" papers, ms. 133, ser. 1 (Walter and Mary Richardson), boxes 1 and 2, National Library of Australia.

2. W. Lindesay Richardson, "Notes on some of the diseases prevalent in Victoria, Australia," p. 803.

3. Ibid., pp. 806, 812.

4. C.-E. A. Winslow, *The Conquest of Epidemic Disease*.

5. Erwin H. Ackerknecht, "Anticontagionism between 1821 and 1867." We would now perhaps more accurately characterize this as a dispute between those who thought that disease was communicable (whether generally infectious or directly contagious) and those who regarded it as generally noncommunicable. "Contagion" was a broader category—including anything communicable—in the nineteenth century than now.

6. Georges Canguilhem, *The Normal and the Pathological*; John Harley Warner, *The Therapeutic Perspective: Medical Practice, Knowledge and Identity in America, 1820–85*.

7. I discuss this tropical exceptionalism in Chapter 3.

8. Winslow, *Conquest of Epidemic Disease*.

9. Owsei Temkin, "An historical analysis of the concept of infection"; John K. Crellin, "The dawn of germ theory: Particles, infection and biology"; and Margaret Pelling, "Contagion/germ theory/specificity."

10. William Bulloch, *The History of Bacteriology*; Winslow, *Conquest of Epidemic Disease*; Gerald L. Gieson, *The Private Science of Louis Pasteur*.

11. Anne Hardy, *The Epidemic Streets: Infectious Disease and the Rise of Preventive Medicine, 1856–1900*; Alan M. Kraut, *Silent Travelers: Germs, Genes and the "Immigrant Menace"*; Judith Walzer Leavitt, *Typhoid Mary: Captive of the Public's Health*; and Nancy Tomes, *The Gospel of Germs: Men, Women and the Microbe in American Life*.

12. George Rosen, *A History of Public Health*; F. B. Smith, *The People's Health, 1830–1910*; John Duffy, *The Sanitarians: A History of American Public Health*; and Dorothy Porter, *Health, Civilisation and the State: A History of Public Health from Ancient to Modern Times*.

13. By this he means the neo-Hippocratic notion that "climate has stamped its indelible mark on racial constitution, not just physiologically, but psychologically and morally." See David N. Livingstone, "Climate's moral economy: Science, race and place in post-Darwinian British and American geography," p. 140.

14. Geoffrey Serle, *The Rush to Be Rich: A History of the Colony of Victoria, 1883–9*; Graeme Davison, *The Rise and Fall of Marvellous Melbourne*; Michael Cannon, *The Land Boomers*.

15. Nehemiah Bartley, *Australia's Pioneers and Reminiscences, 1849–94*, pp. 38–9.

16. Anthony Trollope, *Australia and New Zealand*, vol. 1, p. 25.

17. Richard Twopeny, *Town Life in Australia*, p. 1.

18. Francis W. L. Adams, *Australian Essays*, pp. 2, 61 (Adams's emphasis). "Mark Twain" [Samuel L. Clemens] also thought that the "juvenile city of sixty years and half a million inhabitants" was very American in style (*Following the Equator: A Journey Around the World*, vol. 1, p. 118).

19. Adams, *Australian Essays*, pp. 6, 57.

20. Milton Lewis and Roy MacLeod, "A working man's paradise? Reflections on urban mortality in colonial Australia, 1860–1900"; David Dunstan, *Governing the Metropolis: Politics, Technology and Social Change in a Victorian City: Melbourne, 1850–1901*, esp. chapters 5 and 9; and Bryan Gandevia, *Tears Often Shed: Child Health and Welfare in Australia from 1788*. Sydney was no better; see A.J.C. Mayne, *Fever, Squalor and Vice: Sanitation and Social Policy in Victorian Sydney*; and P. H. Curson, *Times of Crisis: Epidemics in Sydney 1788–1900*.

21. For example, in the 1880s the numbers rose from 202 in 1881 to 420 in 1891, just before the depression caused a contraction of the medical marketplace, forcing many of these doctors to move to other colonies (Davison, *Rise and Fall of Marvellous Melbourne*, p. 97).

22. Diana Dyason, "The medical profession in colonial Victoria, 1834–1901." See also K. F. Russell, "Medicine in Melbourne—the first fifty years"; T. S. Pensabene, *The Rise of the Medical Practitioner in Victoria*; Evan Willis, *Medical Dominance: The Division of Labour in Australian Health Care*; and Milton Lewis and Roy MacLeod, "Medical politics and the professionalisation of medicine in New South Wales, 1850–1901." Bryan Gandevia makes the point that doctors in colonial Victoria had a higher status than in Britain as there were few rivals in the young community as well-educated ("The medico-historical significance of young and developing countries, illustrated by Australian experience").

23. K. S. Inglis, *Hospital and Community: A History of the Royal Melbourne Hospital*; Ann M. Mitchell, *The Hospital South of the Yarra: A History of the Alfred Hospital, Melbourne, from Its Foundation to the 1940s*; Janet McCalman, *Sex and Suffering: Women's Health and a Women's Hospital. The Royal Women's Hospital, 1856–1996*.

24. Dyason, "Medical profession in colonial Victoria"; K. F. Russell, *The Melbourne Medical School, 1862–1962*. The *Australian Medical Journal* in 1896 became the *Intercolonial Medical Journal of Australia*, which in 1910 reverted to the original name. It merged with its Sydney rival, the *Australasian Medical Gazette* (1881), in 1914 to form the *Medical Journal of Australia*. The University of Sydney did not open its medical school until 1883, and Adelaide followed two years later. The Medical Society of Victoria (MSV) was the successor of the Port Phillip Medical Association (1846) and the Victorian Medical Association (1852). Branches of the British Medical Association (BMA) were established in Victoria in 1879 and in New South Wales in 1880; the MSV amalgamated with the BMA (Victorian branch) in 1907. (See Ann Tovell and Bryan Gandevia, "Early Australian medical associations.")

25. *Argus* (27 February 1878), p. 2, quoted in Dunstan, *Governing the Metropolis*, p. 258.

26. It is likely that the category of "typhoid" included some cases of what we would now define as "other gastroenteritis." There are discussions of "infant cholera" during this period, in reference to very severe bouts of diarrhea, but no

evidence that the cholera vibrio was transmitted in Australia. See J.H.L. Cumpston and F. McCallum, *The History of the Intestinal Infections (and Typhus Fever) in Australia, 1788–1923.*

27. J. M. Gunson, "On typhoid fever," p. 107.

28. Bryan Gandevia, "William Thomson and the history of the contagionist doctrine in Melbourne." Thomson (1819–1883) was one of the first supporters of Darwinian evolution in the colonies. He also issued a series of pamphlets claiming that Bacon had written Shakespeare's plays. In Melbourne, James Robertson, at the Melbourne Hospital, had accepted some role for germs in the generation of disease as early as 1865, and William Gillbee introduced a form of Listerian antisepsis in 1867. See also Diana Dyason, "William Gillbee and erysipelas at the Melbourne Hospital: Medical theory and social actions"; and Gregory Tunchon, "Germ theory: Practical implications for medicine in Victoria."

29. William Thomson, *On Typhoid Fever*, p. 64.

30. Ibid., pp. 64, 89, 157. Carl Joseph Eberth identified the germ of typhoid in 1881.

31. Anon., "Review of William Thomson, *On Typhoid Fever*," pp. 220, 220, 223, 228.

32. Patrick Smith, "On the aetiology of typhoid fever."

33. William McCrea, *Observations on Typhoid Fever*, pp. 6, 5.

34. William Thomson, *Contagion Alone the Cause of Typhoid Fever in Melbourne.* For more equivocal support of contagionism, see C. K. Mackellar, "Notes on the aetiology of typhoid fever"; and John Rutherford Ryley, "Notes on the aetiology of typhoid fever."

35. *Argus* (1 May 1879), quoted in Dunstan, *Governing the Metropolis*, p. 258. Not until 1887 did the Board of Health rule unequivocally on the matter, accepting the contagiousness of typhoid and recommending isolation of sufferers, compulsory notification, proper disposal of excreta, protection of milk and water supplies, and general hygiene (Victorian Central Board of Health, *Typhoid Fever*).

36. James W. Barrett, *Typhoid Fever in Victoria*, p. 25. This is probably the first book published by a graduate of the Melbourne medical school.

37. James Jamieson, "Influence of meteorological conditions on the prevalence of typhoid fever," pp. 97, 100.

38. Winslow, *Conquest of Epidemic Disease*; and Leavitt, *Typhoid Mary*.

39. William Thomson, *The Germ Theory of Disease Applied to Eradicate Phthisis from Victoria*, p. 35.

40. Ibid., pp. 35–36.

41. *Royal Commission into Diphtheria.* See also J.H.L. Cumpston, *The History of Diphtheria, Scarlet Fever and Whooping Cough in Australia*; and F. B. Smith, "Comprehending diphtheria." For parallel developments, see Evelynn Hammonds, *Childhood's Deadly Scourge: The Campaign to Control Diphtheria in New York City, 1880–1930.*

42. William Thomson, *Remarks on the Introduction of Diphtheria into Victoria*, pp. 5, 10, 10. See also William Thomson, "Notes on the report of the chairman of the Diphtheria Commission."

43. James Jamieson, "Some points in the pathology of diphtheria," p. 66.

44. Diana Dyason, "James Jamieson and the ladies." Jamieson (1840–1916) was the medical officer for the city of Melbourne between 1885 and 1912.

45. James Jamieson, "Diphtheria and its treatment."

46. James Jamieson, "On the hypothesis of the faecal origin of the contagium of diphtheria," pp. 336, 339.

47. John Blair, "Diphtheria and diphtheritic diseases," p. 298.

48. H. B. Allen, "Notes on the pathology of diphtheria." Allen visited Koch's laboratory in the 1880s and later, as dean of the Melbourne medical school, became the leading advocate of bacteriological research in Victoria. See also Anon., "Diphtheria discussion at the Medical Society."

49. Thomas Cherry, "Diphtheria antitoxin." For local studies that indicated a dramatic fall in case mortality, see T. Cherry and C. H. Mollison, "68 cases of diphtheria"; and J. W. Springthorpe, "Six instances of the use of diphtheria antitoxin." T. Eastoe Abbott reported from Hobart in "Cases of diphtheria treated with antitoxin." In Sydney, W. Camac Wilkinson thought "the effect was truly magical" ("Two cases of diphtheria treated with Behring's antitoxin," p. 233). The antitoxin could also be used to prevent the spread of the disease; but mass immunization against the microorganism did not begin until after 1945.

50. James Jamieson, "On the parasitic theory of disease," p. 317.

51. Ibid., p. 323.

52. James Jamieson, "On the exact role of the pathogenic bacteria," pp. 1, 7.

53. A. Jefferis Turner, "The place of bacteriology in practical medicine," p. 202.

54. See Warwick Anderson, "Excremental colonialism: Public health and the poetics of pollution."

55. For a discussion of hygiene and citizenship, see Warwick Anderson, "Leprosy and citizenship"; and Alison Bashford, "Epidemic and governmentality: Smallpox in Sydney 1881." More generally, on the civic response to smallpox, see Alan Mayne, "'The dreadful scourge': Responses to smallpox in Sydney and Melbourne, 1881–2."

56. H. K. Rusden, "On contagious disease," p. 39. Rusden, a well-known freethinker, was addressing the health section of the Melbourne Social Science Congress.

57. Winslow, *Conquest of Epidemic Disease.*

58. J. W. Springthorpe, *Unseen Enemies and How to Fight Them*, p. 4. On the Australian Health Society and other sources of health education, see Judith Raftery, "Keeping healthy in nineteenth-century Australia."

59. Ibid., pp. 5, 14, 15. See also D. Astley Gresswell, "The management of communicable disease." Gresswell was the chief medical officer in Victoria and was well known for his progressive tendencies.

60. Anon., "Discussion of the report on the prevalence of phthisis in Victoria." For a further reiteration of Bird's opinions, see Samuel Dougan Bird, "On the influence of the Australasian climates on imported phthisis." See also Bryn Thomas and Bryan Gandevia, "Dr Francis Workman, emigrant, and the history of taking the cure for consumption in the Australian colonies"; J. M. Powell, "Medical promotion and the consumptive immigrant to Australia"; A. J. Proust, *History of*

Tuberculosis in Australia, New Zealand and Papua New Guinea. On tuberculosis in the northern hemisphere, see F. B. Smith, *The Retreat of Tuberculosis, 1850–1950*; Shiela Rothman, *Living in the Shadow of Death: Tuberculosis and the Social Experience of Illness in American History*; and Georgina Feldberg, *Disease and Class: Tuberculosis and the Shaping of Modern North American Society.*

61. Samuel Dougan Bird, "On chest complaints in Australia," pp. 41, 129, 130.

62. "Medicus," "The influence of the Victorian climate upon phthisis," pp. 25, 26, 26. James Jamieson also endorsed, with some reservations, the healthfulness of country Victoria and recommended against adopting a town life, in "Victoria as a health-resort."

63. William Thomson, *A Consumptive Voyage to the Medical Society*, pp. 3, 5, 8, 12. Bird responded to earlier criticisms by Thomson, claiming that his critic was a writer "more remarkable for the 'acrimony' of his style, his liberal use of the dictionary of quotations, and his fractious opposition to all that is unconnected to his own limited circle of admirers, than for anything he has done to further the interests of medicine and pathology in this colony" ("On consumption in Australia," p. 80). Charles Evans Reeves, a Melbourne doctor, also warned against travel to Australia in *Consumption in Australia.*

64. William Thomson, *On Phthisis and the Supposed Influence of Climate*, pp. 65, 95.

65. Thomson, *Germ Theory of Disease*, pp. 13, 14, 11.

66. Ibid., pp. 62–3.

67. Ibid., pp. 24, 65.

68. Ibid., p. 52.

69. Bird, "Climate and consumption," p. 123.

70. John Singleton, "Phthisis in Victoria," p. 280. His views had not changed since he wrote "On phthisis in Victoria." For similar views, see Anon., "Report of the special committee of the Medical Society of Victoria on phthisis in Victoria."

71. F. von Mueller, "Phthisis and the eucalypts," p. 53.

72. Robert Koch, "Aetiology of tuberculosis," pp. 424–5. In 1890, Koch announced the discovery of tuberculin, and though there was a brief enthusiasm for this as a treatment of the disease, it soon came to be used only for diagnostic screening. As late as the 1890s a few Melbourne doctors still doubted the contagious character of tuberculosis; see Duncan Turner, *Is Consumption Contagious?* Turner, the physician at the Benevolent Asylum, remained convinced that personal contact posed no danger.

73. Jamieson, "Exact role of the pathogenic bacteria," p. 6.

74. C. F. Coxwell, "A study of phthisis mortality in Victoria"; and D. A. Gresswell, "Prevalence of tuberculosis in Victoria."

75. Springthorpe, *Unseen Enemies*, pp. 4, 12. Springthorpe's diaries are an expression of his overwhelming grief (Springthorpe papers, ms. 9898, bay 11/4, State Library of Victoria).

76. Thomson, *On Typhoid Fever*, p. 108.

77. Twopeny, *Town Life*; see also Andrew Brown-May, *Melbourne Street Life: The Itinerary of Our Days*.

78. Nancy Stepan, "Biology and degeneration: Races and proper places." Daniel Pick describes fears of degeneration within Europe during this period in *Faces of Degeneration: A European Disorder, c.1848–c.1918*.

79. Charles E. Rosenberg, "The bitter fruit: Heredity, disease and social thought."

80. See the correspondence with Agnew in Hobson papers, ms. 8457, box 865/1, State Library of Victoria.

81. Adrian Desmond, *The Politics of Evolution: Morphology, Medicine and Reform in Radical London*, p. 375; and W. F. Bynum, *Science and the Practice of Medicine in the Nineteenth Century*. On Lamarck, see Richard W. Burkhardt Jr., *The Spirit of System: Lamarck and Evolutionary Biology*.

82. James Kilgour, *Effect of the Climate of Australia upon the European Constitution in Health and Disease*, pp. 6, 14, 16.

83. Henry Kingsley, *Recollections of Geoffrey Hamlyn*, vol. 1, p. 295.

84. Samuel Mossman and Thomas Banister, *Australia Visited and Revisited: A Narrative of Recent Travels and Old Experiences in Victoria and New South Wales*, pp. 79, 80, 80–81.

85. Andrew Ross, "The climate of Australia viewed in relation to health," pp. 132, 134.

86. Charles Dilke, *Greater Britain: Charles Dilke Visits Her New Lands, 1866 and 1867*, pp. 87, 151. For other fears of climate-induced physical degeneration in the 1860s and 1870s, see W. F. Mandle, "Cricket and Australian nationalism in the nineteenth century." Historians seem to have held to these notions longer than most: Geoffrey Blainey has suggested that "the physique of the cornstalk was, presumably, shaped partly by climate" ("Climate and Australia's history," p. 8).

87. Anon., "Will the Anglo-Australian race degenerate?" H. Ling Roth, a pioneer anthropologist, thought there had not yet been enough time to determine if the climate would be detrimental; see "The influence of climate and soil on the development of the Anglo-Australian race."

88. Halford (1824–1910) arrived in Melbourne in 1862 and was for many years the mainstay of the tiny medical school. W. A. Osborne believed that "Halford built up a great school of medical teaching, but he did not create a school of research" ("George Britton Halford: His life and work," p. 69.) On Owen and anatomical idealism, see Desmond, *The Politics of Anatomy*. The Australian context is described in Ann Mozley, "Evolution and the climate of opinion in Australia, 1840–76"; Barry W. Butcher, Darwinism and Australia, 1836–1914, and his "Darwin down under: Science, religion and evolution in Australia." More generally, see Thomas F. Glick, ed., *The Comparative Reception of Darwinism*.

89. T. H. Huxley, *Man's Place in Nature and Other Anthropological Essays*; and Charles Darwin, *On the Origin of Species by Means of Natural Selection, of the Preservation of Favoured Races in the Struggle for Life*. See D. R. Oldroyd, *Darwinian Impacts: An Introduction to the Darwinian Revolution*; Peter J. Bowler, *Evolution: The History of an Idea*; and Adrian Desmond and James Moore, *Darwin*.

90. G. B. Halford, *Not Like Man: Bimanous and Biped, nor yet Quadrumanous, but Cheiropodous*, p. 16; and William Thomson, *Not Man, but Man-like*. Halford responded with *Lines of Demarcation between Man, Gorilla and Macaque*. The debate between Halford ("Alferd") and Thomson ("Waldman") was the subject of George Isaacs's "The Burlesque of Frankenstein; or the Man-Gorilla," published in *Rhyme and Prose; and a Burlesque and Its History*. Isaacs has Alferd say: Ah! Doctor Waldman comes: the sceptic Donkey, / Who would have man to be the heir to monkey; / Who *bones* the *feet* of finger-footed apes. / And at the *foetid* members cuts and scrapes / To prove a foot's a hand, as if when proved, / A man would be a monkey once removed. / The infidel! The devil! (p. 1)

91. Charles Darwin, *The Descent of Man and Selection in Relation to Sex*. On the reception of this work, see Nancy Stepan, *The Idea of Race in Science: Great Britain, 1800–1960*, esp. chapter 3.

92. D. A. Gresswell, *Darwinism and the Medical Profession*, p. 42. Gresswell was influenced by William Aitkin, "Darwin's doctrine of evolution in explanation of the coming into being of some diseases"; and James Bland-Sutton, *Evolution and Disease*. See W. F. Bynum, "Darwin and the doctors: Evolution, diathesis and germs in nineteenth-century Britain."

93. The impact of the environment was muted further in the early twentieth century with the development of theories that postulated a harder heredity, especially after August Weissmann proposed the continuity of the germ plasm, that is, the utter imperviousness of all hereditary material to its surroundings. I discuss this in later chapters. See Peter Bowler, *The Eclipse of Darwinism: Anti-Darwinian Theories in the Decades around 1900*.

94. Stepan, "Biology and degeneration."

95. James Bonwick, *Climate and Health in Australasia: New South Wales*, pp. 53, 66.

96. Twopeny, *Town Life*, p. 89.

97. Marcus Clarke, *The Future Australian Race*, pp. 20, 22. For Clarke's satirical comments on the Melbourne medical world, see L. T. Hergenhan, ed., *A Colonial City: High and Low Life. Selected Journalism of Marcus Clarke*. Francis Adams, in *Australian Essays*, agreed with Clarke on the character of the coming Australian, but only if the distinct Melbourne and Sydney types were to merge. For more on the Australian type, see Richard White, *Inventing Australia: Images and Identity, 1688–1980*. It could be argued that earlier medical notions of change of type had licensed speculation on the evolution of a national identity. Russel Ward takes for granted such typological thinking in *The Australian Legend*. J. B. Hirst urges historians to "establish the other legends, stereotypes and symbols Australians have made or adopted" ("The pioneer legend," p. 337).

98. "The Vagabond" [John Stanley James], *Vagabond Country: Australian Bush and Town Life in the Victorian Age*, p. 163. The article first appeared in the Melbourne *Argus,* 20 March 1886.

99. For descriptions of the liberal elite in Melbourne during this period, see F. B. Smith, Religion and Freethought in Melbourne, 1870 to 1890; and Stuart Macintyre, *A Colonial Liberalism: The Lost World of Three Victorian Visionaries*.

100. James C. Scott, *Seeing Like a State: How Certain Schemes to Improve the Human Condition Have Failed*. See also Warwick Anderson, "The natures of culture: Environment and race in the colonial tropics."

101. On the need of modernity for the emergence of "garden cultures," see Ernest Gellner, *Nations and Nationalism*; and Zygmunt Bauman, "Gamekeepers turned gardeners."

102. On social citizenship, see T. H. Marshall, "Citizenship and social class"; and Bryan Turner, "Contemporary problems in the theory of citizenship." On the nexus of hygiene and citizenship, see Anderson, "Leprosy and citizenship"; Porter, *Health, Civilisation and the State*; and Alexandra Minna Stern, "Secrets under the skin: New historical perspectives on disease, deviation and citizenship." As Nancy Tomes points out, to slightly different effect, "adherence to the 'gospel of germs' became the *sine qua non* of modern citizenship" (*The Gospel of Germs*, p. 233).

CHAPTER 3

1. On the mutually productive distinction between the tropical North and the temperate South, see Jon Stratton, "Deconstructing the Territory."

2. Samuel Mossman and Thomas Bannister, *Australia Visited and Revisited: A Narrative of Recent Travels and Old Experiences in Victoria and New South Wales*, pp. 291–2.

3. Anthony Trollope, *Australia and New Zealand*, vol. 1, p. 25.

4. Charles Dilke, *Greater Britain: Charles Dilke Visits Her New Lands, 1866 and 1867*, pp. 92–3.

5. Raymond Williams, "Ideas of nature."

6. I discuss these tropes in greater detail in "The natures of culture: Environment and race in the colonial tropics." See also David Arnold, *The Problem of Nature: Environment, Culture and European Expansion*; and Ann Laura Stoler, *Race and the Education of Desire: Foucault's History of Sexuality and the Colonial Order of Things*. More generally, see Stephen Horrigan, *Nature and Culture in Western Discourses*; and James Duncan, "Sites of representation: Place, time and the discourse of the Other."

7. Ann Laura Stoler and Frederick Cooper, "Between metropole and colony: Rethinking a research agenda," p. 16.

8. Erwin Ackerknecht describes a persisting tropical exceptionalism in medicine in *The History and Geography of the Most Important Diseases*. See also Warwick Anderson, "Immunities of Empire: Race, disease and the new tropical medicine."

9. On the transition from a generic medicine of warm climates to a microbial tropical medicine, see Warwick Anderson, "Disease, race and empire"; John Farley, *Bilharzia: A History of Imperial Tropical Medicine*; David Arnold, *Colonizing the Body: State Medicine and Epidemic Disease in Nineteenth-Century India*; and Mark Harrison, *Public Health in British India: Anglo-Indian Preventive Medicine, 1859–1914*. There are also a number of useful edited collections: David Arnold, ed., *Imperial Medicine and Indigenous Societies*, and *Warm Climates and Western*

Medicine: The Emergence of Tropical Medicine, 1500–1900; Roy MacLeod and Milton Lewis, eds., *Disease, Medicine and Empire: Perspectives on Western Medicine and the Experience of European Expansion*; and Waltraud Ernst and Bernard Harris, eds., *Race, Science and Medicine, 1700–1900*.

10. Charles A. Price makes a similar point in *The Great White Walls Are Built: Restrictive Immigration to North America and Australasia, 1836–88*. Among scientists, "Caucasian" gains in popularity in the 1920s and 1930s, but it never really displaces "white" to become as conventional as in the United States. I discuss this further in Chapter 6. See also Matthew Frye Jacobson, *Whiteness of a Different Color: European Immigrants and the Alchemy of Race*.

11. Randolph Bedford, *Explorations in Civilisation*, pp. 8–9, 9. Bedford (1868–1941) was a contributor to the popular nationalist *Bulletin* and was Labor member for Warrego in the Queensland Legislative Assembly from 1923 until his death.

12. A. M. McIntosh, "Early settlement in northern Australia."

13. Peter G. Spillett, *Forsaken Settlement: An Illustrated History of the Settlement of Victoria, Port Essington, North Australia, 1838–49*. See also Alan Powell, *Far Country: A Short History of the Northern Territory*. For contemporary reports on northern Australia, see C. C. MacKnight, ed., *The Farthest Coast: A Selection of Writings Related to the History of the Northern Coast of Australia*.

14. John McArthur to D. Thomson, colonial secretary, 24 May 1843, NSW Governor's Despatches, January-September 1843, vol. 42, A1231, Dixson Library, pp. 1359, 1361. McArthur attributed most fever and debility to the climate; he was convinced that the common ophthalmia was due to the high winds (to Sir George Gipps, 3 September 1842, NSW Governor's Despatches, August–September 1842, vol. 40, A1229, p. 266). McArthur was concerned to build up the constitutions of whites in such harsh conditions and found that a stimulant such as "beer is very efficacious in preserving the stamina of men subjected to considerable labour and exposure" (to D. Thomson, colonial secretary, 25 April 1845, NSW Governor's Despatches, June–December 1845, vol. 48, A1237, p. 551).

15. John McArthur to D. Thomson, colonial secretary, 24 August 1843, NSW Governor's Despatches, October–December 1843, vol. 43, A1232, pp. 385, 379–80.

16. T. H. Huxley, *Diary of the Voyage of HMS Rattlesnake*, p. 148. The quotation is dated 31 December 1848, some time after leaving Port Essington. Huxley also noted that "there is as much petty intrigue, caballing and mutual hatred as if it were the court of the Great Khan" (p. 149). See also J. McGillivray, *Narrative of the Voyage of HMS Rattlesnake*; and Adrian Desmond, *Huxley: From Devil's Disciple to Evolution's High Priest*.

17. John McArthur to D. Thomson, colonial secretary, 24 August 1843, NSW Governor's Despatches, October–December 1843, vol. 43, A1232, Dixson Library, p. 386.

18. Douglas Gordon, "Sickness and death at the Moreton Bay convict settlement."

19. Ross Patrick, *A History of Health and Medicine in Queensland, 1824–1960.* See also Helen Woolcock, "'Our salubrious climate': Attitudes to health in colonial Queensland."

20. Patrick, *History of Health and Medicine in Queensland.* I discuss the developing medical understanding of malaria and hookworm in later chapters.

21. G. A. Bolton, *A Thousand Miles Away: A History of North Queensland to 1920.*

22. On the history of the labor trade, see B. H. Molesworth, "Kanaka labour in Queensland"; Peter Corris, *Passage, Port and Plantation: A History of the Solomon Islands Labour Migration, 1870–1914*; Kay Saunders, *Workers in Bondage: The Origins of Unfree Labour in Queensland, 1824–1916*; and Ralph Schlomowitz, "Epidemiology of the Pacific labour trade."

23. The Chinese in New South Wales constituted 3.7 percent of the colony's population in 1861, but only 1.4 percent in 1881; in Victoria the figures were 4.6 percent in 1861 and 1.4 percent in 1881. The numbers continued to fall: Of the 40,000 or so in all the colonies in 1880, only 10,000 remained in 1890, mostly working as gardeners, rural laborers, hawkers, shopkeepers, and cooks. See Price, *Great White Walls.* See also Andrew Markus, *Fear and Hatred: Purifying Australia and California, 1850–1901*; and A. T. Yarwood and M. J. Knowling, *Race Relations in Australia: A History.*

24. Cathy May, *Topsawyers: The Chinese in Cairns, 1870–1920,* and "The Chinese in the Cairns district, 1876–1920."

25. Henry Reynolds, "Townspeople and fringe dwellers." On race relations in Queensland generally, see Raymond Evans, Kay Saunders, and Kathryn Cronin, *Exclusion, Exploitation and Extermination: Race Relations in Colonial Queensland.*

26. Powell, *Far Country*; B. R. Davidson, *The Northern Myth: A Study of the Physical and Economic Limits to Agriculture and Pastoral Development in Tropical Australia.* I discuss the Northern Territory in more detail in Chapters 7 and 8.

27. J. Aitken White, "On the fevers of the Gulf of Carpentaria," p. 362 (White's emphasis).

28. Graham Browne, "Charters Towers from 1882 to 1890," pp. 319, 321.

29. Philip James, "Remarks on the fevers and diseases of tropical Queensland," p. 301.

30. David Hardie, *Notes on Some of the More Common Diseases in Queensland in Relation to Atmospheric Conditions, 1887–91*, pp. 104, 113.

31. J. Sidney Hunt, "The evolution of malaria," pp. 77, 76. Hunt had spent five years at Hughenden.

32. T. S. Dyson, "Malarial fevers of tropical Queensland," p. 64.

33. Carl Lumholtz, *Among Cannibals: An Account of Four Years' Travels in Australia and of Camp Life with the Aborigines of Queensland*, pp. 61, 62. Lumholtz (1851–1922) was later associated with the Museum of Natural History in New York and collected extensively in Mexico.

34. Hardie, *Notes on Diseases*, p. 8.

35. Ibid., p. 74.

36. See David N. Livingstone, "Human acclimatisation: Perspectives in a contested field of inquiry in science, medicine and geography"; Dane Kennedy, "The perils of the midday sun: Climatic anxieties in the colonial tropics"; and Mark Harrison, "'The tender frame of man': Disease, climate and racial difference in India and the West Indies, 1760–1860," and *Climates and Constitutions: Health, Race, Environment and British Imperialism in India, 1600–1850.*

37. Joseph Ahearne, "Presidential address, North Queensland Medical Society," p. 293.

38. Ibid., p. 293.

39. J. S. Hunt, "Notes on the demography of North Queensland," pp. 594, 595. Although Hunt cited Darwin, he was obviously most impressed with the more Lamarckian features of Darwin's work.

40. James Hingston, "A coming citizen of the world," p. 91.

41. William J. Sowden, *The Northern Territory As It Is: A Narrative of the South Australian Parliamentary Party's Trip*, pp. 146–7.

42. *Queensland Parliamentary Debates* 40 (1884), p. 52, quoted in Patrick, *History of Health and Medicine in Queensland*, p. 360.

43. *Queensland Parliamentary Debates* 47 (1885), p. 847, quoted in Patrick, *History of Health and Medicine in Queensland*, p. 360.

44. Edmond Marin La Meslée, *The New Australia*, p. 204.

45. R. W. Dale, "Impressions of Australia. II: Speculations about the future," pp. 838–9.

46. Alfred Searcy, *In Australian Tropics*, pp. 363, 366. Searcy was in Darwin from 1882 until 1896.

47. Alfred Deakin, *London Morning Post* (6 March 1907), quoted in John Lack and Jacqueline Templeton, eds., *Sources of Australian Immigration History, Volume 1: 1901–45*, p. 16.

48. Robert Gray, *Reminiscences of India and North Queensland, 1857–1912*, pp. 247, 257.

49. Gilbert White, *Thirty Years in Tropical Australia*, p. 102.

50. Gilbert White, "Some problems of Northern Australia," pp. 57, 58.

51. A.T.H. Nisbet, "Discussion," in the *Transactions of the Ninth Session of the Australasian Medical Congress*, p. 533.

52. J. Langdon Parsons, "Quarterly report on the Northern Territory, March 31, 1885," p. 7.

53. Kay Saunders, "Masters and servants: The Queensland sugar workers' strike, 1911," p. 98. More generally, see Evans, Saunders, and Cronin, *Exclusion, Exploitation and Extermination*. On an earlier climatic rationalization of slavery in North America, see Gary Puckrein, "Climate, health and black labour in the English Americas."

54. Patrick, *History of Health and Medicine in Queensland*, p. 531. Dr. F. Bowe, from Maryborough, assured his medical colleagues that few Kanakas suffered from typhoid, and in general "disease is not accompanied by the usual amount of pain and distress" ("Diseases of Polynesians, as seen in Queensland," p. 59).

55. Matthew Macfie, "How can tropical and sub-tropical Australia be developed?" p. 606.

56. Antill Pockley, "Presidential address," p. 491.

57. Macfie, "Tropical and sub-tropical Australia," p. 602.

58. Baldwin Spencer, quoted in ibid., p. 600. Given his later support for the Australian Institute of Tropical Medicine, Spencer's attitude was probably more ambivalent than Macfie suggested. On Spencer, see D. J. Mulvaney and J. H. Callaby, "*So Much That Is New." Baldwin Spencer, 1860–1929.*

59. Quoted in Macfie, "Tropical and sub-tropical Australia," p. 605. The original is in Benjamin Kidd, *Control of the Tropics*, pp. 48–50. On Kidd, see David P. Crook, *Benjamin Kidd: Portrait of a Social Darwinist.*

60. Macfie, "Tropical and sub-tropical Australia," p. 599. Macfie was probably referring to Woodruff's *The Effects of Tropical Light on White Men*. On Woodruff, see Warwick Anderson, "'The trespass speaks': White masculinity and colonial breakdown."

61. Lt.-Col. Charles E. Woodruff, M.D., to Dr. Richard Arthur, 9 July 1913, reprinted in *Australasian Medical Gazette* (30 August 1913), pp. 206–8.

62. H. Ling Roth, "The influence of climate and soil on the development of the Anglo-Australian race."

63. James Bonwick, *Climate and Health in Australasia: Queensland*, pp. 41, 42.

64. Ibid., p. 57. Like many other observers, Bonwick attributed the high Islander death rate to nostalgia and demoralization. If Chinese died in their natural climate it was because "they are none too clean in their personal habits" (p. 41).

65. A. Norton, "Settling in Queensland and the reasons for doing so—with special reference to droughts," p. 147. Norton's experience of severe droughts in NSW had led him to fear dryness far more than any humidity.

66. W. Lockhart Morton, "Notes of a recent personal visit to the unoccupied Northern District of Queensland."

67. J. A. Panton, "A few days ashore in West Kimberley," p. 70.

68. Ibid., p. 77. See also J. A. Panton, "The discovery, physical geography and resources of the Kimberley District, Western Australia."

69. John Forrest, "The Kimberley District," p. 146.

70. John Mackie, "In the Far North," p. 50.

71. Anon., "Bystander's notebook" (12 May 1888), p. 3, and (24 March 1888), p. 3 (Bystander's emphasis).

72. "Queenslander," "Coloured labour and Queensland sugar," pp. 339, 343, 340.

73. "Killeevy," "Queensland: The colossus of the North," p. 17.

74. Quoted in Harry T. Easterby, *The Queensland Sugar Industry: An Historical Review*, p. 24.

75. On transformations in the sugar industry, see Bolton, *A Thousand Miles Away*; Doug Hunt, "Exclusivism and unionism: Europeans in the Queensland sugar industry, 1900–10"; and Saunders, "Masters and servants." On the economic grounds for the repatriation of Pacific Islanders after 1901, see Adrian

Graves, "The abolition of the Queensland labour trade: Politics or profits?" and "Crisis and change in the Queensland sugar industry, 1863–1906."

76. Anon., "Overflowing China: Travelling through the lands invaded by the Mongol. II: Port Darwin," p. 14.

77. Anon., "Bystander's notebook" (7 January 1888), p. 3.

78. Randolph Bedford, "White, yellow and brown," p. 227.

79. J. Ahearne, "The Australian in the tropics," Red Page, *Bulletin* (29 September 1900).

80. A. G. Stephens, "The Australian in the tropics," Red Page, *Bulletin* (13 October 1900).

81. J.S.C. Elkington, "The Australian in the tropics," Red Page, *Bulletin* (3 October 1900). For more on Elkington, see Chapter 4.

82. "Mitty from Mackay," "The Australian in the tropics," Red Page, *Bulletin* (24 November 1900).

83. S. J. Richards, "The Australian in the tropics," Red Page, *Bulletin* (29 December 1900).

84. Alan Birch, "The implementation of the White Australia Policy in the Queensland sugar industry, 1901–12"; and Peter Corris, "White Australia in action: The repatriation of the Pacific islanders from Queensland." On the survival of the Pacific Islander community in North Queensland, see Clive Moore, *Kanaka: A History of Melanesian Mackay.*

85. Myra Willard, *History of the White Australia Policy to 1920*; N. B. Nairn, "A survey of the white Australia policy in the nineteenth century"; A. C. Palfreeman, "The White Australia Policy."

86. Alfred Deakin, *London Morning Post* (12 November 1901), quoted in Lack and Templeton, eds., *Sources of Australian Immigration History*, vol. 1, p. 11.

87. *Commonwealth Parliamentary Debates* 4 (6 September 1901), p. 4626.

88. Ibid., p. 4633.

89. Ibid., p. 4662.

90. *Commonwealth Parliamentary Debates* 6 (14 November 1901), p. 7246.

91. *Commonwealth Parliamentary Debates* 4 (6 September 1901), p. 4646.

92. Ibid., p. 4649.

93. Ibid., p. 5173.

94. Ibid., p. 4626.

95. Ibid., p. 4654.

96. Ibid., p. 4659. Manifold endorsed the proposal for an empty north (ibid., p. 4663). McDonald also believed that it would be better to leave the north undeveloped than "to attempt to develop [it] by employing colonial labour" (*Commonwealth Parliamentary Debates* 4 [12 September 1901], p. 4848). Bamford, however, argued that there were insufficient data to disparage the north, and he had observed that the children of the tropics compared favorably with those of the temperate south (ibid., p. 4834).

97. J. C. Watson, "Our empty north: An unguarded gate," pp. 425, 426.

98. The phrase is from J.H.L. Cumpston, *Quarantine: Australian Maritime Quarantine and the Evolution of International Agreements Concerning Quarantine*, p. 14.

99. Cumpston, *Quarantine*, p. 12; and W. Perrin Norris, "Report on Quarantine in Other Countries and on the Quarantine Requirements of Australia," p. 32. On the links made between disease and ethnicity in the U.S. quarantine service during this period, see Howard Markel, *Quarantine! East European Jewish Immigrants and the New York City Epidemics of 1892*; and Alan M. Kraut, *Silent Travelers: Germs, Genes and the "Immigrant Menace."*

100. Edward Palmer, *Early Days in North Queensland*, p. 2.

101. Ibid., pp. 163, 164. In the 1880s, Burketown rose from the ashes.

102. "Bill Bowyang" [Alexander Venard], "On the top rail," p. 40.

103. Norris, "Report on Quarantine"; and C. R. Wilburd, "Notes on the history of maritime quarantine in Queensland, 19th century."

104. Alan Mayne, "'The dreadful scourge': Responses to smallpox in Sydney and Melbourne, 1881–2."

105. J.H.L. Cumpston makes this point most strongly in *Quarantine*, where he states that "the Australian population is, from the point of view of the hygienist, an unvaccinated population" (p. 14). See also J.H.L. Cumpston, *The History of Smallpox in Australia, 1788–1908*. Cholera was detected in Australian waters only once, on the *Dorunda* that called at Townsville in 1885. Plague did not become a major concern until the end of the century.

106. Howard Markel has noticed a similar pattern in the United States in *Quarantine!*

107. Desmond Manderson, "'Disease, defilement, depravity': Towards an aesthetic analysis of health. The case of the Chinese in Australia"; and Alan Mayne, "'The dreadful scourge.'"

108. Alison Bashford, "Quarantine and the imagining of the Australian nation," p. 387.

109. Peter Baldwin makes a similar point in *Contagion and the State in Europe, 1830–1930*, pp. 529–36. Baldwin also argues that states deemed closer to the disease source, and those more sparsely populated, tended to favor quarantine in the late nineteenth century. For the origins of the debate on the relations of disease control and styles of governance, see Erwin H. Ackerknecht, "Anticontagionism between 1821 and 1867"; and Roger Cooter, "Anticontagionism and history's medical record."

110. C.E.W. Bean, *The Dreadnought of the Darling*, p. 318.

111. *Commonwealth Parliamentary Debates* (8 October 1903), pp. 5933–34.

112. E. W. Cole, *A White Australia Impossible*, p. 5.

113. Anon., "Are we turning black? The Northern Territory problem. Professor David's opinion," p. 210.

CHAPTER 4

1. "Robert Easterley" and "John Wilbraham" [Robert Potter], *The Germ Growers: An Australian Story of Adventure and Mystery*, p. 138. Potter was the canon of St Paul's Cathedral, Melbourne.

2. Ibid., pp. 177, 184.

3. H. H. Scott, *A History of Tropical Medicine*; and Eli Chernin, "Patrick Manson (1844–1922) and the transmission of filariasis." Murray Verso has related these developments to Australian conditions in "Airs, waters and places."

4. C.-E. A. Winslow, *The Conquest of Epidemic Disease: A Chapter in the History of Ideas*, chapter 16. See also Chapter 2 of this book.

5. Michael Worboys, "The emergence of tropical medicine: A study in the establishment of a scientific specialty"; Philip Manson-Bahr, *History of the School of Tropical Medicine in London, 1899–1949*; B. H. Maegraith, "History of the Liverpool School of Tropical Medicine"; and Helen J. Power, *Tropical Medicine in the Twentieth Century: A History of the Liverpool School of Tropical Medicine, 1898–1990*.

6. Andrew Davidson, ed., *Hygiene and Diseases of Warm Climates*; Patrick Manson, *Tropical Diseases: A Manual of the Diseases of Warm Climates*.

7. On ideas of race during this period, see Nancy Stepan, *The Idea of Race in Science: Great Britain, 1800–1960*; and George M. Frederickson, *The Black Image in the White Mind: The Debate on Afro-American Character and Destiny*. For Australia, see Douglas Cole, "'The crimson thread of kinship': Ethnic ideas in Australia, 1870–1914"; and C. L. Bacchi, "The nature-nurture debate in Australia, 1900–14."

8. Warwick Anderson, "Immunities of empire: Race, disease and the new tropical medicine."

9. Charles E. Rosenberg, "The bitter fruit: Heredity, disease and social thought."

10. Charles Darwin, *The Descent of Man and Selection in Relation to Sex*. I discuss the earlier reception of this work in Melbourne in Chapter 2. See also Michael Adas, *Machines as the Measure of Men: Science, Technology and Ideologies of Western Dominance*.

11. August Weissmann, *The Germ Plasm: A Theory of Heredity*; William Bateson, *Mendel's Principles of Heredity: A Defence*; and Hugo de Vries, *Species and Varieties: Their Origin by Mutation*. See also Stepan, *Idea of Race in Science*; Peter Bowler, *The Eclipse of Darwinism: Anti-Darwinian Evolution Theories around 1900,* and *Evolution: The History of an Idea*.

12. Oswald P. Law and W. T. Gill, "A white Australia: What it means," pp. 146, 149.

13. Ibid., p. 149.

14. Ibid., pp. 151, 154.

15. F. Goldsmith, "The necessity for the study of tropical medicine in Australia."

16. F. Goldsmith, "Tropical disease in Northern Australia."

17. J.S.C. Elkington, *Tropical Australia: Is It Suitable for a Working White Race?*, pp. 7, 5, 6, 7. After graduating in medicine at the University of Melbourne, Elkington studied for a Diploma of Public Health in London. On his way back to Australia he was briefly attached to the Imperial Plague Research Laboratory in Bombay. With his relatives, the Lindsays, he mixed with Melbourne's bohemia

and wrote fiction for the *Bulletin*. He gave the impression that he was as comfortable in the boxing ring as in an art gallery. See Michael Roe, "John Simeon Colebrook Elkington (1871–1955)," *Australian Dictionary of Biography* (*ADB*) 8, pp. 425–6, and *Nine Australian Progressives: Vitalism in Bourgeois Social Thought, 1890–1960*, chapter 4. Jack Lindsay describes Elkington as his surrogate father in *Life Rarely Tells*.

18. T. P. McDonald, "Tropical lands and white races," p. 203.

19. Ibid., pp. 204, 207, 208.

20. Ibid., p. 214.

21. James Cantlie, "Discussion" in ibid., p. 214.

22. McDonald, "Tropical lands and white races," p. 225, 228.

23. Cumpston to Sutton, n.d., Correspondence leading to the establishment of the Australian Institute of Tropical Medicine (AITM), A1928/575/28, National Archives of Australia. Chamberlain had been the British secretary of state for the colonies and a leading supporter of tropical medicine in Britain. The Hospital for Tropical Diseases was attached to the London School of Tropical Medicine.

24. Michael Roe, "John Howard Lidgett Cumpston (1880–1954)," *ADB* 8, pp. 174–6; Roe, *Nine Australian Progressives*, chapter 3; and Margaret Spencer, *John Howard Lidgett Cumpston, 1880–1954: A Biography*. Cumpston had been raised as a Methodist in Box Hill, then a village outside Melbourne, and he retained a narrow evangelical outlook. After graduating in medicine at Melbourne he completed a diploma of public health at London, worked briefly with C. J. Martin at the Lister Institute, and visited the Institut Pasteur in Paris. Cumpston later became the director of the Federal Quarantine Service (1913) and the first director of the Commonwealth Health Department (1921). He was also a historian of the heroic age of Australian exploration and of public health. See his "The evolution of public health administration in Australia"; *The Health of the People: A Study in Federalism*; and *Health and Disease in Australia: A History*. On Heiser, see V. G. Heiser, *An American Doctor's Odyssey: Adventures in Forty-Five Countries*; and Warwick Anderson, "Victor G. Heiser."

25. See Anon., "Richard Alfred O'Brien," *Medical Journal of Australia* (*MJA*) i (1971): 102. O'Brien's move from Cairns to London was aided by C. J. Martin, who briefly had been professor of physiology at Melbourne. Martin encouraged many Australian scientists to work at the Lister Institute, including O'Brien, Cumpston, Henry Priestley, F. Macfarlane Burnet, Hamilton Fairley and Howard Florey. See W. A. Osborne, "C. J. Martin," *MJA* i (1955): 811; and Patricia Morrison, "Sir Charles James Martin," *ADB* 10, pp. 423–5.

26. G. H. Frodsham, *A Bishop's Pleasaunce*, pp. 238–9, 249. The chapter is hemmed in by musings on "the abiding quality of English humour" and "the soul of a savage." On Frodsham, see John C. Vockler, "George Horsfall Frodsham," *ADB* 8, pp. 590–1; and E. C. Rowland, *The Tropics for Christ: Being a History of the Diocese of North Queensland*. J. M. Creed, a member of the Legislative Council of New South Wales, echoed Frodsham's remarks in "The settlement by 'whites' of tropical Australia."

27. The relevant letters and the memorandum are in CP78/5/2, National Archives of Australia. The quotation is from a letter dated 7 March 1907. For a very helpful and detailed account of the establishment of the institute, see R. A. Douglas, "Dr Anton Breinl and the Australian Institute of Tropical Medicine." See also J.H.L. Cumpston, "The Australian Institute of Tropical Medicine"; and Douglas Gordon, *Mad Dogs and Englishmen Went Out in the Queensland Sun: Health Aspects of the Settlement of Tropical Queensland.*

28. On Breinl, see Lori Harloe, White Man in Tropical Australia: Anton Breinl and the Australian Institute of Tropical Medicine, and "Anton Breinl and the Australian Institute of Tropical Medicine"; H. Priestley, "Anton Breinl," *Australian J. Science* 2 (1944): 28; and Douglas, "Dr Anton Breinl."

29. Michael Worboys has attempted to distinguish the approaches to disease control at Liverpool and London in "Manson, Ross and colonial medical policy: Tropical medicine in London and Liverpool, 1899–1914." For a complication of Worboys's argument, see Power, *Tropical Medicine in the Twentieth Century.*

30. G. A. Bolton, *A Thousand Miles Away: A History of North Queensland to 1920*; and Paul Mitchell, "A short medical history of Townsville."

31. Breinl quoted in Anon., "British Medical Association news," p. 88. This is no doubt a reference to the confusing factors in similar physiological research conducted by the American in the Philippines at this time. See Warwick Anderson, "'Where every prospect pleases and only man is vile': Laboratory medicine as colonial discourse."

32. Anton Breinl, "The influence of climate, diseases and surroundings on the white race living in the tropics," p. 996.

33. H. B. Allen, "Second general report on . . . the Institute of Preventive Medicine," p. 76. Allen, the professor of anatomy and pathology and dean of the faculty of medicine, was an excellent administrator but found no time for his own research, though it was said that he could throw a cricket ball more than 100 yards and was a fine swimmer. See K. F. Russell, "Harry Brookes Allen (1854–1926)," *ADB* 7, pp. 42–3. Allen finally succeeded in his efforts to support local medical research with the establishment of the Walter and Eliza Hall Institute in 1916. See Vivienne de Wahl Davis, "Sir Harry Allen and the foundation of the Walter and Eliza Hall Institute of Medical Research."

34. Ernest Scott, *A History of the University of Melbourne*; and Geoffrey Blainey, *A Centenary History of the University of Melbourne.* By contrast, the University of Sydney benefited from a more supportive government, private bequests, and an honest accountant and so recovered more quickly from the 1890s depression. By 1912, the Sydney medical school was enrolling more students than its older rival. See J. A. Young, A. J. Sefton, and Nina Webb, *Centenary Book of the University of Sydney Faculty of Medicine.* Nonetheless, Sydney continued to lag behind Melbourne in medical research.

35. R.J.A. Berry, "The Anatomy Department of the University of Melbourne." I discuss Berry's eugenic enthusiasms in Chapter 6 and his work on Aboriginal skulls in Chapter 7. Berry was dean of the Melbourne medical school from 1925

until 1929; see K. F. Russell, "Richard James Arthur Berry (1867–1962)," *ADB* 7, pp. 276–7. On the Melbourne medical school, see K. F. Russell, *The Melbourne Medical School, 1862–1962.*

36. D. J. Mulvaney and J. H. Callaby, *"So Much That Is New." Baldwin Spencer, 1860–1929: A Biography*; and Len Weickhardt, *Masson of Melbourne.* Spencer became a leading evolutionary anthropologist and an informant of Sir James Frazer and Emile Durkheim (see Chapter 7); Masson became the reluctant father-in-law of Bronislaw Malinowski.

37. John Docker, *The Nervous Nineties: Australian Cultural Life in the 1890s*; and Ken Stewart, ed., *The 1890s: Australian Literature and Literary Culture.*

38. For accounts of university social life, see Audrey Cahn, *University Children*; and Percival Serle, A Life of Good Fortune, typescript, 1948, ms. 2441/2c ii, State Library of Victoria.

39. Among the relevant figures at the University of Melbourne were: Harry Brookes Allen (anatomy and pathology, 1882–1924); W. Baldwin Spencer (biology, 1887–1919); J. W. Springthorpe (hygiene, 1887–1920); James Barrett (special senses, 1897–1937); C. J. Martin (physiology, 1897–1903); J. W. Gregory (geology, 1900–1904); W. A. Osborne (physiology, 1904–1938); and R.J.A. Berry (anatomy, 1906–1929). Allen, Springthorpe, and Barrett were locals; the others were imported from Britain. The relevant medical students included: J.S.C. Elkington (1890–1895); J.H.L. Cumpston (1898–1902), R. O'Brien (1898–1902) and Harvey Sutton (1898–1902). See Russell, *Melbourne Medical School.*

40. David Walker, *Dream and Disillusion: A Search for Australian Cultural Identity.*

41. Alfred Hart, *History of the Wallaby Club*, p. 11. Osborne, Springthorpe, Gregory, and Ernest Scott, the professor of history, were among the more enthusiastic university marsupials. Other prominent early-twentieth-century Wallabies included George Knibbs, the federal statistician; Robert Garran, the head of the federal law department; Frank Tate, the Victorian director of education; Theodore Fink, the owner of the Melbourne *Herald*; and the politicians Lyttleton Groom, J. H. Keating, Dr. Carty Salmon, and Staniforth Smith. A later generation included W. J. Young, R. M. Crawford, David Rivett, John Medley, F. Macfarlane Burnet, and G. L. Wood—all from the university—and the jurist Owen Dixon. The club is still active. See Harold Attwood, ed., *The History of the Wallaby Club*; and Serle, A Life of Good Fortune.

42. Leonie Foster, *High Hopes: The Men and Motives of the Australian Round Table.* Osborne and Barrett were especially keen members of the Round Table.

43. Charles H. Pearson, *National Life and Character: A Forecast*, pp. 67–8, 68, 360–1. See J. M. Tregenza, *Professor of Democracy.* Richard Hofstadter discusses the influence of Pearson on the American scene in *Social Darwinism in American Thought*, pp. 160–1.

44. Alfred Deakin to R. Jebb, 4 June 1908, quoted in Tregenza, *Professor of Democracy*, p. 234. For accounts of Theodore Roosevelt's and William Gladstone's admiration of Pearson, see pp. 231–2.

45. *Commonwealth Parliamentary Debates* 3 (7 August 1901), p. 3503.

46. Osborne to Tregenza, 17 July 1958, quoted in Tregenza, *Professor of Democracy*, p. 233.

47. James Barrett, "White men for the North. The problem of colonization, a plea for research work," Melbourne *Argus* (17 September 1910), p. 4. See also Barrett, *The Twin Ideals: An Educated Commonwealth.* After graduating from Melbourne in 1881, Barrett had studied physiology at King's College, London, and attended a course in bacteriology taught by Koch in Berlin. See Roe, *Nine Australian Progressives*, chapter 3; Stephen Murray-Smith, "Sir James William Barrett (1862–1945)," *ADB* 7, pp. 186–9; and Barrett, *Eighty Eventful Years.* Barrett was a vigorous, if irascible, campaigner against venereal disease and the declining birthrate; he also promoted national parks and imperial unity. In the 1930s, he became chancellor of the University of Melbourne. An obituary recalled his "fine presence and a voice in keeping with his physique, associated with an oracular manner of delivering his quasi-Delphic utterances" (*MJA* ii [1945]: 58–61).

48. Anon., "Tropical Australia: Deputation from Congress to the Prime Minister," pp. 101, 103.

49. Barrett, "White men for the north," p. 4.

50. *Commonwealth Parliamentary Debates* (3 November 1910), pp. 5624, 5629.

51. Ibid., p. 5629.

52. Osborne, a well-built, blue-eyed, athletic Ulsterman, was another who never fulfilled his own research promise, though he became dean of the medical school from 1929 until 1938, as well as a renowned polemicist and author. His writings ranged from "Science and National Efficiency" to a biography of Captain Moonlight, the bushranger, and to *The Laboratory and Other Poems* (Melbourne, 1907). He claimed to be a friend of Buffalo Bill and a master of the art of boomerang throwing. See Barry Jones, "William Alexander Osborne," *ADB* 11, pp. 103–5.

53. Young had trained in biochemistry at Manchester, and then studied the role of phosphorus in carbohydrate metabolism at the Lister Institute, under C. J. Martin. He later became professor of biochemistry at Melbourne and an active Wallaby. See W. A. Osborne, "W. J. Young," *MJA* i (1942): 707–8; Max Marginson, "William John Young," *ADB* 12, p. 601. Priestley, a Sydney medical graduate, had been working at the Lister Institute in the previous year. Tall and athletic, Priestley was a dedicated supporter of the Scouting movement. Despite his appointment at Townsville in bacteriology, he later became the first professor of biochemistry at Sydney. See Anon., "H. Priestley," *MJA* i (1961): 875; and J. Atherton Young, "Henry Priestley," *ADB* 11, pp. 294–5.

54. *Townsville Bulletin* (30 June 1913), quoted in Douglas, "Dr Anton Breinl," p. 751. See also R. A. Douglas, "One day in the medical life of Queensland: The opening of the Australian Institute of Tropical Medicine." The opening ceremony is also described in the *Australasian Medical Gazette* (5 July 1913): 15–16, (12 July 1913): 37, and (9 August 1913): 124–25. For McGregor's opinions on state support for tropical research, see "Some problems of tropical medicine." On McGregor, see R. B. Joyce, *Sir William McGregor.*

55. See, for example, Alfred Searcy, *In Australian Tropics*.

56. Goldsmith, "The necessity for the study of tropical medicine in Australia," p. 178. See also Frodsham, *Bishop's Pleasaunce*, p. 238.

57. Anton Breinl, "Influence of climate, disease and surroundings on the white race living in the tropics," p. 595.

58. A. Duckworth, "Notes on a 'White Australia,'" p. 250.

59. James Barrett, "Tropical Australia discussion," p. 63.

60. Anton Breinl, *Tropical Diseases: Report of Dr Breinl*, p. 1.

61. Anton Breinl, "Report on health and disease in the Northern Territory."

62. Anton Breinl, "The object and scope of tropical medicine in Australia."

63. The reports of the institute indicate that it was generally difficult to obtain sufficient clinical material, but the number of cases of malaria increased enormously when affected soldiers were sent to Townsville during World War I.

64. Breinl, "The object and scope of tropical medicine in Australia," p. 525.

65. Ibid., p. 526.

66. The term is used, for example, by W. J. Young in "Fighting tropical diseases in Australia," p. 34.

67. Aldo Castellani and Albert Chalmers, *Manual of Tropical Medicine*, p. 115.

68. See Warwick Anderson, "Excremental colonialism: Public health and the poetics of pollution."

69. J. V. Danes, "Notes on the suitability of tropical Australia for the white races," p. 417. Beriberi is now believed to be a disease of dietary deficiency.

70. Ibid., pp. 418, 419.

71. Anderson, "Excremental colonialism."

72. Randall M. Packard, *White Plague, Black Labor: Tuberculosis and the Political Economy of Health and Disease in South Africa*; and Saul Dubow, *Scientific Racism in Modern South Africa*.

73. Breinl, "The object and scope of tropical medicine in Australia," p. 526.

74. Young, "Fighting tropical diseases," p. 34.

75. "M. B.," "Correspondence—White Australia Policy," p. 277.

76. James F. Merrillees, "Correspondence—White Australia Policy," p. 345.

77. "Cosmos," "Correspondence—White Australia Policy," p. 43.

78. R.J.A. Berry, "Correspondence—White Australia Policy," p. 93.

79. Breinl, "Tropical medicine in Australia," p. 531. Breinl believed that such research would "prove the necessity of the Institute" and "secure for it more general and liberal support" (*Tropical Diseases*, p. 2).

80. Breinl, "Health and disease in the Northern Territory," p. 37.

81. Young, "Fighting tropical diseases," p. 36.

82. Bruno Latour, "Give me a laboratory and I will raise the world."

83. W. A. Osborne, "Contributions to physiological climatology. Part 1: The relation of loss of water from the skin and lungs to the external temperature in actual climatic conditions." The wet-bulb thermometer had wet fabric around the bulb and indicated the effect of humidity.

84. W. A. Osborne, "Contributions to physiological climatology. Part 2."

85. W. A. Osborne, "The wet-bulb and kata-thermometers," p. 120. Osborne later retired to Townsville, where he continued, at an advanced age, his hammock experiments.

86. J. S. Haldane, "Influence of high air temperatures."

87. A. Breinl and W. J. Young, "Tropical Australia and its settlement," p. 354.

88. Ibid.

89. Ibid, p. 367. The American experiments are reported in Hans Aron, "Investigation on the action of the tropical sun on men and animals"; and H. D. Gibbs, "A study of the effect of tropical sunlight upon men, monkeys, rabbits, and a discussion of the proper clothing for the tropical climate." For an account of the research of the Philippines Bureau of Science during this period, see Anderson, "'Where every prospect pleases and only man is vile.'"

90. C. Eijkman (1895), cited in Breinl and Young, "Tropical Australia," p. 367.

91. W. J. Young, "A note on the black pigment in the skin of an Australian Black."

92. Breinl and Young, "Tropical Australia," p. 367.

93. Anderson, "'Where every prospect pleases.'"

94. John Davy, *Researches, Physiological and Anatomical*, vol. 1, p. 161.

95. Alexander Rattray, "On some of the more important physiological changes induced in the human economy by change of climate, as from temperate to tropical, and the reverse," p. 315. Rattray also drew on his experiences on HMS *Salamander*, traveling regularly between Sydney and the Torres Strait. See also his "Further experiments on the more important physiological changes induced in the human economy by change of climate."

96. Weston P. Chamberlain, "Observations on the influence of the Philippine climate on white men of the blond and brunette type." See also his "Some features of the physiological activity of white races in the Philippine Islands."

97. W. J. Young, "Observations upon the body temperature of Europeans living in the tropics," p. 223.

98. W. E. Musgrave and A. G. Sison, "Blood pressure in the tropics: A preliminary report."

99. Weston P. Chamberlain, "A study of the systolic blood pressure and the pulse rate of healthy adult males in the Philippines."

100. Breinl and Young, "Tropical Australia," p. 379.

101. Davidson, *Hygiene and the Diseases of Warm Climates*; and Charles W. Daniels and E. Wilkinson, *Tropical Medicine and Hygiene*.

102. Weston P. Chamberlain, "The red blood corpuscles and the hemoglobin of healthy adult American males residing in the Philippines," p. 488.

103. A. Breinl and H. Priestley, "Observations on the blood conditions of children of European descent residing in Tropical Australia," p. 606.

104. Luigi Sambon, "Remarks on acclimatization in tropical regions," p. 63. See also L. Westenra Sambon, "Acclimatization of Europeans in tropical lands." In a response that follows the latter paper, Sir Patrick Manson declared that "I now firmly believe in the possibility of tropical colonisation by the white races . . . Now that we

know that the unhealthiness of the tropics depends on the plants and animals of the tropics—the pathological flora and fauna—the situation becomes much more hopeful" (pp. 689–90).

105. Breinl and Young, "Tropical Australia," pp. 389–90.

106. George M. Beard, *A Practical Treatise on Nervous Exhaustion (Neurasthenia) and Its Symptoms, Nature, Sequences, Treatment*. Charles E. Rosenberg has suggested that Beard's work illustrates "the utility of scientific metaphor and authority in helping rationalize a rapidly changing and stress-filled world" ("George M. Beard and American nervousness," p. 98). On the rise of the diagnosis of neurasthenia in America, see also Barbara Sicherman, "The uses of a diagnosis: Doctors, patients and neurasthenia." On neurasthenia in Australia, see David Walker, "Modern nerves, nervous moderns: notes on male neurasthenia."

107. Beard, *Nervous Exhaustion*, p. 189.

108. Valery Havard, "Is mortality necessarily higher in tropical than in temperate climates?" pp. 17, 20.

109. Charles E. Woodruff, "The neurasthenic states caused by excessive light," p. 1006. See also Charles E. Woodruff, *The Effects of Tropical Sunlight Upon the White Man*.

110. Sir Havelock Charles, "Neurasthenia and its bearing on the decay of northern peoples in India," pp. 14, 12, 9. The signs of "Punjab head" were "that an officer, otherwise in every way a good fellow, had become short-tempered; forgetful of names; troubled with sleeplessness; given to feel his work was too much for him; disinclined to take responsibility; given to make molehills into mountains; procrastinating; susceptible on slight exertion, mental or physical, to fatigue; and with a loss of all powers of concentration" (pp. 3–4). Charles noted his debt to Woodruff's "able work on the effects of tropical light" (p. 3).

111. Sir Ronald Ross, "Discussion," in ibid., p. 16.

112. Andrew Balfour, "Discussion," in ibid., pp. 17, 18.

113. F. M. Sandwith, "Discussion," in ibid., p. 28. Charles, in reply, observed that Dr. Sandwith's "urbanity often overwhelms me" (p. 31).

114. Breinl and Priestley, "Tropical Australia," pp. 390–91, 391.

115. Ibid., p. 396.

116. William Nicoll, "The conditions of life in tropical Australia," p. 270. Nicoll had resigned from the institute in 1915.

117. Ibid., p. 287.

118. Ibid., p. 288.

119. Ibid., pp. 289, 290. When Victor Heiser visited Townsville, as director for the east of the International Health Board of the Rockefeller Foundation, he noted in his journal that Nicoll had "succumbed to the alcohol habit" (24 April 1916, Notes of 1916 Trip, 905/Hei 2, 58.5, Rockefeller Archive Center, vol. 1, p. 179). Breinl he found "a most modest and unassuming man" (21 April 1916, ibid., vol. 1, p. 160).

120. Henry Priestley, "Physiological observations in the tropical parts of Australia," pp. 1486, 1488. Priestley left the institute in 1919.

121. Ibid., p. 1491.

122. Ibid., p. 1492.

123. Springthorpe, *Therapeutics, Dietetics and Hygiene*, vol. 1, p. 215, vol. 2, p. 994.

124. A. Breinl, "The influence of climate, disease and surroundings on the white race in the tropics," p. 995. See also A. Breinl to Attlee Hunt, secretary, Home and Territories Department, 22 September 1917, AITM General Correspondence, SP1061/1/350, National Archives of Australia, which explains that "conclusive results cannot be expected until after years of painstaking research." A few years later, Breinl repeated that "the whole question of the physiology of the white man in the tropics is still far from being solved" (to A. Hunt, 27 September 1919, ibid.). He requested further funding of physiological and biochemical research.

125. Australian Institute of Tropical Medicine, *Half-Yearly Report from 1 Jan–30 June 1914*, p. 11.

126. Warwick Anderson, "The trespass speaks: White masculinity and colonial breakdown."

127. Richard Hofstadter, *Social Darwinism*; and John Higham, "The reorientation of American culture in the 1890s." Michael Roe has more broadly identified many of the rising generation of experts as Progressives, in that they sought to avoid radical social change through technical innovation and government action. See *Nine Australian Progressives*.

128. Breinl, "Tropical medicine in Australia," p. 526.

129. Barrett, "The problem of the settlement of tropical Australia," p. 288.

130. Francis Castles, *The Working Class and Welfare: Reflections on the Political Development of the Welfare State in Australia and New Zealand*.

131. Elazar Barkan, *The Retreat of Scientific Racism: Changing Concepts of Race in Britain and the United States Between the Wars*.

132. Bernard O'Dowd, "Race Prejudice," pp. 155, 175.

133. Ibid., pp. 176, 178. See also "Gavah the Blacksmith" [Bernard O'Dowd], "White Australia and qualified democracy." In the early twentieth century, O'Dowd was probably the most vigorous critic of racism from within the Australian labor movement. See Hugh Anderson, *The Poet Militant: Bernard O'Dowd*; and Graeme Osborne, "A socialist dilemma."

CHAPTER 5

1. Anon., "Tropical Australia," p. 45.

2. J.H.L. Cumpston, "Tropical Australia: discussion," p. 49. See also his "Presidential address: Public health and state medicine."

3. The term "medical possibilism" is derived from the related contemporary notion of "geographical possibilism." See P. Vidal de la Blach, *Principles of Human Geography*. I discuss medical possibilism in the tropics more generally in Warwick

Anderson, "The natures of culture: Environment and race in the colonial tropics." See also J. M. Powell, "Taylor, Stefansson and the arid Centre: An historical encounter of 'environmentalism' and 'possibilism.'"

4. On technology and imperialism more generally, see Michael Adas, *Machines as the Measure of Men: Science, Technology and Ideologies of Western Dominance*.

5. Harry Allen, "Public health in Australia: Past and future," p. 5.

6. Ibid., pp. 5, 6.

7. John Powles, "Professional hygienists and the health of the nation." See also Milton Lewis, "Editor's Introduction"; and James Gillespie, *The Price of Health: Australian Governments and Medical Politics, 1910–60*.

8. J.H.L. Cumpston, "The war and public health," p. 193. Cumpston was also frustrated by the lack of national coordination in the efforts to control the 1919 Spanish influenza outbreak. See Humphrey McQueen, "The Spanish influenza pandemic in Australia, 1918–19"; and Anthea Hyslop, "Insidious immigrant: Spanish influenza and border quarantine in Australia, 1919."

9. John Masefield, *Gallipoli*; and C.E.W. Bean, *The Story of the Anzac: From the Outbreak of the War to the End of the First Phase of the Gallipoli Campaign*. See K. S. Inglis, *C.E.W. Bean, Australian Historian;* and *Anzac Remembered: Selected Writings*. Bean pointed out that "the lesson of the war is that by organisation you can do anything" (*In Your Hands, Australians*, p. 36).

10. Gillespie, *Price of Health*, p. 34. Appropriately, the term comes from William James, a founder of American pragmatism, the philosophical foundation of these developments. He was describing the tendency to formulate moral or political issues in medical terms. See William James, *The Varieties of Religious Experience: A Study of Human Nature; Being the Gifford Lectures on Natural Religion Delivered at Edinburgh in 1901–02*. On American progressivism, see Robert H. Wiebe, *The Search for Order 1877–1920*; on the British national efficiency movement, see G. R. Searle, *The Quest for National Efficiency: A Study in British Politics and Political Thought, 1899–1914*.

11. Michael Roe, "The establishment of the Australian Department of Health." According to James Gillespie, Cumpston's Quarantine Service "became the administrative backbone of the department" (*Price of Health*, p. 38).

12. Anton Breinl, "Tropical Australia: Discussion," p. 52.

13. W. A. Osborne, "Tropical Australia: Discussion," pp. 54, 53.

14. A.T.H. Nisbet, "Tropical Australia: Discussion," p. 55.

15. W. A. Osborne, "Physiological factors in the development of an Australian race," p. 72.

16. Ibid., pp. 76, 72.

17. Anon., "White man in the north," p. 315.

18. Ibid., p. 315.

19. Richard Arthur, "Settlement of tropical Australia," p. 345. See also his "The colonisation of tropical Australia."

20. G. L. Wood, "The settlement of northern Australia," pp. 13, 9–10.

21. *Commonwealth Parliamentary Debates* 110 (1925), p. 761.

22. Sir James Barrett, "White Australia policy," p. 681. Barrett did concede that with the "equalisation of all civilisations" the problem of racial differences in disease carriage might be solved, but he thought this was a very distant prospect indeed (p. 683). In this paper, Barrett acknowledges the assistance of W. J. Young, recently appointed a lecturer in biochemistry at the University of Melbourne.

23. J. W. Barrett, "Can tropical Australia be peopled by a white race?" pp. 30, 28.

24. Sir James Barrett, "White colonisation of the tropics," p. 13. In this paper, Barrett thanks Cumpston for his assistance.

25. Attlee Hunt to Breinl, 10 December 1919, AITM General Correspondence, SP1061/1/350, National Archives of Australia (NAA).

26. Breinl to Attlee Hunt, 27 September 1919, ibid.

27. R. A. Douglas, "Dr Anton Breinl and the Australian Institute of Tropical Medicine"; Lori Harloe, White Man in Tropical Australia: Anton Breinl and the Australian Institute of Tropical Medicine, and "Anton Breinl and the Australian Institute of Tropical Medicine"; and Andrew Parker, "A 'complete protective machinery'—classification and intervention through the Australian Institute of Tropical Medicine." Breinl published the last two of his scientific papers in 1921 in the *Medical Journal of Australia*. The more important of them was a study of 180 wharf laborers, in which he found that most indices remained normal, except that rectal temperatures rose a little, but not to a pathological degree. See "An inquiry into the effect of high wet-bulb temperatures upon the pulse rate, rectal temperature, skin-shirt temperature and blood pressure of wharf labourers in North Queensland."

28. P. A. Maplestone, "An evening in tropical Australia," p. 99.

29. Minutes of the Committee, Australian Institute of Tropical Medicine, 18–19 January 1921, SP1061/1/350, NAA.

30. P. A. Maplestone, Memorandum on the Reorganisation of the Institute, 14 Feb. 1921, ibid.

31. P. A. Maplestone, "Research in Australia," p. 476. Maplestone later worked in Sierra Leone (at a branch of the Liverpool School of Tropical Medicine) and in New Guinea, and then taught at a medical school in Calcutta, before retiring to Melbourne.

32. E. S. Sundstroem, *A Summary of Some Studies in Tropical Acclimatisation*, pp. 25, 28. See also Sundstroem, *Contribution to Tropical Physiology: With Special Reference to the Adaptation of the White Man to the Climate of North Queensland*. Sundstroem took up a position at Berkeley in 1925.

33. Sundstroem, *Some Studies in Tropical Acclimatisation*, p. 31.

34. Fedora Gould Fisher, *Raphael Cilento: A Biography*; and A. T. Yarwood, "Sir Raphael Cilento and *The White Man in the Tropics*."

35. "My first objective was to take stock to reorganise, and particularly to restock and transform the AITM from what was formerly a rather haphazard research laboratory to an institution orientated to the needs of both the practitioners and the residents of the north" (Cilento, Memorandum, n.d., SP1061/1/187, NAA).

36. R. W. Cilento, *The White Man in the Tropics, with Especial Reference to Australia and Its Dependencies*, p. 5. For another version of this, see R. W. Cilento, "The conquest of climate." In his article Cilento reiterates the importance of the deportation of "the last few Kanakas, whose fellows for half a century had been demonstrating in the sugar fields of Queensland their extravagant inefficiency as labour machines, and their deadly facility for transmitting malaria, filariasis, hookworm disease and leprosy" (p. 422). W. K. Hancock relies heavily on Cilento in *Australia*, esp. p. 42.

37. Cilento, *White Man in the Tropics*, pp. 8, 10. Cilento repeated the need to exclude "races with lower standards of life and higher rates of disease and reproduction" ("White settlement of tropical Australia," p. 231). He was fond of referring to the Pacific Islanders as "a disease-ridden class of coloured indentured labour," pointing out that, given the widespread distribution of the *Anopheles* mosquito in Australia, it was "fortunate that we have no suitable native population to act as a reservoir of the virus" ("Australia's problems in the tropics," pp. 222, 224).

38. Cilento to C. M. Wenyon, director, Wellcome Bureau of Scientific Research, 17 January 1924, SP1061/1/300, NAA.

39. Cilento, *White Man in the Tropics*, p. 35.

40. Cilento to Elkington, 16 Feb. 1923, SP1061/1/209, NAA. Elkington had prompted this remark, having noted that Sundstroem produced interesting material "wrapped up in a mass of verbiage and irrelevance" (Elkington to Cilento, 5 January 1923, ibid.).

41. Cilento, *White Man in the Tropics*, p. 50.

42. Ibid., p. 57.

43. Ibid., p. 73.

44. Ibid., pp. 73–4. A few years earlier, in a private letter to Andrew Balfour, the director of the Wellcome Bureau of Scientific Research in London, Cilento had been more critical of the emergent type: It was "a tall and rangy type, inclined to be hatchet faced, and somewhat hard-browed and squint eyed from the sun . . . His complexion tends to sallowness, but his skin is healthy looking and firm . . . He is possessed of infinite endurance and has that discontent which some have called divine, but he is becoming quite a distinct and desirable type" (22 October 1923, SP1061/1/300, NAA). For an endorsement of Cilento's argument, see Wood, "Settlement of northern Australia," p. 14.

45. Edwin J. Brady, *Australia Unlimited*, p. 434. For another contemporary prediction of a new Australian type, see W. Ramsay Smith, *On Race-Culture and the Conditions That Influence It in South Australia*.

46. R. Hamlyn-Harris, "'Some anthropological considerations of Queensland and the history of its ethnography,'" pp. 9, 10.

47. Cilento narrowly avoided detention for his overt fascist sympathies and connections during World War II. See Fisher, *Raphael Cilento*.

48. A. H. Baldwin graduated in medicine from the University of Melbourne in 1917 and later, with the support of the Rockefeller Foundation, studied at the Johns Hopkins University and the London School of Hygiene and Tropical Medicine. In

1930, he was appointed deputy director of the School of Public Health and Tropical Medicine at the University of Sydney, where from 1947 until his retirement in 1956 he was professor of tropical medicine. See H. O. Lancaster, "Alec Hutcheson Baldwin (1891–1971)," *ADB* 13, pp. 97–98.

49. John A. Ryle, "Social medicine: Its meaning and scope"; and George Rosen, "What is social medicine: A genetic analysis of the concept." In the late 1940s, Cilento held a number of senior posts at the United Nations, with responsibilities for postwar refugee resettlement. As director of disaster relief in Palestine, he was criticized for his anti-Semitism, and in 1951 he retired to Australia. See Fisher, *Raphael Cilento*.

50. Sir Raphael Cilento and Clem Lack, *Triumph in the Tropics: An Historical Sketch of Queensland*, pp. 421, 437. A copy of their book was sent to all Queensland schools.

51. Sir Raphael Cilento, *Australia's Racial Heritage: A Brief Insight*, pp. 4, 6. On multiculturalism as a Jewish conspiracy, see p. 11.

52. Cilento, *White Man in the Tropics*, p. 106ff.

53. Ibid., p. 153. See also Phyllis Cilento, *You Don't Have to Live with Chronic Ill-Health*.

54. Cilento, *White Man in the Tropics*, p. 152.

55. A. Breinl and W. J. Young, "Tropical Australia and its settlement," p. 392.

56. James M. Phelan, "An experiment with orange-red underwear."

57. H. D. Gibbs, "A study of the effect of tropical sunlight upon men, monkeys and rabbits, and a discussion of the proper clothing for the tropical climate." Gibbs's initial suggestion that one needed nothing more than an umbrella was generally regarded as impractical, as the "natives" might fail to appreciate the physiological soundness of the nakedness of their white "masters."

58. Breinl and Young, "Tropical Australia," p. 394.

59. Cilento, *White Man in the Tropics*, p. 147.

60. Phyllis Cilento, "Women's clothing in the tropics," *Townsville Daily Bulletin*, n.d., SP1061/1/195, NAA. See also Gail Reekie, ed., *On the Edge: Women's Experiences of Queensland*.

61. Breinl and Young, "Tropical Australia," p. 404.

62. Cilento, *White Man in the Tropics*, p. 35.

63. Ibid., pp. 106–24. See also his Report on Plans Submitted to the Under-Secretary, Department of Public Works, Brisbane, 1923, SP1061/1/128, NAA. It was thought that eventually the electric fan might remedy many architectural defects, but for the moment it was impractical, as most north Queensland towns still lacked electric power. On the origins of the Queensland house, see Peter Bell, "Miasma, termites and a nice view of the dam: The development of the highset house in North Queensland"; and Jennifer Craik, "The cultural politics of the Queensland house."

64. Cilento to W. Wynne Williams, 11 December 1922, SP1061/1/128, NAA. Williams, the land commissioner at Cloncurry, later wrote on tropical settlement; see his "Settlement of the tropics."

65. Cilento, *White Man in the Tropics*, p. 68. See James Gillespie, "The Rockefeller Foundation, the hookworm campaign and a national health policy in Australia, 1911–30"; John Ettling, *The Germ of Laziness: Rockefeller Philanthropy and Public Health in the New South*; and William Link, "Privies, progressivism and public schools: Health reform and education in the rural South, 1909–20." The life cycle of hookworm and its mode of entry into the human host were first described by Arthur Looss in Cairo in 1898.

66. T. F. Macdonald, "Experiences of ankylostomiasis in Australia," pp. 69, 71, 70. In 1928, Alec Balfour, then acting director of the Townsville Institute, endorsed Macdonald's findings: "Later stages of degeneration are of the sexual order. Schoolmasters have consulted me as to the cause of general demoralisation among school children. Thymol provided a key to the difficulty with, I am glad to say, happy results" (The Mental Condition in Hookworm Disease, 1928, SP1061/1/83, NAA, p. 4).

67. A. Breinl, "Ankylostomiasis."

68. E. Richard Brown, *Rockefeller Medicine Men: Medicine and Capitalism in America*. James Gillespie points out that, aside from the quarantine service, this was the federal government's first major postwar involvement in public health activities and a stimulus to the establishment of the Commonwealth Department of Health in 1921 ("Rockefeller Foundation").

69. The terms are used frequently: For example, W. Nicoll suggested that "the only remedy appears to be to make promiscuous defecation a serious offence with a heavy penalty" ("The conditions of life in tropical Australia," p. 285). For a more detailed account of the campaign, see Gillespie, "Rockefeller Foundation."

70. Warwick Anderson, "Excremental colonialism: Public health and the poetics of pollution." More generally, on such binary typologies, see Mary Douglas, *Purity and Danger: An Analysis of Concepts of Pollution*.

71. J. H. Waite and I. L. Neilson, "A study of the effects of hookworm infection upon the mental development of North Queensland schoolchildren," p. 4. Waite and Neilson demanded "a sufficient corps of trained sanitarians to penetrate every settlement to teach the people the vital necessity of applied sanitation" (pp. 4–6). See also J. H. Waite, "The Queensland hookworm campaign"; and W. A. Sawyer, "Hookworm disease in relation to the medical profession."

72. H. C. McKay, "Earth-eaters of Queensland."

73. RC to Tropical Institute, 18 June 1925, SP1061/1/5, NAA.

74. DJ to Tropical Institute, 12 March 1925, ibid.

75. EP to Hookworm Office, 26 April 1929, ibid.

76. CGS to Doctor, Government Tropical Institute, 3 April 1928, ibid.

77. Gillespie, "Rockefeller Foundation."

78. R. W. Cilento, "Australia's problems in the tropics." See also G. M. Heydon, "The influence in hookworm infection of the species of worm and the race of man."

79. R. E. Richards, Hookworm Campaign—Malaria and Filaria Survey of the Gulf, 1923, SP1061/1/5, NAA, pp. 4, 3.

80. R. E. Richards to Cilento, 11 January 1923, Hookworm Campaign, Palm Island, SP1061/1/94, NAA.

81. Cilento to R. E. Richards, 15 January 1923, ibid. According to Ross Patrick, mass treatment for hookworm was still a standard procedure in Queensland Aboriginal communities into the 1970s (*A History of Health and Medicine in Queensland, 1824–1960*, p. 251). Recently, Rosalind Kidd has praised Cilento for "finally asserting the centrality of clinical expertise in public health administration" in Aboriginal communities (*The Way We Civilise: Aboriginal Affairs—The Untold Story*, p. 115).

82. J. H. Waite, "Preliminary report of ankylostomiasis in Papua."

83. Cilento, "Australia's problems in the tropics," p. 230. See Donald Denoon with Kathleen Dryan and Leslie Marshall, *Public Health in Papua New Guinea: Medical Possibility and Social Constraint, 1884–1984.* Denoon also has observed that Cilento's perceptions "tied tropical disease to tropical people, ignoring the physical circumstances in which people lived, and stressing hereditary predisposition" ("The idea of tropical medicine and its influence in Papua New Guinea," p. 15).

84. Cilento, *White Man in the Tropics*, p. 95. More generally, on the use of colonial models in domestic settings, see Warwick Anderson, "Where is the post-colonial history of medicine?"

85. William A. Douglass, *From Italy to Ingham: Italians in North Queensland*; and John Lack and Jacqueline Templeton, eds, *Sources of Australian Immigration History, Volume 1: 1901–45*. On immigration history, see also Charles A. Price, *Southern Europeans in Australia*; George Sherrington, *Australia's Immigrants, 1788–1978*; W. D. Borrie, *The Peopling of Australasia: A Demographic History, 1788–1988*; and Michael Roe, *Australia, Britain and Migration, 1915–40: A Study of Desperate Hopes*. The first Italians had settled along the Herbert River in 1891.

86. Gilbert White, "Some problems of Northern Australia," p. 61.

87. T. A. Ferry, "Report of the Royal Commission appointed to inquire into and report on the social and economic effects of increase in the number of aliens in Queensland," p. 42. On popular stereotypes of Italians in North Queensland, see Lyn Henderson, "The truth in stereotype? Italians and criminality in North Queensland between the wars."

88. Ferry, "Report of the Royal Commission," p. 51.

89. Douglass, *From Italy to Ingham*.

90. Cilento, "White settlement," p. 241. Significantly, Cilento (unlike T. F. Macdonald) resisted associating southern Europeans with a biological propensity for hookworm carriage.

91. K. H. Bailey, "Public opinion and population problems," p. 73. On the parallel racialization of Jews in this period, see Jon Stratton, "The colour of Jews: Jews, race and the white Australia policy."

92. Jens Lyng, *Non-Britishers in Australia: Influence on Population and Progress*, pp. 2, 9–11.

93. Ibid., p. 22. Lyng also asserted that the *ancient* Greeks and the founders of Rome must have been Nordic.

94. Ibid., p. 93. In 1928, P. D. Phillips and G. L. Wood observed that "in Australia there is a marked distinction between the homes of the Mediterranean and Asiatic migrants and of the native born" ("The Australian population problem," p. 39).

95. Lyng, *Non-Britishers in Australia*, pp. 212, 222–3.

96. Ibid., p. 225. He thought Alpines would be especially helpful in stagnantly Nordic Tasmania (p. 227).

97. "Report of the Sugar Inquiry Committee 1931," pp. 16, 19. For more favorable views of Italians settlers, see Vance Palmer, "Italians in North Queensland"; and Jean Devanny, *Sugar Heaven*.

98. A. Grenfell Price, *White Settlers in the Tropics*, p. 73. I discuss this work further in Chapter 6.

99. J.H.L. Cumpston, "The depopulation of the Pacific," pp. 1393, 1394.

100. See the material in SP1061/1/65, NAA.

101. On the discovery of the Pacific as a sphere for Australian economic growth, see Nicholas Brown, "Australian intellectuals and the image of Asia: 1920–60."

102. Commonwealth of Australia, *Royal Commission on Health: Minutes of Evidence*, p. 108.

103. Ibid., pp. 109, 102.

104. Ibid., p. 452.

105. Ibid., pp. 455, 456.

106. Milton Lewis, "Editor's introduction"; and Gillespie, *Price of Health*.

107. Elkington to Baldwin, 18 May 1925, SP1061/1/337, NAA. Baldwin's views derived largely from those of Cilento; see "Life in the Queensland tropics. Suitability for whites. Paper by Dr Baldwin," *Townsville Daily Bulletin* (11 September 1928), p. 11.

108. Elkington, Suggestions for Work at the AITM, Townsville, 1925, SP1061/1/337, NAA; and Baldwin to Elkington, 30 January 1925, ibid.

109. Cilento, Report of the Visit of Inspection to the AITM, Townsville, 1928, SP1061/1/337, NAA.

110. "Royal Commission on Health." See Lori Harloe, "From north to south: The translocation of the Australian Institute of Tropical Medicine." On the abolition of the Health Department's Division of Tropical Hygiene in 1932, see Cilento, "Australia's problems in the tropics"; and Sir Raphael Cilento, "Medicine in Queensland."

111. Milton Lewis refers to the earlier resignation of Elkington as a closing of the tropical frontier, in his "Editor's Introduction," p. 12. On the rising interest in the urban child, see Graeme Davison, "The city-bred child and urban reform in Melbourne, 1900–40."

CHAPTER 6

1. R.J.A. Berry, "The menace of the birth-rate," p. 495. On Berry, see K. F. Russell, "Richard James Arthur Berry, 1867–1962." Berry's typescript autobiography, Chance and Circumstance (Bristol, 1954), is held at the Medical History Museum, University of Melbourne.

2. Berry, "The menace of the birth-rate," pp. 492, 495.

3. Commonwealth of Australia, *Royal Commission on Health: Minutes of Evidence*, p. 235.

4. Ibid., pp. 237, 238.

5. Ibid., pp. 260, 261.

6. Ibid., pp. 286, 287.

7. Ibid., p. 285.

8. James C. Scott, *Seeing Like a State: How Certain Schemes to Improve the Human Condition Have Failed*. On public health during this period, see Dorothy Porter, *Health, Civilisation and the State: A History of Public Health from Ancient to Modern Times*.

9. The term "eugenics," meaning "well-born," was coined by Francis Galton, a cousin of Charles Darwin, and an advocate of state control of human breeding to select for desirable features and to eliminate defective characteristics. See Francis Galton, *Hereditary Genius: An Inquiry into Its Laws and Consequences*. For general accounts of eugenics, see G. R. Searle, *Eugenics and Politics in Britain, 1900–14*; Nancy L. Stepan, *The Idea of Race in Science: Great Britain, 1800–1960*; and Daniel Kevles, *In the Name of Eugenics: Genetics and the Uses of Human Heredity*. On the diversity of "eugenics" in Australia, see C. L. Bacchi, "The nature-nurture debate in Australia, 1900–14"; Helen Bourke, "Sociology and the social sciences in Australia"; Michael Roe, *Nine Australian Progressives: Vitalism in Bourgeois Social Thought, 1890–1960*; Stephen Garton, "Sir Charles Mackellar: Psychiatry, eugenics and child welfare in New South Wales, 1900–14"; Mary Cawte, "Craniometry and eugenics in Australia: R. J. A. Berry and the quest for social efficiency"; and James A. Gillespie, *The Price of Health: Australian Governments and Medical Politics, 1910–60*.

10. J. M. Powell, "Protracted reconciliation: Society and the environment."

11. D. R. Walker, "Harvey Sutton," *ADB* 12, pp. 143–4; and Grant Rodwell, "Professor Harvey Sutton: National hygienist as eugenicist and educator." See also Graeme Davison, "The city-bred child and urban reform in Melbourne, 1900–40"; and Gillespie, *Price of Health*. In his lectures to medical students at the University of Sydney, Sutton covered a variety of theories of heredity (including neo-Lamarckism) and discussed the problem of the feeble-minded and the dysgenic influences of low social status. He showed no interest in Aboriginal health.

12. The advisory committee on nutrition, established in 1936, included Sutton, Cumpston, H. Priestley, W. A. Osborne, Cilento, C. Stanton Hicks (from the University of Adelaide), and D.H.K. Lee (from the University of Queensland). See F. W. Clements, *A History of Human Nutrition in Australia*.

13. Harvey Sutton, "The importance of nationality," pp. 508, 510.

14. Harvey Sutton, "Modern development of public health—the child as the test of progress," pp. 356, 357, 363.

15. Christian Bjelke-Petersen, "Growth and development of Hobart school boys, with some notes on anthropometry," p. 826. Bjelke-Peterson also believed that intelligence varied in direct proportion to weight.

16. J.S.C. Elkington, "A plea for the Australian child body," p. 776.

17. Mary Booth, "School anthropometrics: The importance of Australasian measurements conforming to the schedule of the British Anthropometric Committee, 1906," pp. 689–90, 695.

18. On the relations of anthropometric methods and the social program of eugenics in Britain and the United States, see Kevles, *In the Name of Eugenics*.

19. Anon., "Reports of research committees: Anthropometric committee." In 1911, the Australasian Medical Congress set up a committee, including Harvey Sutton, to inquire into the intelligence of schoolchildren. It reported that 4 percent were feeble-minded and a further 12 percent were mentally dull (Anon., "Report of the committee of inquiry into the feeble-minded," p. 703). See also Harvey Sutton, "The feeble-minded—their classification and importance," and "The cure of feeblemindedness."

20. David Kirk and Karen Twigg, "Constructing Australian bodies: Social normalisation and school medical inspection, 1909–19."

21. Sutton, "Importance of nationality," p. 510. See Franz Boas, *Changes in the Bodily Form of Descendants of Immigrants*.

22. Stephen Garton has pointed out that a distinction between curables and incurables meant that environmental interventions and a program of negative eugenics, or sterilization, were not mutually exclusive. He describes the biological and social theories of Cumpston, Elkington, and Barrett as "complex and heterogeneous" ("Sir Charles Mackellar," p. 23). A similar point is made in Roe, *Nine Australian Progressives*, and Davison, "City-bred child." Bacchi, however, describes a more simple transition from prewar Lamarckism to postwar hereditary determinism and eugenics, in "The nature-nurture debate in Australia."

23. Berry, "Menace of the birth-rate"; and W. Ramsay Smith, *On Race-Culture and the Conditions That Influence It in South Australia*. See also Smith, "Australian conditions and problems from the standpoint of present anthropological knowledge." Although Smith generally supported environmental means of race improvement and criticized those who asserted that insanity was hereditary, he was not opposed to encouraging the breeding of the fitter elements of the white population. He was, however, adamantly opposed to sterilization of the unfit. Nancy Leys Stepan and Mark B. Adams have pointed out that virtually any theory of heredity could be reconciled to a program of selective breeding (though some more easily than others) in Stepan, *"The Hour of Eugenics": Race, Gender and Nation in Latin America,* and Adams, "Eugenics in the history of science." Gillespie has also observed that "the language of eugenics . . . could readily accommodate radically different mixtures of environmental and genetic determinism" (*The Price of Health*, p. 34).

24. Sutton, "Modern development of public health," p. 362.

25. C. Harvey Sutton, "Physical education and national fitness," p. 58. On the eve of World War II, Sutton hoped that the democracies would catch up with fascist states that had achieved much greater national fitness.

26. Davison, "City-bred child"; and G. Stedman Jones, *Outcast London: A Study of the Relationship between Classes in Victorian Society*, chapter 6. The classic novel of Australian urban degeneration is Louis Stone, *Jonah*.

27. C.E.W. Bean, *Sydney Morning Herald* (8 June 1907), quoted in Davison, "City-bred child," p. 146.

28. James Barrett, *The Twin Ideals: An Educated Commonwealth*. The description of Barrett is from Davison, "City-bred child," p. 148.

29. James Barrett, "Presidential address."

30. Neville Hicks, *"This Sin and Scandal": Australia's Population Debate, 1891–1911*. Octavius C. Beale, one of the commissioners, published an extract as *Racial Decay: A Compilation of Evidence from World Sources*.

31. See J. A. Kenneth Mackay, *The Yellow Wave: A Romance of the Asiatic Invasion of Australia*; and C. H. Kirmess, *The Australian Crisis*. See Robert Dixon, *Writing the Colonial Adventure: Race, Gender and Nation in Anglo-Australian Popular Fiction, 1875–1914*.

32. Bourke, "Sociology and the social sciences in Australia."

33. V. H. Wallace, "The Eugenics Society of Victoria (1936–61)." Barrett, W. E. Agar and a young F. Macfarlane Burnet were members of this society.

34. R.J.A. Berry and S. D. Porteus, *Intelligence and Social Valuation: A Practical Method for the Diagnosis of Mental Deficiency and Other Forms of Social Inefficiency*. See Cawte, "Craniometry and eugenics in Australia." Porteus later became professor of psychology at the University of Hawaii; see Chapter 7.

35. See Karl Pearson, "On the relationship of intelligence to size and shape of head and to other physical and mental characters"; and R.J.A. Berry and L.W.G. Buchner, "The correlation of size of head and intelligence, as estimated from the cubic capacity of brains of 355 Melbourne criminals."

36. R.J.A. Berry and R. G. Gordon, *The Mental Defective: A Problem in Social Inefficiency*. Berry came to recommend "lethal chambers" for the most serious defectives.

37. W. E. Agar, "Some problems of evolution and genetics." See also W. E. Agar, *A Contribution to the Theory of the Living Organism*.

38. W. E. Agar, "Some eugenic aspects of Australian population problems," pp. 130, 136. In the introduction, Phillips and Wood distance themselves from the more radical aspects of Agar's eugenic program. See also Jens Lyng, "Racial composition of the Australian People."

39. W. E. Agar, *Eugenics and the Future of the Australian Population*, pp. 7, 14. In this pamphlet Agar suggested that immigrants come from "British stock," but attention should focus primarily on the "personal quality" of the applicant (p. 16).

40. Stepan, *The Idea of Race in Science*; and Elazar Barkan, *The Retreat of Scientific Racism: Changing Concepts of Race in Britain and the United States between the World Wars*.

41. Sir Arthur Keith, *Nationality and Race, From an Anthropologist's Point of View*. Keith was based at the Royal College of Surgeons. His views on the hormonal determinants of racial character were influential in Australian medicine in the 1920s and 1930s.

42. See the criticisms by the statistician R. A. Fisher, "The coefficient of racial likeness and the future of craniometry." Fisher remained concerned about dysgenic breeding within populations; see "Eugenics: Can it solve the problem of decay of civilisations?"

43. Boas, *Changes in Bodily Form*. In the United States, the intellectual opposition to racial theory came less from biologists than from Boas and other cultural anthropologists, including his students Ruth Benedict and Margaret Mead.

44. Lancelot Hogben, *Nature and Nurture,* and *Genetic Principles in Medicine and Social Science.* See Gary Wersky, *The Visible College.*

45. Julian S. Huxley and A. C. Haddon, *We Europeans: A Survey of "Racial" Problems*, pp. 7, 8, 220 (emphasis in original).

46. Edwin J. Brady, *Australia Unlimited*, pp. 14, 64, 420, 434. Brady, who based himself at Mallacoota in Victoria, wrote elsewhere that "the people of Queensland—yet few in numbers, but mighty strong in spirit and effort—are holding the frontiers of civilisation for a White Race" (*The Land of the Sun*, p. 15).

47. Fleetwood Chidell, *Australia—White or Yellow?*, p. 145.

48. W. M. Hughes, *The Splendid Adventure: A Review of Empire Relations Within and Without the Commonwealth of Britannic Nations*, pp. 364–65, 366.

49. P. D. Phillips, "Introduction," pp. 10, 12, 17, 28.

50. T. Griffith Taylor, "The evolution and distribution of race, culture and language," p. 55. On Taylor, see his *Journeyman Taylor: The Education of a Scientist*; and J. M. Powell, "National identity and the gifted immigrant: A note on T. Griffith Taylor, 1880–1963," *Griffith Taylor and "Australia Unlimited,"* and "Protracted reconciliation." See also Nancy J. Christie "Environment and race: Geography's search for a Darwinian synthesis."

51. Griffith Taylor, *Environment and Race: A Study of the Evolution, Migration, Settlement and Status of the Races of Man*, p. 45.

52. Ibid., p. 230. Taylor believed that "apart from the Negroes, [there was] no reason for saying that one race, in any important aspect, is better than another" (p. 341). Given a suitable environment, anyone could rise in status. Therefore, Taylor had no objections to race-mixing, as long as Africans had no part in it. Indeed, he took an unpopular stand against white Australia, suggesting that "a small influx of Chinese . . . would greatly stimulate our tropical settlement" (p. 339). But on other occasions he worked within the political constraints of the white Australia policy; see Chapter 8.

53. Griffith Taylor, "Geographical factors controlling the settlement of tropical Australia," p. 17.

54. Ibid., pp. 44, 46. For earlier work along these lines, see Griffith Taylor, *The Control of Settlement by Humidity and Temperatures.* In *Environment and Race*, Taylor suggests that the only reason that Darwin did not show the same death rate as Lagos, the white man's grave, was the absence of a large black population (p. 260).

55. Taylor, *Environment and Race*, p. 266n.

56. Ibid., p. 267.

57. Taylor, "Geographical factors," p. 58.

58. Ibid., pp. 45, 55, 57.

59. Griffith Taylor, "The distribution of future white settlement: A world survey based on physiographic data," p. 400.

60. In *Race and Environment*, Taylor claims that "health is controlled primarily by temperature and humidity" (p. 317).

61. Taylor, "Geographical factors," pp. 63, 65.

62. Taylor, *Race and Environment*, p. 329.

63. Ellsworth Huntington, *Civilization and Climate*, pp. v, 1, 35. For more elaborate charts of the distribution of climatic energy, see his *Character of Races, As Influenced by Physical Environment, Natural Selection and Historical Development.* Taylor wrote to Huntington to tell him that "I know of no one whose good opinion I would rather have on these world problems" (23 June 1920, Taylor papers, ms. 1003/4/127/2E2, National Library of Australia).

64. Huntington, *Civilization and Climate*, pp. 8, 38, 41.

65. Ibid., pp. 134, 298, 294. For a sociological criticism of Huntington's environmental determinism, see P. Sorokin, *Contemporary Sociological Theories Through the First Quarter.*

66. Ellsworth Huntington, *West of the Pacific*, pp. 330, 334, 335, 333.

67. Cilento to Andrew Balfour, 22 October 1923, AITM General Correspondence, SP1061/1/300, National Archives of Australia. Cilento also criticized Huntington for treating Americans in the New England states as the ideal to which Queenslanders must aspire (*White Man in the Tropics*, p. 60). Moreover, Cilento argued that what Huntington attributed to climate, the medical scientist attributed to disease, especially to hookworm.

68. Huntington, *West of the Pacific*, pp. 342, 342–3, 356, 362. Huntington continued to argue that the limited success of white settlement in northern Australia derived from a process of self-selection and natural selection, not from any environmental suitability. For a criticism of his views by the Commonwealth statistician, see C. H. Wickens, "Vitality of white races in low latitudes." For the ensuing debate, see Ellsworth Huntington, "Natural selection and climate in northern Australia"; and C. H. Wickens, "Dr Huntington and low latitudes." Cilento welcomed the modification of Huntington's views but wished he would go further and admit that climate had no bearing on health. Whites were thriving in the tropics because of "adequate measures of preventive medicine" and "the exclusion of races with lower standards of life and higher rates of disease and reproduction" ("Rejoinder to Professor Huntington," p. 130).

69. J. W. Gregory, "White labour in tropical agriculture: a great Australian experiment," p. 379. On Gregory, see David Branagan and Blaine Lim, "J. W. Gregory, traveller in the Dead Heart."

70. J. W. Gregory, *The Menace of Colour*, pp. 18, 11, 159.

71. Ibid., pp. 183, 216, 195, 196.

72. Ibid., pp. 235, 242.

73. H. L. Wilkinson, *The World's Population Problems and a White Australia*, pp. 187, 192–3, 201.

74. Ibid., pp. 254, 258, 261.

75. A. Grenfell Price, *White Settlers in the Tropics*, pp. 241n, 3, 6, 12. Price subscribed to the racial theories of Ales Hrdlicka, "Human races."

76. Price, *White Settlers*, pp. 52, 61, 38.

77. Ibid., pp. 181, 121. In warning against "hybridisation," Price was influenced by the research of C. B. Davenport, the American Mendelian eugenicist. See C. B. Davenport and Morris Steggerda, *Race Crossing in Jamaica.*

78. Price, *White Settlers*, pp. 104, 120.

79. Ibid., p. 69.

80. A. Grenfell Price, "White settlers in the tropics," p. 270.

81. Price, *White Settlers*, p. 238. As the war approached, there were more calls for research on white settlement in the tropics. In 1938, at the International Geographical Congress in Amsterdam, W. Wynne Williams also suggested that "insufficient research has taken place" ("The white man in the Australian tropics: history of colonisation," p. 342). George C. Shattuck, a professor of tropical medicine at Harvard, also urged more investigation of "the problem of colonization of the Tropics by the White Race" ("The possibility of white settlement in the tropics," p. 327). In the same year, L. H. Pike, the agent-general for Queensland, who thought that the white Australia policy was designed to preserve "all the institutions, characteristics and attributes of the British race," concluded that "much work, based upon scientific and medical investigation and governmental administration and assistance, requires still to be done" ("White Australia—tropical Queensland," pp. 720, 733).

82. Douglas H. K. Lee, "The settlement of tropical Australia"; and D.H.K. Lee and R. K. Macpherson, "Tropical fatigue and warfare." See Malcom Whyte, *A Global Scientist: Douglas H. K. Lee.*

83. R. K. Macpherson, "The physiology of adaptation."

84. G. L. Wood, "The immigrant problem in Australia."

85. More generally on the debates about cultural identity and national character during this period, see David Walker, *Dream and Disillusion: A Search for Australian Cultural Identity*; Tim Rowse, *Australian Liberalism and National Character*; and Stephen Alomes, *A Nation at Last? The Changing Character of Australian Nationalism, 1880–1988.*

86. Craig Munro, "Two boys from Queensland: P. R. Stephensen and Jack Lindsay."

87. P. R. Stephensen, *The Foundations of Culture in Australia*, p. 141. Stephensen was a leader of the Australia First movement and interned during World War II for fascist and pro-Japanese sympathies. See Bruce Muirden, *The Puzzled Patriots: The Story of the Australia First Movement*; and Craig Munro, *Wild Man of Letters: The Story of P. R. Stephensen.*

88. P. R. Stephensen, "The foundations of culture in Australia: an essay towards national self-respect."

89. The reference is to the "national mystique" described in Russel Ward, *The Australian Legend*, but Ward was careful to point out that "national character is not, as was once held, something inherited" (p. 1).

CHAPTER 7

1. Edwin J. Brady, *Australia Unlimited*, pp. 630, 593, 584. On Lawson and literary nationalism, see Vance Palmer, *The Legend of the Nineties*; and Colin Roderick, *Henry Lawson, A Life*. For a more general account of Australian responses to arid environments, see Roslynn D. Haynes, *Seeking the Centre: The Australian Desert in Literature, Art and Film.*

2. J. W. Gregory, *The Menace of Colour*, pp. 152, 150. See also his *The Dead Heart of Australia*.

3. Griffith Taylor, *Environment and Race: A Study of the Evolution, Migration, Settlement and Status of the Races of Man*; and Ellsworth Huntington, *Civilization and Climate*.

4. Jens Lyng, *Non-Britishers in Australia: Influence on Population and Progress*. I will use the terms "full-blood" and "half-caste" without quotation marks in the rest of this work, as they were used by the historical actors.

5. Ernestine Hill, *The Great Australian Loneliness*, p. 54. Hill became the ghost-writer for Daisy Bates, whom she met on this trip. Katharine Susannah Prichard, a friend, thought the Sydney travel writer wrote well but was incapable of logic. At the time of her death in 1972, Hill was still working on her novel about an albino Aboriginal.

6. Ibid., pp. 43, 121.

7. A. Grenfell Price, *White Settlers in the Tropics*, p. 120.

8. Russell McGregor, "An Aboriginal Caucasian: Some uses for racial kinship in early twentieth century Australia." See also Russell McGregor, *Imagined Destinies: Aboriginal Australians and the Doomed Race Theory, 1880–1939*.

9. A. Grenfell Price, "'Scandalous history' of the Aborigines. Whites brought death and disease. Investigator's proposals. Infiltration of half-castes," *Adelaide Advertiser* (18 April 1934).

10. Matthew Frye Jacobson, *Whiteness of a Different Color: European Immigrants and the Alchemy of Race*. Jacobson argues that "Caucasian" replaced notions of "divisible whiteness," but evidently in Australia it might undermine surface definitions of whiteness altogether, at the same time as it reinscribed internal divisions through qualifiers such as "archaic."

11. E. J. Brady, *The Land of the Sun*, pp. 246, 248, 251.

12. I discuss the scientific management of the "half-caste problem" in Chapter 8.

13. H. L. Wilkinson, *The World's Population Problems and a White Australia*, p. 221.

14. Frederic Wood Jones, "The claims of the Australian Aborigine," p. 505. Wood Jones later claimed that "the 'civilising' experiment has failed utterly" ("Black and white. Our responsibility to the native. Science demands new regime," *Adelaide Advertiser* [10 April 1934]).

15. Charles Darwin, *A Naturalist's Voyage: Journal of Researches*, p. 417. See also the references to Aboriginal people, based on the research of T. H. Huxley and Armand de Quatrefages, in his *The Descent of Man, and Selection in Relation to Sex*, pp. 38–9, 264, 848.

16. Of course, theories of race struggle antedated Darwin's principal publications. See Robert Knox, *The Races of Men: A Fragment*.

17. McGregor, *Imagined Destinies*; and Henry Reynolds, *Frontier: Aborigines, Settlers and Land*. See David Collins, *An Account of the English Colony in New South Wales*; and Peter Cunningham, *Two Years in New South Wales*. For other early accounts of Aboriginal people in New South Wales, see W.E.H. Stanner, "The history of indifference thus begins." For Victoria, see Thomas Francis Bride,

ed., *Letters from Victorian Pioneers, Being a Series of Papers on the Early Occupation of the Colony, the Aborigines, etc.*

18. William Westgarth, *A Report on the Condition, Capabilities and Prospects of the Australian Aborigines*, pp. 22, 23.

19. Ibid., p. 16. On the facial angle and its significance, see Nancy L. Stepan, *The Idea of Race in Science: Great Britain, 1800–1960.*

20. Westgarth, *Report*, pp. 36, 35–6. Westgarth also claimed that "the Australian savage has been suited to the circumstances which surround him" (p. 35).

21. Ibid., pp. 5, 39.

22. R. Brough Smyth, *The Aborigines of Victoria, and Other Parts of Australia and Tasmania*, pp. xix, xx. An agnostic and a rationalist, Brough Smyth was secretary of the Board for the Protection of Aborigines and active in the Royal Society of Victoria.

23. Ibid., p. xxxix.

24. Ibid., pp. 257, 259.

25. Ibid., pp. xvii, lxix.

26. T. H. Huxley, "On the geographical distribution of the chief modifications of mankind," p. 404.

27. Paul Topinard, "Etudes sur les Tasmaniens," p. 307. The other leading French anthropologists later more or less agreed with Huxley; see Armand de Quatrefages de Breau and Ernest T. Hamy, *Crania Ethnica: Les Crânes des Races Humaines*; and Quatrefages, *Histoire Générale des Races Humaines: Introduction à l'étude des races humaines*, esp. pp. 368–69.

28. H. Ling Roth, *The Aborigines of Tasmania*, p. 227.

29. N.J.B. Plomley, *Friendly Mission: The Tasmanian Journals and Papers of George Augustus Robinson, 1829–34.*

30. Roth, *Aborigines of Tasmania*, pp. 4, 5.

31. Edward B. Tylor, "Preface," in ibid., p. v.

32. Tom Griffiths, *Hunters and Collectors: The Antiquarian Imagination in Australia*; and Paul Turnbull, *Science, National Identity and Aboriginal Body Snatching in Nineteenth Century Australia,* and "Ramsay's regime: The Australian Museum and the procurement of Aboriginal bodies, c.1874–1900."

33. The anthropology section (section F) of the Australasian Association for the Advancement of Science was founded in 1888, but few of the contributors to its proceedings would have identified themselves primarily as anthropologists until the next century.

34. Darwin, *Descent of Man*. On nineteenth-century racial theory, see Stepan, *The Idea of Race in Science*. More specifically, see Barry Butcher, "Darwinism, social Darwinism and the Australian Aborigines: A re-evaluation."

35. Edward M. Curr, *The Australian Race: Its Origin, Languages, Customs, Place of Landing in Australia and the Routes by Which It Spread Itself over That Continent*, vol. 1, pp. 36, 38, 42.

36. Ibid., vol. 1, pp. 152, 188. Friedrich Blumenbach had claimed that Australians were Malayan; Barron Field regarded them as degenerate Ethiopians, in *Geographical Memoirs of New South Wales.*

37. Curr, *Australian Race*, vol. 1, p. 105. Curr notes that "the subject of the diseases generally of our Aborigines and the peculiarities of their constitutions have heretofore failed to attract the attention of the gentlemen of the medical profession in these colonies" (vol. 1, p. 234).

38. T. H. Huxley, "On the ethnology and archaeology of India." James Cowles Pritchard had previously asserted that Aborigines were Negrito in origin, arriving from New Guinea; see *Researches into the Physical History of Mankind*, vol. 4, p. 214. Darwin seems to have accepted Huxley's claim that the Australians were homogeneously Caucasian; see *Descent of Man*, pp. 38–9.

39. W. H. Flower and R. Lydekker, *An Introduction to the Study of Mammals, Living and Extinct*, p. 748. See also G. W. Rusden, *The History of Australia*.

40. Alfred R. Wallace, *Australasia, Volume 1: Australia and New Zealand*, pp. 149, 152, 157.

41. John Mathew, *Eaglehawk and Crow: A Study of the Australian Aborigines*. Mathew was moderator-general of the Presbyterian Church in Australia (1922–1924).

42. John Mathew, *Two Representative Tribes of Queensland, with an Inquiry Concerning the Origin of the Australian Race*, pp. 35, 143. Mathew quoted a letter from Daisy Bates confirming that social classes correspond to Aboriginal skin color (p. 32).

43. Mathew, *Eaglehawk and Crow*, p. 78.

44. Mathew, *Two Representative Tribes*, p. 81. He believed that "the partial adoption of European habits both aggravated that maladies they were naturally liable to and induced others of a more serious nature, such as syphilis and phthisis" (p. 110).

45. A. W. Howitt, "On the origin of the Aborigines of Tasmania and Australia."

46. M. H. Walker, *Come Wind, Come Weather: A Biography of Alfred Howitt*. See especially A. W. Howitt, *The Native Tribes of Southeast Australia*.

47. L. H. Morgan, "Preface," in Lorimer Fison and A. W. Howitt, *Kamilaroi and Kurnai*, p. 2. See Lewis Henry Morgan, *Ancient Society: or, Researches in the Lines of Human Progress, from Savagery Through Barbarism to Civilisation*, esp. chapter 1. See also Thomas R. Trautmann, *Lewis Henry Morgan and the Invention of Kinship*; and Adam Kuper, *The Invention of Primitive Society: Transformations of an Illusion*.

48. W. Baldwin Spencer, "The Aboriginals of Australia," p. 33. Spencer conducted his most important fieldwork in the 1890s with F. J. Gillen, the telegraph officer, magistrate, and subprotector of Aborigines at Alice Springs; see W. Baldwin Spencer and F. J. Gillen, *The Native Tribes of Central Australia*. Spencer, a north country Nonconformist, had attended Tylor's anthropology lectures at Oxford; he took up the chair of biology at Melbourne in 1887. On Spencer, see D. J. Mulvaney and J. H. Callaby, *"So Much That Is New." Baldwin Spencer, 1860–1929: A Biography*. On Gillen, see John Mulvaney, Howard Morphy, and Alison Petch, eds., *"My Dear Spencer": The Letters of F. J. Gillen to Baldwin Spencer*.

49. W. Baldwin Spencer and F. J. Gillen, *Across Australia*, vol. 1, p. 132.

50. Spencer, "The Aboriginals of Australia."

51. W. Baldwin Spencer, "Preliminary report on the Aborigines of the Northern Territory," p. 41. See also Tony Austin, *Simply the Survival of the Fittest: Aboriginal Administration in South Australia's Northern Territory, 1863–1910*; and Russell McGregor, "The idea of racial degeneration: Baldwin Spencer and the Aborigines of the Northern Territory."

52. Paul Topinard, *Anthropology*; and Quatrefages and Hamy, *Crania Ethnica*. See J. G. Garson, "Osteology."

53. W. Turner, "Report on the human crania and other bones of the skeletons collected during the voyage of *HMS Challenger*, in the years 1873–76. Part 1: The crania."

54. H. Klaatsch, "The skull of the Australian Aboriginal."

55. R.J.A. Berry, A.W.D. Robertson and K. Stuart Cross, "A biometrical study of the relative degree of purity of race of the Tasmanian, Australian and Papuan," p. 27. See also R.J.A. Berry and A.W.D. Robertson, "The place in nature of the Tasmanian Aboriginal as deduced from a study of his calvarium." For surveys of Aboriginal craniometry, see G. M. Morant, "A study of the Australian and Tasmanian skulls, based on previously published measurements"; and Tasman Brown, *Morphology of the Australian Skull, Studied by Multivariate Analysis*.

56. Gregory, *Dead Heart*, pp. 171, 61.

57. Ibid., pp. 62, 132, 180, 61.

58. Ibid., p. 34.

59. Elsie Masson, *An Untamed Territory: The Northern Territory of Australia*, pp. 23–4, 156, 152–3. Masson's father was the professor of chemistry at the University of Melbourne.

60. On evolutionary primitivism, see Kuper, *Invention of Primitive Society*; and Marianna Torgovnick, *Gone Primitive: Savage Intellects, Modern Lives*. On the creation of ambivalence from fragmented, modern efforts to order social life, see Zygmunt Bauman, *Modernity and Ambivalence*.

61. Douglas Pike, *Paradise of Dissent: South Australia, 1829–57*.

62. On the history of the Adelaide medical school, see A. A. Lendon, *Jubilee of the Medical School, 1885–1935*; A. A. Abbie, *The University of Adelaide School of Medicine*; and V. A. Edgeloe, The Medical School of the University of Adelaide: A Brief History from an Administrative Viewpoint (1991), typescript in the Adelaide University Archives. On the history of medicine in South Australia more generally, see K. N. White, "Negotiating science and liberalism: Medicine in nineteenth-century Australia."

63. W. Ramsay Smith, "Australian conditions and problems from the standpoint of present anthropological knowledge," p. 374. Smith graduated in medicine from the University of Edinburgh and migrated to Adelaide in 1896. An unusually sympathetic observer of Aboriginal customs and habits, he was the author of *Myths and Legends of the Australian Aborigines*.

64. W. Ramsay Smith, *In Southern Seas: Wanderings of a Naturalist*, p. 166. See also his "The place of the Australian Aboriginal in recent anthropological research." For a similar plea for studies in physical anthropology, see R. Hamlyn-

Harris, "Some anthropological considerations of Queensland and the history of its ethnography." Hamlyn-Harris was especially interested in "the effect of civilisation on the natives constitutionally" (p. 24.).

65. Smith, *Southern Seas*, pp. 223, 239, 273.

66. Though born in Adelaide, Stirling had trained in England. See Bryan Gandevia, "The Sir Edward Stirling Memorial Lecture"; and E. C. Stirling, "Anthropology of the central Australian Aborigines," and "Preliminary report on the discovery of native remains at Swanport, River Murray; with an enquiry into the alleged occurrence of a pandemic among the Australian Aboriginals." On the Horn expedition, see S. R. Morton and D. J. Mulvaney, eds., *Exploring Central Australia: Society, the Environment and the 1894 Horn Expedition*.

67. P. G. Jones, "South Australian anthropological history: The Board for Anthropological Research and its early expeditions." The unusually close connection of the medical school with the museum helped to sustain a natural history tradition in biomedical research at Adelaide.

68. When Wood Jones moved to the Melbourne medical school in 1930, many of his colleagues, including W. A. Osborne and Wilfred Agar, regarded him with suspicion.

69. Wood Jones, "The claims of the Australian Aborigine." Wood Jones graduated in medicine from the University of London and worked with Grafton Elliot Smith, the Australian anatomist, before his appointment as professor of anatomy at the Royal Free Hospital in London (1915–1919). After Adelaide, Wood Jones was Rockefeller professor of physical anthropology at the University of Hawaii. He was later professor of anatomy at Melbourne (1930–1937), at Manchester (1938–1944), and at the Royal College of Surgeons, London (1945–1951). See Monica Macallum, "Frederic Wood Jones (1879–1954)," *ADB 9*, pp. 510–12.

70. F. Wood Jones and T. D. Campbell, "Anthropometric and descriptive observations on some South Australian Aboriginals, with a summary of previously recorded anthropometric data," p. 303.

71. T. D. Campbell and Aubrey J. Lewis, "The Aborigines of South Australia: Anthropometric, descriptive and other observations recorded at Ooldea," pp. 185, 190.

72. T. D. Campbell and Cecil J. Hackett, "Adelaide University field anthropology. Central Australia No.1. Introduction: Descriptive and anthropometric observations."

73. T. D. Campbell, J. H. Gray, C. J. Hackett, "Physical anthropology of the Aborigines of central Australia," pp. 111, 138, 253, 255. For an anthropometrical study that challenges Aboriginal homogeneity, see F. J. Fenner, "Adelaide University field anthropology. Central Australia No. 13. Anthropometric observations on South Australian Aborigines of the Diamantina and Cooper Creek regions." Fenner was honorary craniologist to the South Australian Museum.

74. T. D. Campbell, "Food, food values and food habits of the Australian Aborigines in relation to their dental conditions." But see J. B. Cleland and H. K. Fry, "An outbreak of scurvy with joint lesions in Australian Aborigines in central Australia."

75. F. Wood Jones, "Black and white. Our responsibility to the native. Science demands new regime," Adelaide *Advertiser* (10 April 1934).

76. Wood Jones, "Claims of the Australian Aborigine," pp. 498, 501, 505. Wood Jones further remarked that "the white colonists of Australia have contracted a huge debt; they are under a moral obligation of no less magnitude than that of making some reparation for the filching of a whole vast continent from its real owners" (p. 497).

77. Frederic Wood Jones, *Australia's Vanishing Race*, pp. 9. 11.

78. Ibid., pp. 26, 29.

79. Ibid., pp. 17, 40. One might also align Wood Jones with the more evolutionist Herbert Basedow on many of these issues. See especially Herbert Basedow, *The Australian Aboriginal*. Basedow deplored the "demoralisation of primitive ethics" and claimed that to have communed with the nomadic full-bloods was "to have hobnobbed with Nature's aristocrats" (*Knights of the Boomerang: Episodes from a Life Spent Among the Native Tribes of Australia*, pp. 14, 19).

80. William K. Gregory to Madison Grant, 22 November 1923, Rockefeller Foundation, RG 1.1 (Projects), series 410D (Australia), box 3, folder 23, Rockefeller Archive Center (RAC). Gregory was the secretary of the Galton Society, a eugenics discussion group; Grant was the author of *The Passing of the Great Race*, which warned of the mongrelization of Nordics.

81. C. B. Davenport to Edwin R. Embree, 3 March 1924, RG 1.1, series 410D, box 3, folder 23, RAC. Davenport was the most influential Mendelian eugenicist in the United States; see Daniel J. Kevles, *In the Name of Eugenics: Genetics and the Uses of Human Heredity*. Clark Wissler, the curator of anthropology at the American Museum of Natural History, was also a strong supporter of the proposal.

82. For a fuller explanation of Smith's decision, see G. E. Smith to E. R. Embree, 30 September 1924, RG 1.1, series 410D, box 3, folder 24, RAC. See also A. P. Elkin and N.W.G. Macintosh, eds., *Grafton Elliot Smith: The Man and His Work*.

83. See Australia—Studies in Anthropology, RG 1.1, series 410D, box 3, folder 25, RAC. See also E. R. Embree to G. E. Smith, 7 May 1924, ibid., box 3, folder 23. For other accounts of the establishment of the Board, see Jones, "South Australian anthropological history"; Nicolas Peterson, "'Studying man and man's nature': The history of the institutionalisation of Aboriginal anthropology"; and D. J. Mulvaney, "Australian anthropology: Foundations and funding." In Chapter 8 I briefly consider the work conducted at Sydney under Radcliffe-Brown's successor, A. P. Elkin.

84. On the naturalist in medicine, a career path favored at Adelaide, see J. B. Cleland, "The naturalist in medicine with particular reference to Australia."

85. J. B. Cleland, "An objection to the direct continuity of the germ plasm, with a suggestion as to the part possibly played by hormones in heredity," p. 34. Cleland's theories parallel those of Sir Arthur Keith.

86. J. B. Cleland, "Complexities of evolution: Interesting, if puzzling, phases of development in forms of life."

87. J. B. Cleland, "Disease among the Australian Aborigines," p. 53.

88. The principal Adelaide expeditions during this period were Wilgena 1925; Ooldea 1926; Macumba 1927; Koonibba 1928; Hermannsburg 1929; Macdonald

Downs 1930; Cockatoo Creek 1931; Mt. Liebig 1932; Mann Range and Ernabella 1933; Diamantina 1934; Warburton Range 1935; and The Granites 1936. The parties often used Alice Springs, an administrative center with a population of 400, or Hermannsburg, a Lutheran mission established in 1877, as staging posts. Although the Coniston massacre took place outside Alice Springs in 1928, the scientists made no reference to it. Travel became much easier after the extension of the railway from Oodnadatta to Alice Springs in 1929. In the late 1920s, there were probably no more than six medical doctors in central Australia, so the expeditions were often called on to provide medical care to the white and Aboriginal communities they passed through. For an evocative account of travel through the region in the early 1930s, see A. Grenfell Price, "Pioneer reactions to a poor tropical environment: A journey through central and north Australia in 1932." On the history of the area, see Andrew Markus, *Governing Savages*.

89. L. and H. Hirszfeld, "Serological differences between the blood of different races."

90. A. H. Tebbutt, "Comparative iso-agglutinin index of Australian Aborigines and Australians," and "Second report on the comparative iso-agglutinin index of Australian Aborigines and Australians"; and D.H.K. Lee, "Blood groups of North Queensland Aborigines, with a statistical collection of some published figures for various races."

91. H. Woollard and J. B. Cleland, "Anthropology and blood grouping with special reference to Australian Aborigines," p. 184.

92. Ibid., pp. 186, 187. Lucy Bryce refers to postwar blood grouping, led in the 1950s by R. T. Simmons at the Commonwealth Serum Laboratories and J. J. Graydon at the Victorian Blood Transfusion Service, intended to "tell us something of the migrations and long history of our Aboriginal race" (*An Abiding Gladness*, p. 254).

93. J. B. Cleland, "Further results in blood grouping central Australian Aborigines," p. 80. See also his "Blood grouping of Australian Aboriginals." (I use the various names given to Aboriginal groups by the investigators, not the current versions, such as Arrente.)

94. Anon., "Anthropological expedition to the north-west of South Australia, 1933," p. 99.

95. J. B. Cleland, "Ecology of the Aboriginal inhabitants of Tasmania and South Australia," pp. 97, 98.

96. Cedric Stanton Hicks, Just in Time: A Physiologist among the Nomad Tribes of Central Australia, 1929–39, 2 vols. (1974), unpublished ms., Cedric Stanton Hicks papers, series 1, box 1, University of Adelaide Archives, pp. 1, 5.

97. Ibid., p. 16. Hicks's assistant was R. F. Matters.

98. C. S. Hicks, R. F. Matters, M. L. Mitchell, "The standard metabolism of Australian Aboriginals," p. 69. The authors note that detribalized Aborigines are "a curious people, giving the impression that they are superlatively lazy and inactive, but the fact remains that the men can and do form most successful football teams, in which their success is due entirely to their running speed, in which . . . they surpass their white opponents" (pp. 72–3).

99. Ibid., pp. 81, 82. The Lutheran missionaries assisted with experiments.

100. See C. S. Hicks and R. F. Matters, "The standard metabolism of Australian Aboriginals."

101. Hicks, Just in Time, p. 20.

102. Ibid., pp. 29, 31, 34, 38. Hicks later described his work as "searching for some explanation of the apparently 'normal' European basal metabolism of native Aborigines" (p. 49). See also C. S. Hicks et al., "The respiratory exchange of the Australian Aborigine."

103. Hicks, Just in Time, p. 34.

104. F. Goldby, C. S. Hicks, W. J. O'Connor, D. A. Sinclair, "A comparison of the skin temperature and skin circulation of naked whites and Australian Aboriginals exposed to similar environmental changes," p. 36. See also C. Stanton Hicks, "The Australian Aboriginal: A study in comparative physiology."

105. Hicks, Just in Time, p. 77. Hicks later became an expert on nutrition and a pioneer ecologist who warned of the dangers of urbanization. See his *Soil, Food and Life*.

106. Henry Priestley and Ellen M. Hindmarsh, "The blood urea and nitrogen output of Australian students"; and H. S. Halcro Wardlaw, "The energy consumption of Australian students."

107. See Rockefeller Foundation, RG 1.1, Series 410A, box 3, folder 20 (University of Sydney, Physiology), RAC.

108. H. S. Halcro Wardlaw and C. H. Horsley, "The basal metabolism of some Australian Aborigines," pp. 263, 265, 269. Variations in technique, and in the nutritional status and lifestyle of the subjects, may have accounted for the disparity of the Adelaide and Sydney results. Few would now regard the fact that many of these people were underweight and inactive as an inherent racial characteristic.

109. H. S. Halcro Wardlaw, H. Whitridge Davies, M. R. Joseph, "Energy metabolism and insensible perspiration of Australian Aborigines."

110. H. S. Halcro Wardlaw, H. C. Barry, I. W. McDonald, and A. K. Macintyre, "The haemoglobin and solids of the blood of Australian Aborigines and whites."

111. J. B. Cleland, Visits to Native Institutions in Western Australia, c. 1940, Cleland papers, box 2, folder 2, University of Adelaide Archives, p. 7.

112. J. B. Cleland, The Rocket-Bomb Range and the Natives of South Australia, 1946, Cleland papers, box 2, folder 3, University of Adelaide Archives, p. 1.

113. J. B. Cleland, The Place of the Aborigines in Australia's Society, c. 1957, Cleland papers, box 2, folder 5, University of Adelaide Archives, pp. 3, 4.

114. Ibid., pp. 1, 7. The second statement is hand-written in the margins of the typescript.

115. Hill, *Great Australian Loneliness*, p. 157. Later, Hill developed a more favorable image of Aborigines, claiming that "if quick adaptability to environment is the test of intelligence, they are the equal of any race on earth" (*The Territory*, p. 345).

116. R.J.A. Berry, Chance and Circumstance (Bristol, 1954), Medical History Museum, University of Melbourne, p. 132.

117. S. D. Porteus, "Mental tests with delinquents and Australian Aboriginal children"; and R.J.A. Berry and S.D. Porteus, *Intelligence and Social Valuation: A Practical Method for the Diagnosis of Mental Deficiency and Other Forms of Social Inefficiency*.

118. Berry, Chance and Circumstance, pp. 143, 145.

119. Stanley D. Porteus, *A Psychologist of Sorts: The Autobiography and Publications of the Inventor of the Porteus Maze Tests*, p. 51.

120. Porteus claimed that Berry lacked the "brilliance" of Wood Jones, in *A Psychologist of Sorts*, p. 51. Referring to Berry's research, Porteus, in the 1960s, judged that "the equating of achievement with physical characters was a most attractive game for thinkers who lacked the disciplinary control of sufficient facts" (p. 54). But even if he later deplored the work of "race dogmatists" (p. 83) like Berry, Griffith Taylor, and Ellsworth Huntington, Porteus continued to believe in definite racial capacities for intelligence. Thus Filipinos and Hawaiians "have lived too long in the tropics to attain toughness of mental fibre" (p. 85).

121. Frederic Wood Jones and Stanley D. Porteus, *The Matrix of the Mind*, pp. 413, 414, 419. On "primitive mentality," see Lucien Lévy-Bruhl, *Primitive Mentality*.

122. Stanley D. Porteus, *The Psychology of a Primitive People: A Study of the Australian Aborigine*, p. v.

123. Géza Róheim, *The Children of the Desert: The Western Tribes of Central Australia*.

124. Porteus, *Psychology of a Primitive People*, pp. 354, 359, 360.

125. Ibid., pp. 374, 389. Porteus returned to central Australia in 1962, and worked with A. James McGregor and other Adelaide researchers at Yuendamu.

126. R. Pulleine and H. Woollard, "Physiology and mental observations on the Australian Aborigines," p. 62. But later H. K. Fry and Pulleine do admit a positive, but not "perfect," correlation between intelligence and cranial capacity ("The mentality of the Australian Aborigine," p. 154).

127. Pulleine and Woollard, "Physiology and mental observations," pp. 70, 71.

128. H. K Fry, "Adelaide University field anthropology: Central Australia. Physiological and psychological observations." On the Torres Straits expedition, see Anita Herle and Sandra Rouse, eds., *Cambridge and the Torres Strait: Centenary Essays on the 1898 Anthropological Expedition*.

129. See H. K. Fry, "Aboriginal mentality." Later studies showed a gradual increase in average "mental age" and a greater range. See, for example, H. L. Fowler, "Report on psychological tests on natives in the north-west of Western Australia." Fowler argued that his results indicated that "numbers of our natives are capable of considerable mental development" (p. 127).

130. Natalie Robarts, "The Victorian Aborigine as he is," p. 445.

131. Herbert Pitts, *The Australian Aboriginal and the Christian Church*, pp. 20, 55.

132. R. Hamlyn-Harris, "Some anthropological considerations of Queensland and the history of its ethnography," pp. 26, 25.

133. Fry and Pulleine, "Mentality of the Australian Aborigine," p. 162. It seems that Fry also tested their response to scalding water ("Aboriginal mentality," p. 355).

134. Fry, "Physiological and psychological observations," p. 91.

135. Porteus, *Psychology of a Primitive People*, p. 122.

136. James Barnard, "Aborigines of Tasmania," p. 597.

137. On notions of the "dressed native" in South Africa, see Randall Packard, *White Plague, Black Labor: Tuberculosis and the Political Economy of Health and Disease in South Africa*. Charles E. Rosenberg discusses diseases of civilization—and the persistence of notions of "fit" and "stress" in medicine—in "Pathologies of progress: The idea of civilization as risk."

138. Spencer and Gillen, *Across Australia*, vol. 2, pp. 300–1.

139. Spencer and Gillen, *Native Tribes*, p. 17.

140. J. Burton Cleland, "Disease amongst the Australian Aborigines," p. 53. See Ernest Hunter, *Aboriginal Health and History: Power and Prejudice in Remote Australia*.

141. Cleland, "Disease amongst the Australian Aborigines," pp. 55, 56.

142. Warwick Anderson, "Immunities of empire: Race, disease and the new tropical medicine."

143. Cleland, "Disease amongst the Australian Aborigines," p. 57.

144. Ibid., pp. 58, 59.

145. See Chapter 8 for a discussion of half-caste destinies.

146. Cleland, "Disease amongst the Australian Aborigines." See also Cecil J. Hackett, "A critical survey of some references to syphilis and yaws among the Australian Aborigines."

147. See Chapter 5 for Cilento's studies of hookworm.

148. Raphael Cilento, Report of the Federal Health Council, 5th Session, 1931, and Report of the Federal Health Council, Appendix III, 1934, both quoted in Suzanne Parry, "Tropical medicine and northern identity," p. 93.

149. C. E. Cook, "The native in relation to the public health," p. 569.

150. C. E. Cook, "Leprosy problems," p. 802.

151. Cook, "Native in relation to public health," pp. 571, 569, 571. For more on Cook and his policies of absorption, see Chapter 8.

152. Torgovnick, *Gone Primitive*. See also Griffiths, *Hunters and Collectors*.

153. S. L. Larnach, "A scientific expedition to central Australia," p. 9.

154. R. H. Croll, *I Recall: Collections and Recollections*, pp. 95, 103. See also his *Wide Horizons: Wanderings in Central Australia*.

155. Katharine Susannah Prichard, *Coonardoo: The Well in the Shadow*, pp. 223, 224. Prichard cites Herbert Basedow on Caucasian affinities and the existence of tribes with fair hair.

156. T.G.H. Strehlow, *Aranda Traditions* and *Songs of Central Australia*. See Tim Rowse, "The collector as outsider—T. G. H. Strehlow as 'public intellectual.'" Strehlow's father was the Lutheran pastor at Hermannsburg. The Anthropological Board of Study supported Strehlow's early research. On 18 March 1935,

Rex Ingamells wrote to Strehlow, assuring him that "your criticism has a special value for me in that you know the things I endeavour to write about as well as— and, in many instance, far better—than I do myself" (Strehlow Research Centre Archives, Alice Springs). Strehlow later called for "the achievement of harmonious coexistence by the various nations and races of mankind" (*Dark and White Australians*, p. 28). Bruce Chatwin admired Strehlow's writings, and was smitten with the "nomads"; see *The Songlines*.

157. See P. R. Stephensen, *The Foundations of Culture in Australia: An Essay Towards National Self-Respect*. Stephensen was involved with the Aborigines Progressive Association, founded the Aboriginal Citizenship Committee in 1937, and helped to promote an Aboriginal day of mourning in 1938. See Bruce Muirden, *The Puzzled Patriots: The Story of the Australia First Movement*; and Craig Munro, *Wild Man of Letters: The Story of P. R. Stephensen*. Ian Mudie, the Jindyworobak most closely associated with Stephensen's Australia First movement, narrowly escaped internment during World War II. See Brian Elliott, "Jindyworobaks and Aborigines," and *The Jindyworobaks*.

158. Rex Ingamells, "Statement," p. 66.

159. Rex Ingamells, *Handbook of Australian Literature*, p. 2. In contrast, A. D. Hope, a cosmopolitan poet, argued that "a poet who writes life a second-hand Abo is no more likely to produce sincere work than the poet who writes like a second-hand Englishman." He was disturbed that some of the Jindyworobak work "has traces of the fanaticism of the Hitler Youth Movement" (quoted in Elliott, *Jindyworobaks*, pp. 249, 251).

160. Rex Ingamells, "Unknown land," p. 22. The poet Les Murray has called himself the last of the Jindyworobaks.

161. George W. Stocking Jr., has described the parallel dehistoricization of social anthropology in *After Tylor: British Social Anthropology, 1888–1951*.

CHAPTER 8

1. F. T. Macartney, ed., *The Collected Verse of A. B. Paterson*; and Clement Semmler, *The Banjo of the Bush: The Life and Times of A. B. Paterson*. More generally, see Russel Ward, *The Australian Legend*; J. B. Hirst, "The pioneer legend"; and Graeme Davison, "Sydney and the bush: An urban context for the Australian legend."

2. H. H. Finlayson, *The Red Centre: Man and Beast in the Heart of Australia*, pp. 74, 88, 76. Frederic Wood Jones wrote the foreword.

3. Charles P. Mountford, *Brown Men and Red Sand: Wanderings in Wild Australia*, pp. ix, 174, 176–7. Mountford had accompanied J. B. Cleland to central Australia in the 1930s. For similar attitudes, see W. E. Harney, *Taboo*, and *North of 23°: Ramblings in Northern Australia*. Harney, a well-known Territory bushman and a former member of the International Workers of the World, was an associate of A. P. Elkin, the professor of anthropology at Sydney. Harney later advised on the making of the film *Jedda* (1955).

4. Charles Chewings, *Back in the Stone Age: Native Tribes of Central Australia*, pp. 9, 10, 13, 45. Chewings, the son of a South Australian pastoralist, had received a Ph.D. in geology from the University of Heidelberg.

5. Ibid., pp. 145, 150. Still, in the introduction Chewings thanks Cleland and Finlayson for their advice.

6. Ibid., pp. 152, 153, 154.

7. On Aboriginal labor practices in central Australia, see Tim Rowse, *White Flour, White Power: From Rations to Citizenship in Central Australia*.

8. See Russell McGregor, *Imagined Destinies: Aboriginal Australians and the Doomed Race Theory, 1880–1939*.

9. It may now appear surprising that plans were made to absorb Aboriginal Australians into white Australia at the same time as other scientists expressed reservations about whether Mediterraneans were white enough to be allowed to join the nation's breeding population. But then, Aborigines were there already, and Greeks mostly were not. See Chapter 6.

10. Patrick Wolfe makes the argument that "repressive authenticity" licenses half-caste absorption, through the logic of the elimination of the "in-between" (*Settler Colonialism and the Transformation of Anthropology: The Politics and Poetics of an Ethnographic Event*, p. 186). On the construction of Aboriginal authenticity, see Jeremy R. Beckett, ed., *Past and Present: The Construction of Aboriginality*; and Bain Attwood, *The Making of Aborigines*.

11. The Adelaide research thus provides another example, though perhaps a more muted one, of how even those with some Lamarckian sensitivities might still support a human breeding program. See Nancy Stepan, *"The Hour of Eugenics": Race, Gender and Nation in Latin America*.

12. R. Brough Smyth, *The Aborigines of Victoria, and Other Parts of Australia and Tasmania*, vol. 1, p. 21. Just a few years earlier, Charles Darwin had pondered whether Australian and European crosses might be sterile and decided they were not (*The Descent of Man, and Selection in Relation to Sex*, p. 264).

13. Natalie Robarts, "The Victorian Aborigine as he is," pp. 445–6.

14. Jens Lyng estimated that there were more than 15,000 half-castes and 60,000 full-bloods in the 1920s, at a time when the European population of Australia was 6 million or so. He believed the half-caste numbers would increase as the detribalized full-blood males "lose their energy, virility and whatever racial pride they once possessed; they become indolent and apathetic toward life, and guard with less jealousy than formerly their women folk from associating with the whites" (*Non-Britishers in Australia: Influence on Population and Progress*, p. 203).

15. Ernestine Hill, *The Great Australian Loneliness*, pp. 138, 205.

16. Ibid., pp. 203, 204, 207. Hill was much more convinced by Daisy Bates, the great white queen of the Never-Never, ranting at Ooldea about savagery and cannibalism and condemning the propagation of half-castes (see esp. p. 227). In her later work, Hill moderated her own opinions considerably.

17. Xavier Herbert, *Capricornia*, p. 238. P. R. Stephensen was the first publisher of *Capricornia*, and for a time Herbert was attracted to Stephensen's blend of fascism, anti-Semitism, and support for Aboriginal rights. For Stephensen, the lesson

of *Capricornia* was that Australians could be either children of the soil or mere citizens of the world; see *The Publicist* (1 January 1939). On Herbert's relations with Cecil Cook, see Suzanne Saunders, "Another dimension: Xavier Herbert in the Northern Territory."

18. Herbert, *Capricornia*, pp. 327–8.

19. Ibid., pp. 417, 187.

20. Herbert Basedow, *The Possibilities of the Northern Territories of Australia, with Special Reference to Development and Migration*, p. 17. See also his *The Australian Aboriginal*.

21. W. Ramsay Smith, *In Southern Seas: Wanderings of a Naturalist*, pp. 172–3. Earlier, Smith had argued that "the Australian Aboriginal, racially, would be the uncle of the Caucasian" ("The place of the Australian Aboriginal in recent anthropological research," p. 574).

22. Smith, "Place of the Australian Aboriginal," p. 575.

23. S. L. Larnach, "'They sink and show no trace,'" p. 15. Larnach, who had accompanied the 1932 Sydney physiology expedition, deplored "the grim war of extermination which was waged against the blacks" (p. 13). Larnach became the curator of the anatomy museum at the University of Sydney. See his *Australian Aboriginal Craniology*.

24. A. Grenfell Price, "'Scandalous history' of the Aborigines. Whites brought death and disease. Investigator's Proposals. Infiltration of half-castes," Adelaide *Advertiser* (18 April 1934). Price remained cautious about mixtures of more disparate racial types, such as Chinese and Europeans.

25. Griffith Taylor, *Environment and Race: A Study of the Evolution, Migration, Settlement and Status of the Races of Man*, pp. 339, 340.

26. J. W. Gregory, *The Menace of Colour*, p. 235.

27. H. L. Wilkinson, *The World's Population Problems and a White Australia*, pp. 187, 192–3.

28. Charles B. Davenport, "Notes on the physical anthropology of Australian Aborigines and black-white hybrids," p. 88. Davenport was especially concerned with preventing the entry into the United States of defective germ plasm and with the segregation of the feeble-minded. See his *Heredity in Relation to Eugenics*. On Davenport, see Charles E. Rosenberg, "Charles Benedict Davenport and the irony of American eugenics"; and Daniel J. Kevles, *In the Name of Eugenics: Genetics and the Uses of Human Heredity*.

29. Charles B. Davenport and Morris Steggerda, *Race Crossing in Jamaica*, p. 469.

30. W. E. Castle, *Genetics and Eugenics: A Textbook for Students of Biology and a Reference Book for Animal and Plant Breeders*, p. 234. In this text, Castle examines Norfolk Islanders as a natural experiment in race crossing (pp. 235–7). For ideas about race during this period in the United States, see George W. Stocking Jr., *Race, Culture and Evolution: Essays in the History of Evolution*.

31. W. E. Castle, "Biological and social consequences of race-crossing," pp. 147, 151, 153. It is interesting that few of the American experts report the "throwbacks" with African-European crosses that the Australian investigators claimed

were common. Castle also alluded to the rapid biological absorption of American Indians (p. 156)—even though he did not assign them a Caucasian identity.

32. H. S. Jennings, *The Biological Basis of Human Nature*, p. 203. See also his *Prometheus, or Biology and the Advancement of Man*. The idea that closely allied races might mate with good results—the notion of "eugenesic" crosses—derives from Paul Broca, *On the Phenomenon of Hybridity in the Genus Homo*, pp. 54–60.

33. Jennings, *Biological Basis*, pp. 276, 277, 288.

34. Griffith Taylor and F. Jardine, "Kamilaroi and white: A study of racial mixture in New South Wales," p. 289. Soon after publication of this paper, Taylor received a letter from Roland B. Dixon, a professor of anthropology at Harvard University, pointing out that "only by a large accumulation of such material can we get any certainty as to the effects of race mixtures" (28 June 1925, Taylor papers, ms. 1003/4/404, National Library of Australia). Dixon had earlier proposed that he and Taylor "wake up" anthropologists "to the importance of the larger view, and to the need of considering problems of racial distribution in mankind, on the same basis as biologists do for other animals" (8 March 1925, ibid., ms. 1003/4/406).

35. G. Pitt Rivers, "The effect on native races of contact with European civilisation," pp. 3–4, 7.

36. N. B. Tindale, "A South Australian looks at some beginnings of archaeological research in Australia." Tindale later returned to archaeological work; he retired from the South Australian Museum in 1965 and taught in the United States. See Philip Jones, "Obituary for Norman Barnett ('Tinny') Tindale."

37. N. B. Tindale, 7 October 1936, Journal of Anthropological Visit to United States and Europe, 1936–7, 3 vols., Tindale collection, AA 338/1/46/1, South Australian Museum Archives, vol. 1, p. 383. Hooton had studied at Oxford with H. K. Fry, one of the older generation of Adelaide investigators. Tindale had earlier visited S. D. Porteus in Hawaii and argued with him about the intelligence of Aboriginal Australians (ibid., 23 July 1936, vol. 1, p. 98). Later he met with Clark Wissler at the American Museum of Natural History, Carleton Coon at Harvard, Ellsworth Huntingdon and Arnold Gesell at Yale, and Griffith Taylor in Toronto.

38. Tindale reported to J. B. Cleland that Hooton was especially interested in studying first-generation hybrids (7 May 1937, Cleland papers, box 1, file 1, University of Adelaide Archives). Clark Wissler had previously written to Cleland urging the physical study of "natives in contact with civilization" (23 February 1937, ibid.).

39. J. B. Birdsell, Joint research of the University of Adelaide and the Division of Anthropology of Harvard University, with the cooperation of the Museum of South Australia, 5 May 1938, Hooton papers, 995–1, box 22, folder: Birdsell—Australian Project, Peabody Museum Archives, Harvard University. See also Birdsell, A project for the investigation of the black-white hybrids of Australia, n.d., ibid.

40. E. A. Hooton to James B. Conant, 6 December 1937, ibid.

41. Hooton papers, box 3, folder 7: Birdsell. Until the end of World War II, Harvard was the only major American center for graduate work in physical

anthropology. In the postwar years, Hooton's students, S. L. Washburn and Birdsell among them, held most of the senior physical anthropology positions in the United States. Hooton's more important works include *Up from the Ape*; *Apes, Men and Morons*; and *Crime and the Man*. See W. W. Howells, "Memoriam—Earnest Albert Hooton." For Hooton's earlier views of race crossing, see "Race mixture in the United States."

42. C. B. Davenport to E. A. Hooton, 16 May 1938, Hooton papers, box 7, folder 1: C. B. Davenport Correspondence, 1931–44.

43. J. B. Birdsell to E. A. Hooton, 4 July 1938, Hooton papers, box 22. Hooton warned "it will require a certain amount of tact to deal with his [Cleland's] official manner" (Hooton to Birdsell, 13 February 1939, ibid.).

44. Tindale, 13 May 1938, Harvard and Adelaide Universities' Anthropological Expedition Journal, 1938–9, 2 vols., Tindale Collection, AA 338/1/15/1, South Australian Museum Archives, vol. 1, p. 5. This is a reference to the people of the Deccan plateau and implied a Caucasian relationship.

45. Tindale to Cleland, 20 May 1938, Cleland papers, box 1, file 1.

46. Tindale, 25 May 1938, Harvard and Adelaide Universities' Anthropological Expedition Journal, vol. 1, p. 93.

47. Tindale and Birdsell to Cleland, 16 July 1938, Cleland papers, box 1, file 1.

48. Tindale, 26 July 1938, Harvard and Adelaide Universities' Anthropological Expedition Journal, vol. 1, p. 215.

49. Tindale to Cleland, 23 October 1938, Cleland papers, box 1, file 1.

50. Birdsell, Interim report of the Harvard-Adelaide study of Australian-white hybrids, 19 January 1939, Hooton papers, box 22.

51. Hooton to Birdsell, 13 July 1939, Hooton papers, box 22. War priorities meant that the material did not arrive at the Peabody until 1950. See Accession file 51–32, Peabody Museum Archives.

52. Birdsell to Hooton, 20 April 1938, Hooton papers, box 22.

53. Birdsell, 20 April 1938, Australian Daily Field Journal, 1938–9, 2 vols., Birdsell collection, AA 689, South Australian Museum Archives, vol. 1, p. 1. Birdsell was passing through La Perouse in Sydney (emphasis in original).

54. Birdsell to Hooton, 4 July 1938, Hooton papers, box 22.

55. Birdsell, 4 July 1938, Australian Daily Field Journal, vol. 1, p. 19.

56. Birdsell to Hooton, 28 December 1938, Hooton papers, box 22. Birdsell repeated describes "bagging" full-bloods and others; see, for example, Birdsell to Hooton, 20 April 1939, ibid.

57. Birdsell to Hooton, 13 Feb. 1939, ibid.

58. Hooton to Birdsell, 25 April 1939, ibid.

59. Hooton to Cleland, 25 April 1939, ibid.

60. Birdsell, 15 May 1938, Australian Daily Field Journal, vol. 1, p. 3.

61. Tindale, 18 September 1938, Harvard and Adelaide Universities' Anthropological Expedition Journal, vol. 1, p. 425.

62. Tindale, 24 October 1938, ibid., vol. 1, p. 587.

63. Tindale, 25 January 1939, Harvard and Adelaide Universities' Anthropological Expedition Journal, 2 vols., Tindale collection AA 338/1/15/2, South Australian Museum Archives, vol. 2, p. 107 (insert).

64. Ibid., 31 March 1939, vol. 2, p. 859. I discuss the policies of Neville, the protector of Aborigines in Western Australia, later in this chapter. In general, Tindale and Birdsell regarded Neville as a fanatic. For example, Birdsell wrote that he thought that Neville was "a bit touched on the 'American Negro' blood in the south west" of Western Australia—which Birdsell denied was "Negro" at all (Birdsell, 30 June 1939, Australian Daily Field Journal, vol. 2, p. 18).

65. Tindale, 19 January 1939, Harvard and Adelaide Universities' Anthropological Expedition Journal, vol. 2, p. 69 (insert).

66. Ibid., 28 January 1939, vol. 2, pp. 135–7, 137, 137 (insert).

67. N. B. Tindale, "Survey of the half-caste problem in South Australia," p. 67. The other major report was his "Distribution of Aboriginal tribes: A field survey." This formed the basis of modern tribal maps of Australia.

68. Tindale, "Survey of the half-caste problem," p. 67.

69. Ibid., pp. 68, 120–1.

70. Ibid., pp. 122, 128, 129. For surveys of previous colonial and state Aboriginal policies, see Bain Attwood, *The Making of Aborigines*; Anna Haebich, *Broken Circles: Fragmenting Indigenous Families, 1800–2000*.

71. Tindale, "Survey of the half-caste problem," p. 124. Hooton wrote to Tindale (7 June 1944) to tell him that the paper on the half-caste problem "makes a perfectly swell introduction to this subject which, after all, was the primary purpose of the whole expedition" (Hooton papers, box 25, folder 10: Tindale, 1944–5). Birdsell's support for half-caste absorption is reported in Anon., "Views of American anthropologist back from long trip. 'Do not isolate them—help them,'" Adelaide *Mail* (8 July 1939). (The clipping is attached to Tindale, Harvard and Adelaide Universities' Anthropological Expedition Journal, vol. 2.) Birdsell is quoted as saying that "with proper encouragement the half-caste as a group seem well fitted to assume an independent and self-sustaining position in the lower economic categories of white society."

72. Birdsell to Hooton, 27 October 1950, Hooton papers, box 3, folder 7: Birdsell. See also Birdsell to Hooton, 12 August 1952, ibid.

73. The "discovery" of this type in Queensland is announced in Norman B. Tindale and Joseph B. Birdsell, "Tasmanoid types in North Queensland." More generally, see J. B. Birdsell, "Preliminary data on the trihybrid origin of Australian Aborigines"; and Malcolm D. Prentis, "From Lemuria to Kow Swamp: The rise and fall of tri-hybrid theories of Aboriginal origins." Manning Clark accepted Birdsell's trihybrid theory; see C.M.H. Clark, *A History of Australia,* vol. 1, p. 3. Hooton promoted it internationally in works such as *Up from the Ape*, from the second edition onwards.

74. Joseph B. Birdsell, "The racial origin of the extinct Tasmanians," p. 108.

75. Ibid., p. 111. Birdsell argued that the Tasmanians had been a dihybrid race, an amalgam of Oceanic Negritos and Murrayians.

76. Lyng, *Non-Britishers in Australia*. (Lyng's work was among the books that Birdsell stored at the Peabody during the war; see Accession file 51–32, Peabody Museum.) See Chapter 5.

77. F. J. Fenner, "The Australian Aboriginal skull: Its non-metrical morphological characters." Frank Fenner's father, Charles, a geographer, was involved in

many of the research projects of the Adelaide Board for Anthropological Research. Frank Fenner later became professor of microbiology at the Australian National University and one of the leaders of the global smallpox eradication program.

78. Birdsell, "The racial origin of the extinct Tasmanians," p. 114. In the 1940s and 1950s, A. A. Abbie, the professor of anatomy at Adelaide, criticized hybrid theories and reiterated arguments for Aboriginal homogeneity ("Physical characteristics of Australian Aborigines," and "The homogeneity of Australian Aborigines"). Not surprisingly, Abbie emphasized the plasticity of heredity, and the importance of environmental influences, even on the germ plasm; see his "Sterilisation of the unfit." More generally, see Prentis, "From Lemuria to Kow Swamp."

79. Conventionally, it has been argued that "social context, not empirical research or internal logic, determined the contours of hereditarian thought" (Charles E. Rosenberg, "The bitter fruit: Heredity, disease and social thought," p. 32). William Provine has claimed that opinions about race crossing and racial classification changed between 1938 and 1946, even though "there simply was not a decisive study of race crossing during this time," and he attributes this shift to revulsion at Nazi race policies ("Geneticists and the biology of race crossing," p. 795). But in this case, at least, scientists seem to have become skeptical about racial analysis for a combination of local social, political and *scientific* reasons—that is, "empirical research and internal logic" did seem to some degree to shape, and to challenge, their hereditarian thought. See also William B. Provine, *The Origins of Theoretical Population Genetics*; and Elazar Barkan, *The Retreat of Scientific Racism: Changing Concepts of Race in Britain and the United States between the World Wars*. For the half-caste studies conducted in South Africa in the 1940s, see Saul Dubow, *Scientific Racism in Modern South Africa*, pp. 180–9.

80. Joseph B. Birdsell, "The problem of the evolution of human races: Classification or clines?" p. 136.

81. Ibid., pp. 140, 138, 139.

82. J. B. Birdsell, *Human Evolution: An Introduction to the New Physical Anthropology*, pp. 505, 533.

83. J. B. Birdsell, *Microevolutionary Patterns in Aboriginal Australia: A Gradient Analysis of Clines*, n.p. This was the culmination of fifty years of research. Previously, Tindale had published a work that also used the tribe as a unit of analysis: *Aboriginal Tribes of Australia: Their Terrain, Environmental Controls, Distribution, Limits and Proper Names*.

84. Tindale to Birdsell, 30 July 1980, Birdsell papers, AA 689, box 28, South Australian Museum Archives.

85. Cecil Cook, 1930, quoted in McGregor, *Imagined Destinies*, p. 163. On Cook, see Andrew Markus, *Governing Savages*; Tony Austin, "Cecil Cook, scientific thought and 'half-castes'"; Austin, *I Can Picture the Old Home so Clearly: The Commonwealth and "Half-Caste" Youth in the Northern Territory, 1911–39*; Austin, *Never Trust a Government Man: Northern Territory Aboriginal Policy, 1911–39*; and Suzanne Saunders, "A duly qualified medical practitioner: Health services in the Northern Territory, 1911–39."

86. C. E. Cook, "Leprosy problems." See also Suzanne Saunders, "Isolation: The development of leprosy prophylaxis in Australia."

87. C. E. Cook, "The native in relation to public health." See Chapter 7.

88. Cook to Weddell (Administrator of the Northern Territory), 27 June 1933, A659/40/1/408, National Archives of Australia, quoted in Austin, "Cecil Cook," p. 113.

89. Ibid., pp. 114–15.

90. C.E.A. Cook, "The native problem—why is it unsolved?" pp. 11, 19.

91. Ibid., pp. 21, 24.

92. Aboriginal Affairs Planning Authority, *Aboriginal Welfare: The Initial Conference of Commonwealth and State Aboriginal Authorities*, p. 1.

93. Ibid., pp. 10, 11.

94. A. O. Neville, *Australia's Coloured Minority: Its Place in the Community*, p. 25. See also Patricia Jacobs, "Science and veiled assumptions: Miscegenation in W.A., 1930–37," and her *Mister Neville*; and Anna Haebich, *For Their Own Good: Aborigines and Government in the South West of Western Australia, 1900–40*.

95. Neville, *Australia's Coloured Minority*, pp. 57, 63.

96. Ibid., p. 42.

97. Ibid., pp. 133, 135, 132.

98. Ibid., pp. 130, 131.

99. Ibid., pp. 120, 141.

100. Ibid., pp. 168, 174, 179.

101. Ibid., p. 182.

102. J. W. Bleakley, *The Aborigines of Australia*.

103. *Bringing Them Home: Report of the National Inquiry into the Separation of Aboriginal and Torres Strait Islander Children from Their Families*, p. 37. Robert Manne estimates that one in ten Aboriginal children were separated from their families between 1910 and 1970; see his "In denial: The Stolen Generations and the right." See also Peter Read, *The Stolen Generations: The Removal of Aboriginal Children in New South Wales, 1833–1969*; Paul Hasluck, *Shades of Darkness: Aboriginal Affairs, 1925–65*; and Haebich, *Broken Circles*. For Aboriginal accounts, see Coral Edwards and Peter Read, *The Lost Children*; and Carmel Bird, *The Stolen Generation: Their Stories*. The Australian policy of absorption has some affinities with the less forcible policies of racial amalgamation pursued in Latin America during this period, especially the "matrimonial eugenics" of the Brazilian Estada Nova. Nancy Stepan concludes that the emphasis on "national homogeneity through biological amalgamation was as much a mystification of the social and political realities of their very poor societies as was the reverse theory that warned against racial heterogeneity and hybrid degeneration" ("*The Hour of Eugenics,*" p. 170). See also Thomas E. Skidmore, *Black into White: Race and Nationality in Brazilian Thought*; Richard Graham, ed., *The Idea of Race in Latin America, 1870–1940*; Dain Borges, "Puffy, ugly, slothful and inert: Degeneration in Brazilian social thought, 1880–1940"; and Jeffrey Lesser, *Negotiating National Identity: Immigrants, Minorities and the Struggle for Ethnicity in Brazil*.

104. A. P. Elkin, "Introduction," in Neville, *Australia's Coloured Minority*, pp. 11, 15–16, 17. Elkin had been a student of the Australian diffusionist Grafton Elliot Smith. See Tigger Wise, *The Self-Made Anthropologist: A Life of A. P. Elkin*; and Russell McGregor, "The concept of primitivity in the writings of A. P. Elkin,"

and "Intelligent parasitism: A. P. Elkin and the rhetoric of assimilation." More generally, on race and Australian social anthropology in the twentieth century, see Gillian Cowlishaw, "Colour, culture and the Aboriginalists."

105. Raymond Firth, "Anthropology in Australia, 1926–32—and after," p. 2. See also his "Anthropology and native administration."

106. A. P. Elkin, "Anthropology in Australia, past and present," pp. 199, 197.

107. A. P. Elkin, "Anthropology and the future of the Australian Aborigines," pp. 2, 3.

108. Ibid., pp. 7, 18.

109. S. D. Porteus, *The Psychology of a Primitive People: A Study of the Australian Aborigine*. See also his "Mentality of Australian Aborigines."

110. Ralph Piddington, "Psychological aspects of culture contact," pp. 324, 323.

111. A. P. Elkin, "The social life and intelligence of the Australian Aborigine: A review of S. D. Porteus's *Psychology of a Primitive People*," p. 112. Porteus in response conceded that some Aborigines "may equal average white status" ("Correspondence," p. 109). For an elaboration of Elkin's ideas on Aboriginal educability, see his "Native education, with special reference to the Australian Aborigines."

112. For a more extensive discussion, see Russell McGregor, "Representations of the half-caste in the Australian scientific literature of the 1930s."

113. A. P. Elkin, "Civilised Aborigines and native culture," pp. 119, 124.

114. Ibid., pp. 136, 145.

115. More generally, on notions of hybridity and identity, see Robert J. C. Young, *Colonial Desire: Hybridity in Theory, Culture and Race*. On the ambiguities of post-war Aboriginal hybridity, see Ian Anderson, "Black bit, white bit," and "I, the 'hybrid' Aborigine: Film and representation."

116. Marie Reay, "A half-caste Aboriginal community in north-western New South Wales"; R. M. and C. H. Berndt, *From Black to White in South Australia*; and Catherine H. Berndt, "Mateship or success: An assimilation dilemma." See also A. P. Elkin, "Reaction and interaction: A food-gathering people and European settlement in Australia."

117. A. P. Elkin, *Citizenship for the Aborigines: A National Aboriginal Policy*, pp. 12, 90. See also Geoffrey Gray, "From nomadism to citizenship: A. P. Elkin and Aboriginal advancement."

118. On notions of Aboriginal citizenship, see John Chesterman and Brian Galligan, *Citizens Without Rights: Aborigines and Australian Citizenship*; and Peterson and Sanders, eds., *Citizenship and Indigenous Australians*.

CONCLUSION

1. Anon., "Prolific Australia: The continent of the British race," pp. 67, 68, 68.

2. Walter Murdoch, *The Australian Citizen: An Elementary Account of Civic Rights and Duties*, p. 148. E. J. Hobsbawm has claimed that between 1870 and

1918 "ethnicity and language became the central, increasingly the decisive or even the only criteria of potential nationhood" (*Nations and Nationalism Since 1780: Programme, Myth, Reality*, p. 102). Benedict Anderson tends, though, to understate the importance of the racial imaginary of nationalism in *Imagined Communities: Reflections on the Origin and Spread of Nationalism*.

3. Theodore Roosevelt, "National life and character," pp. 270, 271, 278, 279. On the tension between "racial nationalism" and "civic nationalism" in Roosevelt's thinking, see Gary Gerstle, *American Crucible: Race and Nation in the Twentieth Century*.

4. Theodore Roosevelt, *Biological Analogies in History*, pp. 4, 33, 34, 39. See also Richard Hofstadter, *Social Darwinism in American Thought*.

5. Others have argued that the relational aspects of whiteness make it an empty category. See Richard Dyer, *White*; and Toni Morrison, *Playing in the Dark: Whiteness and the Literary Imagination*. G. W. Fredrickson has described whiteness in South Africa and the United States as "a fluid, variable and open-ended process" (*A Comparative Study of American and South African History*, p. xviii). In contrast, John Cell detects some stable features of whiteness in *The Highest Stage of White Supremacy: The Origins of Segregation in South Africa and the American South*. For a philosophical account of the fluidity of race, see David Theo Goldberg, *Racist Culture: Philosophy and the Politics of Meaning*.

6. Nancy Stepan, "Biology and degeneration: Races and proper places."

7. Zygmunt Bauman, *Modernity and Ambivalence*.

8. James C. Scott, *Seeing Like a State: How Certain Schemes to Improve the Human Condition Have Failed*.

9. Leszek Kolakowski, *Modernity on Endless Trial*.

10. Ken Gelder and Jane M. Jacobs, *Uncanny Australia: Sacredness and Identity in a Postcolonial Nation*.

11. For a popular revision of Taylor's theories, see Tim Flannery, *The Future Eaters: An Ecological History of the Australasian Lands and People*. Flannery claims that "the environment shapes more than people's bodies; for it shapes their culture, their beliefs and their economy" (p. 302). He regards Taylor as "one of the greatest and most courageous scientists that Australia has ever produced" (p. 363).

12. David Catcheside at Adelaide and Michael White at Melbourne were largely responsible for the institutionalization of population genetics in Australia during the 1950s. See D. A. McCann and P. Batterham, "Australian genetics: A brief history."

13. A. P. Elkin, "Is white Australia doomed?" pp. 195–6.

14. Ibid., pp. 197, 198. But in the same publication, G. L. Wood, recalling Wilfred Agar's advice, was still hoping to breed a "superior race" of whites in Australia ("Australia's empty cradles," p. 87). In the early 1960s many of Elkin's arguments were taken up in Immigration Reform Group, *Immigration: Control or Colour Bar? The Background to "White Australia" and a Proposal for Change*. By this stage, "the colour-prejudiced man, like the anti-Semite, is an insecure man, an ignorant man, to speak plainly an inferior man, who, in the circumstances of the

second half of this century, is a nuisance to his country and an embarrassment to his fellow citizens" (p. 123).

15. Jon Strattan, *Race Daze: Australia in Identity Crisis*; Ghassan Hage, *White Nation: Fantasies of White Supremacy in a Multicultural Society*; and John Docker and Gerhard Fischer, eds., *Race, Culture and Identity in Australia and New Zealand*.

Bibliography of Works Cited

Primary Sources

Manuscript Collections

Dixson Library, Sydney, NSW.
New South Wales Governor's Despatches, A1229, A1231, A1232, A1237.

Medical History Museum, University of Melbourne, Vic.
R.J.A. Berry, Chance and Circumstance (c. 1954).

Mitchell Library, Sydney, NSW.
John Dickson Loch, Information in Regard to Adelaide and South Australia, ms. A2755.

National Archives of Australia, Canberra, ACT.
Institute of Tropical Medicine—Townsville, A461.
Institute of Tropical Medicine/School of Public Health and Tropical Medicine, A1928.
Tropical Medicine—Australian Institute, A11804.

National Archives of Australia, Sydney, NSW.
AITM—General Correspondence, etc. (1916–32), SP1060/1.
AITM—General Correspondence, etc. (1908–55), SP1061/1.
School of Public Health and Tropical Medicine—General Correspondence (1930–65), SP1063/1.
Correspondence re Staff, etc. (1911–69), SP1064/1.

National Library of Australia, Canberra, ACT.
J.H.L. Cumpston papers, mss. 434, 613.
S. T. Haslett papers, ms. 7385.
C. S. Hicks papers, ms. 5623.
G. T. Howard papers, ms. 3121.

"Henry Handel Richardson" papers, ms. 133.
T. Griffith Taylor papers, ms. 1003.

Northern Territory Archives, Darwin, NT.

Peabody Museum Archives, Harvard University, USA.
E. A. Hooton papers, ms 995–1.
Accession File 51–32.

Rockefeller Archive Center, USA.
RG 1.1 (Projects), series 410D (Australia).
Heiser Trip Diaries, 905/Hei 2, 58.5.

South Australian Museum Archives, Adelaide, SA.
N. B. Tindale collection, AA 338.
J. B. Birdsell collection, AA 689.

State Library of Victoria, Melbourne, Vic.
E. C. Hobson papers, ms. 8457.
George Wakefield papers, ms. 6331.
David Henry Wilsone papers, ms. 9825.
James Selby papers, ms. 9866.
T. L. McMillan papers, ms. 11634.
J. W. Springthorpe papers, ms. 9898.
Percival Serle, A Life of Good Fortune, ms. 2441/2c ii.

Strehlow Research Centre Archives, Alice Springs, NT.
T.G.H. Strehlow papers.

**University of Adelaide Archives, Barr-Smith Library,
University of Adelaide, SA.**
A. A. Abbie papers, 572.994/A124M.
J. B. Cleland papers, 572/C61.
C. S. Hicks papers, 572.9942/H631P.
Anthropology Board of Study.
V. A. Edgeloe, The Medical School of the University of Adelaide:
    A Brief History from an Administrative Viewpoint.

University of Melbourne Archives, Vic.
H. B. Allen papers.
James Barrett papers.
W. A. Osborne papers.

Periodicals

Australian Journal of Experimental Biology and Medical Science (1924–34)
Australian Medical Journal (1856–90)
AMG (1881–96)

MJA (1914–22)
Oceania (1930–40)
The Publicist (1936–9)

Books and Articles

Abbie, A. A. "Sterilisation of the unfit." *Phoenix* [Adelaide University Union] (1946): 9–19.

_____. "Physical characteristics of Australian Aborigines." In *Australian Aboriginal Studies: A Symposium of Papers Presented at the 1961 Research Conference*, eds. W.E.H. Stanner and Helen Shiels, 90–116. Melbourne: Oxford University Press, 1963.

_____. "The homogeneity of Australian Aborigines." *Archaeology and Physical Anthropology in Oceania* 3 (1968): 223–31.

Abbott, T. Eastoe. "Cases of diphtheria treated with antitoxin." *AMG* 14 (1895): 234–6.

Aboriginal Affairs Planning Authority. *Aboriginal Welfare: The Initial Conference of Commonwealth and State Aboriginal Authorities*. Canberra: Government Printer, 1937.

Adams, Francis W. L. *Australian Essays*. London: Griffith, Farran, 1886.

_____. *The Australians—A Social Sketch*. London: T. Fisher Unwin, 1893.

Agar, W. E. "Some problems of evolution and genetics" [Presidential Address, Section D, Zoology]. *Report of the 17th Meeting AAAS, Adelaide, 1924*, 347–58. Adelaide: Government Printer, 1926.

_____. "Some eugenic aspects of Australian population problems." In *The Peopling of Australia*, eds. P. D. Phillips and G. L. Wood, 128–44. Melbourne: Macmillan, 1928.

_____. *Eugenics and the Future of the Australian Population*. Melbourne: Eugenics Society of Victoria, 1939.

_____. *A Contribution to the Theory of the Living Organism*. Melbourne: Melbourne University Press, 1943.

Ahearne, Joseph. "Presidential address, North Queensland Medical Society." *AMG* 9 (1890): 292–5.

Aitkin, William. "Darwin's doctrine of evolution in explanation of the coming into being of some diseases." *Glasgow Medical J.* 24 (1885): 98–107, 160–72.

Allen, H. B. "Notes on the pathology of diphtheria." *AMJ* 2ns (1880): 311–16.

_____. "Second general report on . . . the Institute of Preventive Medicine." *Victorian Parliamentary Papers* 4 (1891).

_____. "Public health in Australia: Past and future." *Health* 1 (1923): 1–6.

Anon. "Local topics." *AMJ* 14 (1869): 193.

_____. "Review of William Thomson, *On Typhoid Fever*." *AMJ* 20 (1875): 219–28.

_____. "Report of the special committee of the Medical Society of Victoria on phthisis in Victoria." *AMJ* 22 (1877): 358–60.

_____. "Discussion of the report of the prevalence of phthisis in Victoria." *AMJ* 22 (1877): 373–8.

_____. "Will the Anglo-Australian race degenerate?" *Victorian Review* 1 (1879): 114–23.

_____. "Diphtheria discussion at the Medical Society." *AMJ* 2ns (1880): 367–8.

_____. "Bystander's notebook." *Boomerang* [Brisbane] (24 March, 12 May 1888).

_____. "Overflowing China: Travelling through the lands invaded by the Mongol. II. Port Darwin." *Boomerang* [Brisbane] (19 May 1888): 13–14.

_____. "Prolific Australia: The continent of the British race." *Lone Hand* 1 (May 1907): 67–78.

_____. "Tropical Australia: Deputation from Congress to the Prime Minister." *Transactions of the Australasian Medical Congress, 11th Session, Melbourne, 1908*, vol. 4, 101–3. Melbourne: J. Kemp, 1909.

_____. "Are we turning black? The Northern Territory problem. Professor David's opinion." *Science of Man* 13 (1911): 209–10.

_____. "British Medical Association news." *AMG* 20 (1911): 88.

_____. "Reports of research committees: Anthropometric committee." *Report of the 14th Meeting AAAS, Melbourne, 1913*, 605–21. Melbourne: Government Printer, 1914.

_____. "Tropical Australia." *Transactions of the Australasian Medical Congress, 11th Session, Brisbane, 1920*, 41–69. Brisbane: Anthony James Cumming, 1921.

_____. "White man in the north." *MJA* i (1921): 315–16.

_____. "Anthropological expedition to the northwest of South Australia, 1933." *Oceania* 4 (1933): 99–101.

Aron, Hans. "Investigation on the action of the tropical sun on men and animals." *PJS* 6 (1911): 101–23.

Arthur, Richard. "Settlement of tropical Australia." *MJA* i (1921): 345.

_____. "The colonisation of tropical Australia." *Transactions of the Australasian Medical Congress, 12th Session, Melbourne, 1922*, vol. 2, 93–7. Melbourne: Government Printer, 1923.

Australian Institute of Tropical Medicine. *Half-Yearly Report from 1 Jan.–30 June 1914*. Melbourne: Government Printer, 1914.

Bailey, K. H. "Public opinion and population problems." In *The Peopling of Australia*, eds. F. W. Eggleston et al., 69–103. Melbourne: Melbourne University Press, 1933.

Balfour, A. "The problem of acclimatisation." *Lancet* 205 (1923): 84–7.

Ballantyne, James. *Homes and Homesteads in the Land of Plenty: A Handbook of Victoria as a Field of Emigration*. Melbourne: Mason, Firth and McCutcheon, 1871.

Barnard, James. "Aborigines of Tasmania." *Report of the 2nd Meeting AAAS, Melbourne, 1890*, 597–611. Melbourne: AAAS, 1891.

Barrett, James W. *Typhoid Fever in Victoria*. Melbourne: George Robertson, 1883.

_____. "Presidential address." *MJA* i (1901): 10–27.

_____. "The problem of the settlement of tropical Australia." In *Twin Ideals: An Educated Commonwealth*, vol. 1, 286–91. London: H. K. Lewis, 1918.

_____. "Tropical Australia discussion." *Transactions of the Australasian Medical Congress, 11th Session, Brisbane, 1920*, 63. Brisbane: Anthony James Cumming, 1921.

_____. "White Australia policy." *United Empire* 13 (1922): 679–83.

_____. "Can tropical Australia be peopled by a white race?" *The Margin: Journal of the Commerce Students' Society* [University of Melbourne] 1 (1925): 28–35.

_____. "White colonisation of the tropics." In *Comptes rendus du 15ème Congrès international de Géographie, Amsterdam, 1938*, vol. 2, 3–38. Leiden: E. J. Brill, 1938.

_____. *Eighty Eventful Years*. Melbourne: J. C. Stephens, 1945.

Bartlett, Thomas. *New Holland: Its Colonisation, Productions and Resources*. London: Longman, Brown, Green and Longmans, 1843.

Bartley, Nehemiah. *Australia's Pioneers and Reminiscences, 1849–94*. Sydney: John Ferguson, 1978 [1896].

Basedow, Herbert. *The Australian Aboriginal*. Adelaide: F. W. Preece and Sons, 1925.

_____. *The Possibilities of the Northern Territories of Australia, with Special Reference to Development and Migration*. London: Empire Parliamentary Association, 1932.

_____. *Knights of the Boomerang: Episodes from a Life Spent among the Native Tribes of Australia*. Sydney: Endeavour Press, 1935.

Bateson, William. *Mendel's Principles of Heredity: A Defence*. Cambridge: Cambridge University Press, 1902.

Beale, Octavius C. *Racial Decay: A Compilation of Evidence from World Sources*. Sydney: Angus and Robertson, 1910.

Bean, C.E.W. *The Dreadnought of the Darling*. London: Alston Rivers, 1911.

_____. *In Your Hands, Australians*. London: Cassell, 1919.

_____. *The Story of the Anzac: From the Outbreak of the War to the End of the First Phase of the Gallipoli Campaign*. Sydney: Angus and Robertson, 1940 [1921].

Beard, George M. *A Practical Treatise on Nervous Exhaustion (Neurasthenia) and Its Symptoms, Nature, Sequences, Treatment*. 2nd edn. New York: William Wood, 1880.

Bedford, Randolph. *Explorations in Civilisation*. Sydney: Angus and Robertson, c. 1914.

_____. "White, yellow and brown." *Lone Hand* 9 (July 1911): 224–48.

Bennett, George. *Wanderings in New South Wales, Batavia, Pedir Coast, Singapore and China*. 2 vols. London: Richard Bentley, 1834.

_____. *Gatherings of a Naturalist in Australia: Being Observations Principally on the Animal and Vegetable Productions of New South Wales, New Zealand and Some of the Austral Islands*. London: John van Voorst, 1860.

Berndt, Catherine H. "Mateship or success: An assimilation dilemma." *Oceania* 23 (1962): 71–89.

Berndt, R. M. and C. H. *From Black to White in South Australia*. Melbourne: Cheshire, 1951.

Berry, R.J.A. "Correspondence—White Australia Policy." *MJA* ii (1915): 93.

————. "The menace of the birth-rate." *MJA* ii (1917): 491–6.

————. "The Anatomy Department of the University of Melbourne." *MJA* i (1923): 409–10.

Berry, R.J.A., A.W.D. Robertson, and K. Stuart Cross. "A biometrical study of the relative degree of purity of race of the Tasmanian, Australian and Papuan." *Proceedings Royal Society of Edinburgh* 31 (1910–11): 17–40.

Berry, R.J.A., and A.W.D. Robertson. "The place in nature of the Tasmanian Aboriginal as deduced from a study of his calvarium." *Proceedings Royal Society of Edinburgh* 31 (1910–11): 41–69.

Berry, R.J.A., and L.W.G. Buchner. "The correlation of size of head and intelligence, as estimated from the cubic capacity of brains of 355 Melbourne criminals." *Proceedings Royal Society of Victoria* 25 (1913): 229–53.

Berry, R.J.A., and S. D. Porteus. *Intelligence and Social Valuation: A Practical Method for the Diagnosis of Mental Deficiency and Other Forms of Social Inefficiency.* Vineland NJ: Resident Publication of the Training School, 1920.

Berry, R.J.A., and R. G. Gordon. *The Mental Defective: A Problem in Social Inefficiency.* London: Kegan Paul, 1931.

Bird, S. D. *On Australasian Climates and Their Influence on the Prevention and Arrest of Pulmonary Consumption.* London: Longman, 1863.

————. "On consumption in Australia." *AMJ* 10 (1865): 276–83.

————. "On chest complaints in Australia." *AMJ* 12 (1867): 33–50, 130–7.

————. "Climate and consumption." *AMJ* 15 (1870): 110–25.

————. "On the influence of the Australasian climates on imported phthisis." *AMJ* 23 (1878): 34–40.

Birdsell, J. B. "The racial origin of the extinct Tasmanians." *Records of the Queen Victoria Museum* 2 (1949): 105–22.

————. "Preliminary data on the trihybrid origin of Australian Aborigines." *Archaeology and Physical Anthropology in Oceania* 2 (1967): 100–55.

————. "The problem of the evolution of human races: Classification or clines?" *Social Biology* 19 (1972): 136–62.

————. *Human Evolution: An Introduction to the New Physical Anthropology,* 2nd edn. Chicago: Rand McNally College Publishing, 1975 [1972].

————. "Some reflections on fifty years in biological anthropology." In *The Excitement and Fascination of Science,* ed. Joshua Lederberg, vol. 3, part 1, 125–36. Palo Alto, CA: Annual Reviews Inc., 1990.

————. *Microevolutionary Patterns in Aboriginal Australia: A Gradient Analysis of Clines.* New York: Oxford University Press, 1993.

Bjelke-Petersen, Christian. "Growth and development of Hobart school boys, with some notes on anthropometry." *Report of the 9th Meeting AAAS, Hobart, 1902,* 823–9. Hobart: Government Printer, 1903.

Blair, John. "Diphtheria and diphtheritic diseases." *AMJ* 22 (1877): 298–301.

Bland-Sutton, James. *Evolution and Disease.* London: Scott, 1890.

Bleakley, J. W. *The Aborigines of Australia.* Brisbane: Jacaranda Press, 1961.

Boas, Franz. *Changes in the Bodily Form of Descendents of Immigrants.* Washington: Government Printing Office, 1911.

"Boldrewood, Rolf" [T. H. Browne]. *Old Melbourne Memories,* 2nd edn. London: Macmillan, 1896.

Bonwick, James. *Climate and Health in Australasia: New South Wales.* London: Street, 1886.

————. *Climate and Health in Australasia: Victoria.* London: Street, 1886.

Booth, Mary. "School anthropometrics: The importance of Australasian measurements conforming to the schedule of the British Anthropometric Committee, 1906." *Report of the 13th Meeting AAAS, Sydney, 1911,* 689–96. Sydney: Government Printer, 1912.

Bowe, F. "Diseases of Polynesians, as seen in Queensland." *Intercolonial Medical Congress of Australasia, 2nd Session, Melbourne, 1889,* 59–63. Melbourne: Stillwell and Co, 1889.

"Bowyang, Bill" [Alexander Venard]. "On the top rail." *North Queensland Register* (14 December 1946): 40.

Brady, Edwin J. *Australia Unlimited.* Melbourne: George Robertson, n.d. [c. 1918].

————. *The Land of the Sun.* London: Edward Arnold, 1924.

Breinl, Anton. *Tropical Diseases: Report of Dr Breinl.* Melbourne: Parliament of Australia, 1910.

————. "Report on health and disease in the Northern Territory." *Bulletin of the Northern Territory* 1 (1912): 32–53.

————. "The object and scope of tropical medicine in Australia." *Transactions of the Australasian Medical Congress, 9th Session, Sydney 1911,* vol. 1, 534–5. Sydney: Government Printer, 1913.

————. "Ankylostomiasis." *Transactions of the Australasian Medical Congress, 9th Session, Sydney, 1911,* vol. 1, 536–42. Sydney: Government Printer, 1913.

————. "The influence of climate, diseases and surroundings on the white race living in the tropics." In *Therapeutics, Dietetics and Hygiene,* ed. J. W. Springthorpe, vol. 2, 994–6. Melbourne: James Little, 1914.

————. "Influence of climate, disease and surroundings on the white race living in the tropics." *MJA* i (1915): 595–600.

————. "An inquiry into the effect of high wet-bulb temperatures upon the pulse rate, rectal temperature, skin-shirt temperature and blood pressure of wharf labourers in North Queensland." *MJA* i (1921): 303–12.

Breinl, A., and H. Priestley. "Observations on the blood conditions of children of European descent residing in Tropical Australia." *Annals of Tropical Medicine and Parasitology* 8 (1914): 591–608.

Breinl, A., and W. J. Young. "Tropical Australia and its settlement." *American J. Tropical Medicine and Parasitology* 13 (1920): 351–412.

Bride, Thomas Francis, ed. *Letters from Victorian Pioneers, Being a Series of Papers on the Early Occupation of the Colony.* Melbourne: Heinemann, 1969 [1898].

Broca, Paul. *On the Phenomenon of Hybridity in the Genus Homo,* ed. C. Carter Blake, 54–60. London: Anthropological Society, 1864.

Brown, Isaac Baker Jr. *Australia for the Consumptive Invalid: The Voyage, Climates and Prospects for Residence.* London: Robert Hardwicke, 1865.

Brown, Tasman. *Morphology of the Australian Skull, Studied by Multivariate Analysis* [Australian Aboriginal Studies No. 49]. Canberra: Australian Institute of Aboriginal Studies, 1973.

Browne, Graham. "Charters Towers from 1882 to 1890." *AMG* 9 (1890): 318–23.

Bryce, Lucy. *An Abiding Gladness.* Melbourne: Georgian House, 1965.

Butler, Samuel. *Handbook for Australian Emigrants.* Glasgow: W. R. McPhun, 1839.

Campbell, T. D. "Food, food values and food habits of the Australian Aborigines in relation to their dental conditions." *Australian J. Dentistry* 43 (1939): 1–15, 45–55, 73–87.

Campbell, T. D., and Aubrey J. Lewis. "The Aborigines of South Australia: Anthropometric, descriptive and other observations recorded at Ooldea." *Transactions Royal Society of South Australia* 50 (1926): 183–91.

Campbell, T. D., and Cecil J. Hackett. "Adelaide University field anthropology. Central Australia No.1: Introduction: Descriptive and anthropometric observations." *Transactions Royal Society of South Australia* 51 (1927): 65–75.

Campbell, T. D., J. H. Gray, and C. J. Hackett. "Physical anthropology of the Aborigines of central Australia." *Oceania* 7 (1936): 106–39, 246–61.

Castellani, Aldo, and Albert Chalmers. *Manual of Tropical Medicine.* New York: Ballière, Tindall and Cox, 1920.

Castle, W. E. *Genetics and Eugenics: A Textbook for Students of Biology and a Reference Book for Animal and Plant Breeders.* Cambridge MA: Harvard University Press, 1916.

————. "Biological and social consequences of race-crossing." *American J. Physical Anthropology* 9 (1926): 145–56.

Centenary Celebrations Council. *Victoria, the First Century: An Historical Survey.* Melbourne: Robertson and Mullens, 1934.

Chamberlain, Weston P. "Observations on the influence of the Philippine climate on white men of the blond and brunette type." *PJS* 6 (1911): 427–63.

————. "A study of the systolic blood pressure and the pulse rate of healthy adult males in the Philippines." *PJS* 6 (1911): 467–81.

————. "The red blood corpuscles and the hemoglobin of healthy adult American males residing in the Philippines." *PJS* 6 (1911): 483–8.

————. "Some features of the physiological activity of white races in the Philippine Islands." *American J. Tropical Disease and Preventive Medicine* 1 (1913): 12–32.

Charles, Havelock. "Neurasthenia and its bearing on the decay of northern peoples in India." *Transactions of the Society Tropical Medicine and Hygiene* 7 (1913–14): 2–28.

Chatwin, Bruce. *The Songlines.* London: Vintage, 1998 [1987].

Cherry, Thomas. "Diphtheria antitoxin." *AMJ* 17ns (1895): 101–6.

Cherry, T., and C. H. Mollison. "68 cases of diphtheria." *AMJ* 17ns (1895): 388–403.

Chewings, Charles. *Back in the Stone Age: Native Tribes of Central Australia*. Sydney: Angus and Robertson, 1936.

Chidell, Fleetwood. *Australia—White or Yellow?* London: William Heinemann, 1926.

Cilento, Phyllis. *You Don't Have to Live with Chronic Ill-Health*. Sydney: Whitcombe and Tombs, 1977.

Cilento, R. W. *The White Man in the Tropics, with Especial Reference to Australia and Its Dependencies* [Department of Health Service Publication No. 7]. Melbourne: Government Printer, c. 1925.

————. "White settlement of tropical Australia." In *The Peopling of Australia*, eds. P. D. Phillips and G. L. Wood, 222–45. Melbourne: Macmillan, 1928.

————. "Rejoinder to Professor Huntington." *Economic Record* 6 (1930): 127–32.

————. "Australia's problems in the tropics" [Presidential Address, Section I, Medical Science and National Health]. *Report of the 21st Meeting ANZAAS, Sydney, 1932*, 216–33. Sydney: Government Printer, 1933.

————. "The conquest of climate." *MJA* i (1933): 421–32.

————. *Australia's Racial Heritage: A Brief Insight*. Fitzroy, Vic.: League of Rights, n.d. [c. 1971].

Cilento, Raphael, and Clem Lack. *Triumph in the Tropics: An Historical Sketch of Queensland*. Fortitude Valley, Qld.: Smith and Patterson, 1959.

Clark, James. *The Sanative Influence of Climate*. 4th edn. London: John Murray, 1846.

Clarke, Marcus. *The Future Australian Race*. Melbourne: A. H. Massima, 1877.

Cleland, J. B. "An objection to the direct continuity of the germ plasm, with a suggestion as to the part possibly played by hormones in heredity." *West Australian Natural History Society* 6 (1909): 34–7.

————. "Blood grouping of Australian Aboriginals." *Australian J. Experimental Biology and Medical Science* 3 (1926): 33.

————. "Disease among the Australian Aborigines." *J. Tropical Medicine and Hygiene* 31 (1928): 53–9, 65–70, 125–30, 141–5, 157–60, 173–7, 196–8, 202–6, 216–20, 232–5, 262–6, 281–2, 290–4, 307–13, 326–30.

————. "Further results in blood grouping central Australian Aborigines." *Australian J. Experimental Biology and Medical Science* 7 (1930): 79–90.

————. "Complexities of evolution: Interesting, if puzzling, phases of development in forms of life." In *Science for All*, eds. Kerr Grant et al., 81–4. Adelaide: Advertiser Newspapers, 1937.

————. "Ecology of the Aboriginal inhabitants of Tasmania and South Australia." *Australian J. Science* 2 (1940): 97–101.

————. "The naturalist in medicine with particular reference to Australia." *MJA* i (1950): 549–65.

Cleland, J. B., and H. K. Fry. "An outbreak of scurvy with joint lesions in Australian Aborigines in central Australia." *MJA* i (1930): 410–2.

Clutterbuck, James B. *An Essay in the Nature and Treatment of Australian Diseases, Including More Especially Dysentery and Fever*. Melbourne: Stillwell and Knight, 1868.

Cole, E. W. *A White Australia Impossible*. Melbourne: Coles Book Arcade, 1903.

Collins, David. *An Account of the English Colony in New South Wales*, 2 vols., ed. Brian H. Fletcher. Sydney: A. H. and A. W. Reed, 1975 [1798].

Commonwealth of Australia. *Royal Commission on Health: Minutes of Evidence*. Melbourne: Government Printer, 1925.

Cook, C. E. "Leprosy problems." *MJA* ii (1926): 801–3.

_____. "The native in relation to the public health." *MJA* i (1949): 569–71.

_____. "The native problem—why is it unsolved?" *Australian Quarterly* 22 (1950): 11–24.

"Cosmos." "Correspondence—White Australia Policy." *MJA* ii (1915): 43–4.

Coxwell, C. F. "A study of phthisis mortality in Victoria." *AMJ* 15ns (1893): 185–206.

Creed, J. M. "The settlement by 'whites' of tropical Australia." *United Empire* 3ns (1912): 569–80.

Croll, R. H. *Wide Horizons: Wanderings in Central Australia*. Sydney: Angus and Robertson, 1937.

_____. *I Recall: Collections and Recollections*. Melbourne: Robertson and Mullens, 1939.

Cumpston, J.H.L. *Quarantine: Australian Maritime Quarantine and the Evolution of International Agreements Concerning Quarantine* [Quarantine Service Publication No. 2]. Melbourne: Government Printer, 1913.

_____. *The History of Smallpox in Australia, 1788–1908* [Quarantine Service Publication No. 3]. Melbourne: Government Printer, 1914.

_____. "The war and public health." In *University of Melbourne War Lectures*, 185–98. Melbourne: George Robertson, 1916.

_____. "Tropical Australia: Discussion." *Transactions of the 1920 Australasian Medical Congress, 11th Session, Brisbane, 1920*, 49. Brisbane: Anthony James Cumming, 1921.

_____. "Presidential address: Public health and state medicine." *Transactions of the 1920 Australasian Medical Congress, 11th Session, Brisbane, 1920*, 77–87. Brisbane: Anthony James Cumming, 1921.

_____. "The depopulation of the Pacific." *Proceedings of the Pan-Pacific Science Congress, Australia, 1923*, vol. 2, 1389–94. Melbourne: Government Printer, 1924.

_____. *The History of Diphtheria, Scarlet Fever and Whooping Cough in Australia*. Canberra: Government Printer, 1927.

_____. "The Australian Institute of Tropical Medicine." *MJA* ii (1928): 398–400.

_____. "The evolution of public health administration in Australia." *MJA* i (1932): 194–8.

_____. "The culture of human life." *Australian and New Zealand J. Surgery* 16 (1946): 3–13.

Cumpston, J.H.L., and F. McCallum. *The History of the Intestinal Infections (and Typhus Fever) in Australia, 1788–1923*. Melbourne: Government Printer, 1927.

Cunningham, Peter. *Two Years in New South Wales*, ed. David S. Macmillan. Sydney: Angus and Robertson, 1966 [1827].

Curr, Edward M. *Recollections of Squatting in Victoria, Then Called the Port Phillip District, from 1841 to 1851*. Melbourne: George Robertson, 1883.

_____. *The Australian Race: Its Origin, Languages, Customs, Place of Landing in Australia and the Routes by Which It Spread Itself over That Continent*, 4 vols. Melbourne: John Ferres, 1886.

Dale, R. W. "Impressions of Australia. II: Speculations about the future." *Contemporary Review* 54 (1888): 836–60.

Danes, J. V. "Notes on the suitability of tropical Australia for the white races." *J. and Proceedings Royal Society of NSW* 44 (1910): 416–9.

Daniels, Charles W., and E. Wilkinson. *Tropical Medicine and Hygiene*, 2nd edn., 2 vols. New York: Wood, 1913–14.

Darwin, Charles. *On the Origin of Species by Means of Natural Selection, of the Preservation of Favoured Races in the Struggle for Life*. London: Murray, 1859.

_____. *The Descent of Man and Selection in Relation to Sex*, 2 vols. London: Murray, 1871.

_____. *A Naturalist's Voyage: Journal of Researches*, 2nd edn. London: John Murray, 1889 [1845].

Davenport, Charles B. *Heredity in Relation to Eugenics*. New York: Henry Holt, 1911.

_____. "Notes on the physical anthropology of Australian Aborigines and black-white hybrids." *American J. Physical Anthropology* 8 (1925): 73–94.

Davenport, Charles B., and Morris Steggerda. *Race Crossing in Jamaica*. Washington, DC: Carnegie Institution, 1929.

Davidson, Andrew, ed. *Hygiene and Diseases of Warm Climates*. Edinburgh: Pentland, 1893.

Davy, John. *Researches, Physiological and Anatomical*, 2 vols. London: Smith, Elder, 1839.

Deakin, Alfred. "Science and empire." *Nature* 76 (9 May 1907): 37.

Devanny, Jean. *Sugar Heaven*. Sydney: Modern Publishers, 1936.

Dilke, Charles. *Greater Britain: Charles Dilke Visits Her New Lands, 1866 and 1867*, ed. Geoffrey Blainey. North Ryde, NSW: Methuen Hayes, 1985 [1868].

Divorty, P. "The influence of an Australian climate on the constitution of the western European." *Sydney Magazine of Science and Art* 1 (1858): 83–91.

Duckworth, A. "Notes on a 'White Australia.'" *J. and Proceedings Royal Society of NSW* 44 (1910): 226–51.

Dyson, T. S. "Malarial fevers of tropical Queensland." *Intercolonial Medical Congress of Australasia, 2nd Session, Melbourne, 1889*, 64–6. Melbourne: Stillwell, 1888.

"Easterley, Robert," and "John Wilbraham" [Robert Potter]. *The Germ Growers: An Australian Story of Adventure and Mystery*. Melbourne: Melville, Mullen and Slade, 1892.

Elkin, A. P. "The social life and intelligence of the Australian Aborigine: A review of S. D. Porteus's *Psychology of a Primitive People*." *Oceania* 3 (1932–3): 101–13.

_____. "Anthropology and the future of the Australian Aborigines." *Oceania* 5 (1934): 1–18.

_____. "Civilised Aborigines and native culture." *Oceania* 6 (1935): 117–46.

_____. "Anthropology in Australia, past and present" [Presidential Address, Section F, Anthropology]. *Report of the 22nd Meeting ANZAAS, Melbourne, 1935*, 196–207. Melbourne: Government Printer, 1935.

_____. "Native education, with special reference to the Australian Aborigines." *Oceania* 7 (1936): 459–500.

_____. *Citizenship for the Aborigines: A National Aboriginal Policy*. Sydney: Australasian Publishing Co., 1944.

_____. "Is white Australia doomed?" In *A White Australia: Australia's Population Problem*, eds. W. D. Borrie et al., 195–6. Sydney: Australasian Publishing Co., 1947.

_____. "Introduction." In *Australia's Coloured Minority: Its Place in the Community*, by A. O. Neville, 1–17. Sydney: Currawong Publishing Co., n.d.

Elkington, J.S.C. *Tropical Australia: Is It Suitable for a Working White Race?* Melbourne: Government Printer, 1905.

_____. "A plea for the Australian child body." *Report of the 12th Meeting AAAS, Brisbane, 1909*, 774–9. Brisbane: Government Printer, 1910.

Faber, C. "Australasia and South Africa as health resorts, especially for consumptive immigrants." *Practitioner* 20 (1878): 17–30.

_____. "Australasia, South Africa and South America as health resorts, comprising a medical climatology of the southern hemisphere." *Practitioner* 20 (1878): 346–66.

Fenner, F. J. "Adelaide University field anthropology. Central Australia No. 13: Anthropometric observations on South Australian Aborigines of the Diamantina and Cooper Creek regions." *Transactions Royal Society of South Australia* 55 (1936): 46–54.

_____. "The Australian Aboriginal skull: Its non-metrical morphological characters." *Transactions Royal Society of South Australia* 63 (1939): 248–306.

Ferry, T. A. "Report of the Royal Commission appointed to inquire into and report on the social and economic effects of increase in the number of aliens in Queensland." *Queensland Parliamentary Papers* 3 (1925): 25–52.

Field, Barron. *Geographical Memoirs of New South Wales*. London: John Murray, 1825.

Finlayson, H. H. *The Red Centre: Man and Beast in the Heart of Australia*. Sydney: Angus and Robertson, 1936.

Firth, Raymond. "Anthropology and native administration." *Oceania* 2 (1931): 1–8.

_____. "Anthropology in Australia, 1926–1932—and after." *Oceania* 3 (1932): 1–12.

Fisher, R. A. "Eugenics: Can it solve the problem of decay of civilisations?" *Eugenics Review* 18 (1926): 128–36.

_____. "The coefficient of racial likeness and the future of craniometry." *J. Royal Anthropological Institute* 66 (1936): 57–63.

Flower, W. H., and R. Lydekker. *An Introduction to the Study of Mammals, Living and Extinct*. London: Adam and Charles Black, 1891.

Forrest, John. "The Kimberley District." *Transactions and Proceedings Royal Geographical Society of Australasia (Victorian Branch)* 3–4 (1885–6): 137–49.

Fowler, H. L. "Report on psychological tests on natives in the northwest of Western Australia." *Australian J. Science* 2 (1940): 124–7.

Frodsham, G. H. *A Bishop's Pleasaunce.* London: Smith Elder, 1915.

Fry, H. K "Adelaide University field anthropology: Central Australia. Physiological and psychological observations." *Transactions and Proceedings Royal Society of South Australia* 54 (1930): 76–104.

————. "Aboriginal mentality." *MJA* i (1935): 353–60.

Fry, H. K., and R. Pulleine. "The mentality of the Australian Aborigine." *Australian J. Experimental Biology and Medical Science* 8 (1931): 153–167.

Galton, Francis. *Hereditary Genius: An Inquiry into Its Laws and Consequences.* London: Macmillan, 1869.

Garson, J. G. "Osteology." In *The Aborigines of Tasmania,* by H. Ling Roth, 2nd edn., 191–220. Hobart: Fuller's Bookshop, 1899 [1890].

"Garryowen" [Edmund Finn]. *The Chronicles of Early Melbourne, 1835–52: Historical, Anecdotal and Personal,* 3 vols. Melbourne: Heritage Publications, n.d.

"Gavah the Blacksmith" [Bernard O'Dowd]. "White Australia and qualified democracy." *Tocsin* (25 April 1901): 4.

Gibbs, H. D. "A study of the effect of tropical sunlight upon men, monkeys, rabbits, and a discussion of the proper clothing for the tropical climate." *PJS* 7B (1912): 91–114

Gilchrist, Ebenezer. *The Use of Sea-Voyages in Medicine, and Particularly in Consumption, with Observations on That Disease.* London: T. Cadell, 1771.

Goldby, F., C. S. Hicks, W. J. O'Connor, and D. A. Sinclair. "A comparison of the skin temperature and skin circulation of naked whites and Australian Aboriginals exposed to similar environmental changes." *Australian J. Experimental Biology and Medical Science* 16 (1938): 29–37.

Goldsmith, F. "Tropical disease in Northern Australia." *Transactions of the Intercolonial Medical Congress of Australasia, 5th Session, Brisbane, 1899,* 106–8. Brisbane: E. Gregory, 1901.

————. "The necessity for the study of tropical medicine in Australia." *Transactions of the Intercolonial Medical Congress of Australasia, 6th Session, Hobart, 1902,* 178–9. Hobart: John Vail, 1903.

Grant, Madison. *The Passing of the Great Race, or The Racial Basis of European History.* New York: C. Scribner, 1916.

Gray, Robert. *Reminiscences of India and North Queensland, 1857–1912.* London: Constable, 1913.

Gregory, J. W. *The Dead Heart of Australia.* London: John Murray, 1909.

————. "White labour in tropical agriculture: A great Australian experiment." *Nineteenth Century and After* 67 (1910): 368–80.

————. *The Menace of Colour.* London: Seeley Service, 1925.

Gresswell, D. Astley. "The management of communicable disease." *AMJ* 12ns (1890): 564–75.

————. *Darwinism and the Medical Profession.* Melbourne: Stillwell, 1895.

_____. "Prevalence of tuberculosis in Victoria." *Victorian Year Book 1903*, 232–41. Melbourne: Government Printer, 1904.

Gunson, J. M. "On typhoid fever." *AMJ* 17 (1872): 103–11.

Hackett, Cecil J. "A critical survey of some references to syphilis and yaws among the Australian Aborigines." *MJA* i (1936): 733–48.

Haldane, J. S. "Influence of high air temperatures." *J. Hygiene* 5 (1905): 494–513.

Halford, G. B. *Not Like Man: Bimanous and Biped, nor yet Quadrumanous, but Cheiropodous*. Melbourne: Wilson and Mackinnon, 1863.

_____. *Lines of Demarcation between Man, Gorilla and Macaque*. Melbourne: Wilson and Mackinnon, 1864.

Hamlyn-Harris, R. "Some anthropological considerations of Queensland and the history of its ethnography." *Proceedings Royal Society of Queensland* 29 (1917): 1–44.

Hancock, W. K. *Australia*. London: Ernest Benn, 1945 [1930].

Hardie, David. *Notes on Some of the More Common Diseases in Queensland in Relation to Atmospheric Conditions, 1887–91*. Brisbane: Government Printer, 1893.

Harney, W. E. *Taboo*. Sydney: Australasian Publishing Co., 1943.

_____. *North of 23°: Ramblings in Northern Australia*. Sydney: Australasian Publishing Co., n.d. [c. 1948].

Havard, Valery. "Is mortality necessarily higher in tropical than in temperate climates?" *American Medicine* 9 (7 January 1905): 16–20.

Heiser, V. G. *An American Doctor's Odyssey: Adventures in Forty-Five Countries*. London: Cape, 1936.

Herbert, Xavier. *Capricornia*. Sydney: Angus and Robertson, 1996 [1938].

Heydon, G. M. "The influence in hookworm infection of the species of worm and the race of man." *MJA* ii (1927): 206–8.

Hicks, C. Stanton. "The Australian Aboriginal: A study in comparative physiology." *Swiss Medical J.* 71 (1941): 509–18.

_____. *Soil, Food and Life*. Melbourne: Royal Australasian College of Physicians, 1945.

Hicks, C. S., and R. F. Matters. "The standard metabolism of Australian Aboriginals." *Australian J. Experimental Biology and Medical Science* 11 (1933): 177–84.

Hicks, C. S., R. F. Matters, and M. L. Mitchell. "The standard metabolism of Australian Aboriginals." *Australian J. Experimental Biology and Medical Science* 8 (1931): 69–82.

_____. "The respiratory exchange of the Australian Aborigine." *Australian J. Experimental Biology and Medical Science* 12 (1934): 79–90.

Hill, Ernestine. *The Great Australian Loneliness*. London: Jarrolds, 1937.

_____. *The Territory*. Sydney: Angus and Robertson, 1951.

Hingston, James. "A coming citizen of the world." *Victorian Review* 1 (1879): 76–93.

Hirszfeld, L. and H. "Serological differences between the blood of different races." *Lancet* ii (1919): 675–9.

Hogben, Lancelot. *Genetic Principles in Medicine and Social Science.* London: Williams and Norgate, 1931.

_____. *Nature and Nurture.* New York: Norton, 1933.

Hooton, E. A. "Race mixture in the United States." *Pacific Review* 2 (1921): 116–27.

_____. *Up from the Ape.* London: Allen and Unwin, 1931.

_____. *Apes, Men and Morons.* New York: G. P. Putnam's Sons, 1937.

_____. *Crime and the Man.* New York: Greenwood Press, 1968 [1939].

Howitt, A. W. "On the origin of the Aborigines of Tasmania and Australia." *Report of the 7th Meeting AAAS, Sydney, 1898,* 723–58. Sydney: AAAS, 1899.

_____. *The Native Tribes of Southeast Australia.* London: Macmillan, 1904.

Howitt, William. *Land, Labour and Gold, or Two Years in Victoria with Visits to Sydney and van Diemen's Land.* Kilmore, Vic.: Lowden, 1972 [1855].

Hrdlicka, Ales. "Human races." In *Human Biology and Racial Welfare,* ed. E. V. Cowdry, 156–83. New York: P. B. Hoeber, 1930.

Hughes, W. M. *The Splendid Adventure: A Review of Empire Relations Within and Without the Commonwealth of Britannic Nations.* London: Ernest Benn, 1929.

Hunt, Edward. "On colonial fever and on some recent cases of remittent fever." *AMJ* 14 (1869): 166–85.

Hunt, J. Sidney. "The evolution of malaria." *AMG* 10 (1890): 75–8.

_____. "Notes on the demography of North Queensland." *Transactions of the Intercolonial Medical Congress, 3rd session, Sydney, 1892,* 594–9. Sydney: Government Printer, 1893.

Hunter, John. *An Historical Journal of Events at Sydney and at Sea, 1787–92,* ed. John Bach. Sydney: Angus and Robertson, 1968 [1793].

Huntington, Ellsworth. *Civilization and Climate.* New Haven: Yale University Press, 1915.

_____. *Character of Races, as Influenced by Physical Environment, Natural Selection and Historical Development.* New York: Charles Scribner's Sons, 1924.

_____. *West of the Pacific.* New York: Charles Scribner's Sons, 1925.

_____. "Natural selection and climate in northern Australia." *Economic Record* 5 (1929): 185–201.

Huxley, Julian S., and A. C. Haddon. *We Europeans: A Survey of "Racial" Problems.* Harmondsworth: Penguin 1939 [1935].

Huxley, T. H. "On the ethnology and archaeology of India." *J. Ethnological Society* 1ns (1869): 89–93.

_____. *Man's Place in Nature and Other Anthropological Essays.* London: Macmillan, 1894.

_____. "On the geographical distribution of the chief modifications of mankind." *J. Ethnological Society* 2ns (1870): 404–12.

_____. *Diary of the Voyage of HMS Rattlesnake,* ed. Julian Huxley. London: Chatto and Windus, 1935.

Ingamells, Rex. "Statement." In *Jindyworobak Anthology, 1948,* ed. Roland E. Robinson. Melbourne: Jindyworobak, 1948.

_____. *Handbook of Australian Literature*. Melbourne: Jindyworobak, 1949.

_____. "Unknown land." In *Jindyworobaks*, by Brian Elliot. St Lucia: University of Queensland Press, 1979.

Isaacs, George. "The Burlesque of Frankenstein; or the Man-Gorilla." In *Rhyme and Prose; and a Burlesque and Its History*. Melbourne: Clarson, Shallard, 1865.

James, Philip. "Remarks on the fevers and diseases of tropical Queensland." *AMG* 10 (1891): 300–4.

James, William. *The Varieties of Religious Experience, a Study of Human Nature; Being the Gifford Lectures on Natural Religion Delivered at Edinburgh in 1901–02*. New York: Modern Library, 1926 [1902].

Jameson, R. G. *Australia and Her Gold Regions*. New York: Cornish, Lamport, 1852.

Jamieson, James. "Some points in the pathology of diphtheria." *AMJ* 16 (1871): 65–7.

_____. "Diphtheria and its treatment." *AMJ* 18 (1873): 331–37.

_____. "On the hypothesis of the faecal origin of the contagium of diphtheria." *AMJ* 19 (1874): 332–46.

_____. "On the parasitic theory of disease." *AMJ* 21 (1876): 256–62, 287–300, 315–24.

_____. "Victoria as a health-resort." *British Medical Journal* ii (1879): 933–6.

_____. "On the exact role of the pathogenic bacteria." *AMJ* 5ns (1883): 1–8.

_____. "Influence of meteorological conditions on the prevalence of typhoid fever." *AMJ* 12ns (1890): 97–110.

Jennings, H. S. *Prometheus, or Biology and the Advancement of Man*. London: Kegan, Paul, Trench, Trubner, 1925.

_____. *The Biological Basis of Human Nature*. London: Faber and Faber, 1930.

Jones, Frederic Wood. "The claims of the Australian Aborigine." *Report of the 18th Meeting AAAS, Perth, 1926*, ed. A. Gibb Maitland, 497–519. Perth: Government Printer, 1928.

_____. *Australia's Vanishing Race*. Sydney: Angus and Robertson, 1934.

Jones, F. Wood, and T. D. Campbell. "Anthropometric and descriptive observations on some South Australian Aboriginals, with a summary of previously recorded anthropometric data." *Transactions Royal Society of South Australia* 48 (1924): 303–12.

Jones, Frederic Wood, and Stanley D. Porteus, *The Matrix of the Mind*. London: Edward Arnold, 1929.

Keating, John H. *White Australia: Men and Measures in Its Making*. Launceston, Tas.: Examiner, 1924.

Keith, Arthur. *Nationality and Race, from an Anthropologist's Point of View*. Oxford: Oxford University Press, 1919.

Kelly, William. *Life in Victoria, or Victoria in 1853, and Victoria in 1858*, 2 vols. Kilmore, Vic.: Lowden Publishing, 1977 [1859].

Kidd, Benjamin. *The Control of the Tropics*. New York: Macmillan, 1898.

Kilgour, James. *Effect of the Climate of Australia upon the European Constitution in Health and Disease.* Geelong: William Vale, 1855.

"Killeevy." "Queensland: The colossus of the North." *Freeman's Journal* [Special Queensland Number] (7 October 1899): 17–41.

Kingsley, Henry. *Recollections of Geoffrey Hamlyn.* London: J. M. Dent, 1876 [1859].

Kirmess, C. H. *The Australian Crisis.* Melbourne: Lothian, 1909.

Klaatsch, H. "The skull of the Australian Aboriginal." *Reports from the Pathological Laboratory of the Lunacy Department, NSW* 1 (1908): 43–167.

Knox, Robert. *The Races of Men: A Fragment.* Philadelphia: Lee and Blanchard, 1850.

Koch, Robert. "Aetiology of tuberculosis." *AMJ* 4ns (1882): 409–26.

La Meslée, Edmond Marin. *The New Australia*, trans. Russel Ward. London: Heinemann, 1973 [1883].

Lancelott, F. *Australia as It Is: Its Settlements, Farms and Goldfields.* London: Colburn, 1852.

Lang, John Dunmore. *Emigration; Considered Chiefly in Reference to the Practicability and Expediency of Importing and of Settling Throughout the Territory of New South Wales, a Numerous, Industrious and Virtuous Agricultural Population.* Sydney: E. S. Hall, 1833.

_____. *Cooksland in Northeastern Australia; the Future Cotton Field of Great Britain: Its Characteristics and Capabilities for European Colonisation.* London: Longman, Brown, Green and Longmans, 1847.

Larnach, S. L. "A scientific expedition to central Australia." *Australian Outlook* 1 (1933): 9, 12.

_____. "'They sink and show no trace.'" *Australian Outlook* 2 (1934): 9, 13, 15.

_____. *Australian Aboriginal Craniology* [*Oceania* Monographs], 2 vols. Sydney: University of Sydney, 1978.

Law, Oswald P., and W. T. Gill. "A white Australia: what it means." *Nineteenth Century and After* 55 (1904): 146–54.

Lee, D.H.K. "Blood groups of North Queensland Aborigines, with a statistical collection of some published figures for various races." *MJA* ii (1926): 401–10.

_____. "The settlement of tropical Australia." *MJA* ii (1936): 707–12.

Lee, D.H.K., and R. K. Macpherson. "Tropical fatigue and warfare" *J. Applied Physiology* 1 (1948): 60–72.

Lévy-Bruhl, Lucien. *Primitive Mentality*, trans. Lilian A. Clare. London: George Allen and Unwin, 1923.

Lindsay, Jack. *Life Rarely Tells.* London: Bodley Head, 1958.

Lumholtz, Carl. *Among Cannibals: An Account of Four Years' Travels in Australia and of Camp Life with the Aborigines of Queensland.* Firle, Sussex: Caliban Books, 1979 [1889].

Lyng, Jens. *Non-Britishers in Australia: Influence on Population and Progress.* Melbourne: Macmillan, 1927.

_____. "Racial composition of the Australian People." In *The Peopling of Australia*, eds., P. D. Phillips and G. L. Wood, 145–64. Melbourne: Macmillan, 1928.

Macartney, F. T., ed. *The Collected Verse of A. B. Paterson*. Sydney: Angus and Robertson, 1921.

Macdonald, T. F. "Experiences of ankylostomiasis in Australia." *Transactions Society of Tropical Medicine and Hygiene* 1 (1907–08): 68–75.

Macfie, Matthew. "How can tropical and sub-tropical Australia be developed?" *Report of the 11th Meeting AAAS, Adelaide, 1907*, 593–616. Adelaide: AAAS, 1908.

MacGillivray, P. H. "Notes of dissections of colonial fever." *AMJ* 9 (1864): 238–42.

Mackay, J. A. Kenneth. *The Yellow Wave: A Romance of the Asiatic Invasion of Australia*. London: R. Bentley, 1897.

Mackellar, C. K. "Notes on the aetiology of typhoid fever." *AMG* 1 (1881–2): 117–19.

Mackenna, J. W. "On the comparative effect of climate on certain diseases." *AMJ* 5 (1860): 14–20.

Mackie, John. "In the Far North." *Sydney Quarterly Magazine* 2 (1885).

Mackin, C. Travers. "Sunstroke, or *coup de soleil*: Its causes, consequences and pathology." *AMJ* 1 (1856): 5–13, 81–8.

Macpherson, R. K. "The physiology of adaptation." *MJA* i (1964): 905–07.

Magarey, S. J. "Our climate and infant mortality." *Transactions, Proceedings and Report of the Philosophical Society of Adelaide, South Australia, for 1878–9*, 1–9. Adelaide: Webb, Vardon and Pritchard, 1879.

Manson, Patrick. *Tropical Diseases: A Manual of the Diseases of Warm Climates*. London: Cassell, 1898.

Maplestone, P. A. "An evening in tropical Australia." *Melbourne University Magazine* 7 (1913): 99–100.

_____. "Research in Australia." *MJA* i (1922): 476–77.

Masefield, John. *Gallipoli*. London: W. Heinemann, 1916.

Masson, Elsie. *An Untamed Territory: The Northern Territory of Australia*. London: Macmillan, 1915.

Mathew, John. *Eaglehawk and Crow: A Study of the Australian Aborigines*. Melbourne: Melville, Mullen and Slade, 1899.

_____. *Two Representative Tribes of Queensland, with an Inquiry Concerning the Origin of the Australian Race*. London: T. Fisher Unwin, 1910.

"M. B." "Correspondence—White Australia Policy." *MJA* i (1915): 277–8.

McCrea, William. *Observations on Typhoid Fever*. Melbourne: Samuel Mullen, 1879.

McDonald, T. P. "Tropical lands and white races." *Transactions Society of Tropical Medicine and Hygiene* 1 (1907–8): 201–28.

McGillivray, J. *Narrative of the Voyage of HMS Rattlesnake*, 2 vols. London: Boone, 1852.

McGregor, William. "Some problems of tropical medicine." *Lancet* (13 October 1900): 1055–61.

McKay, H. C. "Earth-eaters of Queensland." *Smith's Weekly* (16 June 1923).

McKenna, J. William. *Mortality of Children in Victoria*. Melbourne: W. Fairfax, 1858.

"Medicus." "Correspondence." *AMJ* 15 (1870): 156–7.

_____. "The influence of the Victorian climate upon phthisis." *AMJ* 23 (1878): 25–7.

Merrillees, James F. "Correspondence—White Australia Policy." *MJA* i (1915): 345–6.

Morant, G. M. "A study of the Australian and Tasmanian skulls, based on previously published measurements." *Biometrika* 19 (1927): 417–40.

Morgan, Lewis Henry. *Ancient Society: or, Researches in the Lines of Human Progress, from Savagery Through Barbarism to Civilisation*. London: Macmillan, 1877.

_____. "Preface." In *Kamilaroi and Kurnai*, by Lorimer Fison and A. W. Howitt. Melbourne: G. Robertson, 1880.

Morton, W. Lockhart. "Notes of a recent personal visit to the unoccupied Northern District of Queensland." *Transactions Philosophical Institute of Victoria* 4 (1859): 188–99.

Mossman, Samuel, and Thomas Banister. *Australia Visited and Revisited: A Narrative of Recent Travels and Old Experiences in Victoria and New South Wales*. Sydney: Ure Smith, 1974 [1853].

Mountford, Charles P. *Brown Men and Red Sand: Wanderings in Wild Australia*. Melbourne: Robertson and Mullens, 1948.

Mueller, F. von. "Phthisis and the eucalypts." *AMJ* 1ns (1879): 53–4.

Murdoch, Walter. *The Australian Citizen: An Elementary Account of Civic Rights and Duties*. Melbourne: Whitcomb and Tombs, 1912.

Musgrave, W. E., and A. G. Sison. "Blood pressure in the tropics: A preliminary report." *PJS* 5 (1910): 325–9.

Neild, James E. "Some remarks on the diarrhoea and dysentery of this colony." *AMJ* 8 (1863): 8–10.

_____. "The medical profession." In *Victoria and Its Metropolis: Past and Present*, 3 vols., ed. Alexander Sutherland, vol. 1, 779–85. Melbourne: McCarron Bird, 1888.

Neville, A. O. *Australia's Coloured Minority: Its Place in the Community*. Sydney: Currawong Publishing Co., n.d.

Nicoll, W. "The conditions of life in tropical Australia." *J. Hygiene* 16 (1917): 269–90.

Norris, Perrin W. "Report on quarantine in other countries and on the quarantine requirements of Australia." *Commonwealth Parliamentary Papers* 28 (1912).

Norton, A. "Settling in Queensland and the reasons for doing so—with special reference to droughts." *Proceedings Royal Society of Queensland* 17 (1903): 147–60.

O'Dowd, Bernard. "Race prejudice." *Theosophy in Australasia* (2 September 1912): 153–6; (1 October 1912): 175–9.

Osborne, W. A. "Contributions to physiological climatology. Part 1: The relation of loss of water from the skin and lungs to the external temperature in actual climatic conditions." *J. Physiology* 41 (1910–11): 345–54.

————. "Contributions to physiological climatology. Part 2." *J. Physiology* 49 (1914–15): 133–8.

————. "The wet-bulb and kata-thermometers." *Proceedings of the Royal Society of Victoria* 29ns (1916): 119–22.

————. "Physiological factors in the development of an Australian race." *Transactions of the Australasian Medical Congress, 11th session, Brisbane, 1920,* 71–82. Brisbane: Anthony James Cumming, 1921.

Palmer, Edward. *Early Days in North Queensland.* Sydney: Angus and Robertson, 1983 [1903].

Palmer, Vance. "Italians in North Queensland." Melbourne *Punch* (22 October 1925).

Panton, J. A. "The discovery, physical geography and resources of the Kimberley District, Western Australia." *Proceedings of the Geographical Society of Australasia (NSW and Victorian Branches)* 1 (1883–4): 119–32.

————. "A few days ashore in West Kimberley." *Transactions and Proceedings Royal Geographical Society of Australasia (Victorian Branch)* 3–4 (1885–6): 67–80.

Parsons, J. Langdon. "Quarterly report on the Northern Territory, 31 March 1885." *South Australian Parliamentary Papers* 54 (1885).

Pearson, Charles H. *National Life and Character: A Forecast.* London: Macmillan, 1894.

Pearson, Karl. "On the relationship of intelligence to size and shape of head and to other physical and mental characters." *Biometrika* 5 (1906–7): 105–46.

Phelan, James M. "An experiment with orange-red underwear." *PJS* 5 (1910): 525–46.

Phillips, P. D. "Introduction." In *The Peopling of Australia,* eds. F. W. Eggleston et al., 9–31. Melbourne: Melbourne University Press, 1933.

Phillips, P. D., and G. L. Wood. "The Australian population problem." In *The Peopling of Australia,* eds. Phillips and Wood, 1–47. Melbourne: Macmillan, 1930.

Piddington, Ralph. "Psychological aspects of culture contact." *Oceania* 3 (1932–3): 312–24.

Pike, L. H. "White Australia—tropical Queensland." *J. Royal Society of Arts* 86 (1938): 719–39.

Pitts, Herbert. *The Australian Aboriginal and the Christian Church.* London: Society for Promoting Christian Knowledge, 1914.

Pockley, Antil. "Presidential address." *AMG* 30 (1911).

Porteus, Stanley D. "Mental tests with delinquents and Australian Aboriginal children." *Psychological Review* 24 (1917): 32–42.

_____. *The Psychology of a Primitive People: A Study of the Australian Aborigine.* London: Edward Arnold, 1931.

_____. "Mentality of Australian Aborigines." *Oceania* 4 (1933–4): 30–6.

_____. "Correspondence." *Oceania* 4 (1933–4): 107–9.

_____. *A Psychologist of Sorts: The Autobiography and Publications of the Inventor of the Porteus Maze Tests.* Palo Alto, CA: Pacific Books, 1969.

Price, A. Grenfell. "Pioneer reactions to a poor tropical environment: A journey through central and north Australia in 1932." *Geographical Review* 23 (1933): 353–71.

_____. "White settlers in the tropics." In *Comptes rendus du 15ème Congrès international de Géographie, Amsterdam 1938,* vol. 2, 267–71. Leiden: E. J. Brill, 1938.

_____. *White Settlers in the Tropics.* New York: American Geographical Society, 1939.

Prichard, Katharine Susannah. *Coonardoo: The Well in the Shadow.* Sydney: Angus and Robertson, 1957 [1929].

Priestley, Henry. "Physiological observations in the tropical parts of Australia." In *Proceedings of the Pan-Pacific Science Congress,* ed. Gerald Lightfoot, vol. 2, 1486–92. Melbourne: Government Printer, 1923.

Priestley, Henry, and Ellen M. Hindmarsh. "The blood urea and nitrogen output of Australian students." *MJA* i (1924): 234–5.

Pritchard, James Cowles. *Researches into the Physical History of Mankind,* 3rd edn., 4 vols. London: Houlston and Stoneman, 1841–47.

Pulleine, R., and H. Woollard. "Physiology and mental observations on the Australian Aborigines." *Transactions and Proceedings Royal Society of South Australia* 54 (1930): 62–75.

Quatrefages de Breau, Armand de. *Histoire Générale des Races Humaines: Introduction à l'étude des races humaines.* Paris: J. B. Ballière, 1887.

Quatrefages de Breau, Armand de, and Ernest T. Hamy. *Crania Ethnica: Les Crânes des Races Humaines,* 2 vols. Paris: J. B. Ballière et fils, 1882.

"Queenslander." "Coloured labour and Queensland sugar." *Sydney Quarterly Magazine* 2 (1885): 339–44.

Rattray, Alexander. "On some of the more important physiological changes induced in the human economy by change of climate, as from temperate to tropical, and the reverse." *Proceedings of the Royal Society of London* 18 (1869–70): 513–29; 19 (1870–1): 295–316.

_____. "Further experiments on the more important physiological changes induced in the human economy by change of climate." *Proceedings of the Royal Society of London* 21 (1872–3): 2–10.

Read, C. R. *What I Heard, Saw and Did at the Australian Goldfields.* London: T. and W. Boone, 1853.

Reay, Marie. "A half-caste Aboriginal community in north-western New South Wales." *Oceania* 15 (1944–5): 296–323.

Reeves, Charles Evans. *Consumption in Australia.* Melbourne: J. Brookes, 1874.

"Report of the Sugar Inquiry Committee, 1931." *Commonwealth Parliamentary Papers* 240 (1929–31), part III, pp. 7–192.

"Resident" [John Hunter Kerr]. *Glimpses of Life in Victoria*. Melbourne: Melbourne University Press, 1996 [1872].

"Richardson, Henry Handel" [Ethel Florence Robertson]. *The Fortunes of Richard Mahony*. Melbourne: Heinemann, 1946 [1930].

Richardson, W. Lindesay. "Notes on some of the diseases prevalent in Victoria, Australia." *Edinburgh Medical Journal* 14 (1869): 802–12.

Rivers, G. Pitt. "The effect on native races of contact with European civilisation." *Man* 27 (1927): 2–10.

Robarts, Natalie. "The Victorian Aborigine as he is." *Report of the 14th Meeting AAAS, Melbourne, 1913*, 444–6. Melbourne: Government Printer, 1914.

Robertson, James. "On the nature or essence of disease in Victoria." *AMJ* 13 (1868): 247–53.

Róheim, Géza. *The Children of the Desert: The Western Tribes of Central Australia*. New York: Basic Books, 1974.

Rolleston, Christopher. "The sanitary condition of Sydney." *Sydney Magazine of Science and Art* 1 (1858): 37–40.

Roosevelt, Theodore. "National life and character" [1894]. In *American Ideals and Other Essays, Social and Political*, 261–92. New York and London: G. P. Putnam's Sons, 1907.

—————. *Biological Analogies in History* [Romanes Lecture, 1910]. Oxford: Clarendon Press, 1910.

Ross, Andrew. "The climate of Australia viewed in relation to health." *NSW Medical Gazette* 1 (1870–71): 131–8, 163–7, 195–202, 227–34, 259–66.

Roth, H. Ling. "The influence of climate and soil on the development of the Anglo-Australian race." *Victorian Review* 2 (1880): 840–9.

—————. *The Aborigines of Tasmania*, 2nd edn. Hobart: Fuller's Bookshop, 1899 [1890].

"Royal Commission into Diphtheria." *Victorian Parliamentary Papers* 3 (1872), part II.

"Royal Commission on Health." *Commonwealth Parliamentary Papers* 3 (1926–8), part IV.

Rusden, G. W. *The History of Australia*, 2nd edn. Melbourne: Melville, 1897.

Rusden, H. K. "On contagious disease." *AMJ* 3ns (1881): 39–40.

Ryle, John A. "Social medicine: Its meaning and scope." *British Medical Journal* ii (1943): 633–36.

Ryley, John Rutherford. "Notes on the aetiology of typhoid fever." *AMG* 1 (1881–2): 159–60.

Sambon, Luigi Westenra. "Remarks on acclimatization in tropical regions." *British Medical Journal* i (9 January 1897): 61–6.

—————. "Acclimatisation of Europeans in tropical lands." *Geographical J.* 12 (1898): 589–606.

Sawyer, W. A. "Hookworm disease in relation to the medical profession." *Health* 1 (1923): 11–13.

Scoresby-Jackson, R. E. *Medical Climatology*. London: John Churchill, 1862.

Searcy, Alfred. *In Australian Tropics*. London: George Robertson, 1907.

Shattuck, George C. "The possibility of white settlement in the tropics." In *Comptes rendus du 15ème Congrès international de Géographie, Amsterdam, 1938*, vol. 2, 327. Leiden: E. J. Brill, 1938.

Singleton, John. "On phthisis in Victoria." *AMJ* 16 (1871): 206–9.

————. "Phthisis in Victoria." *AMJ* 21 (1876): 279–86.

Smith, Patrick. "On the aetiology of typhoid fever." *AMJ* 22 (1877): 202–15.

Smith, W. Ramsay. "The place of the Australian Aboriginal in recent anthropological research." *Report of the 11th Meeting AAAS, Adelaide, 1907*, 558–77. Adelaide: AAAS, 1908.

————. *On Race-Culture and the Conditions that Influence It in South Australia*. Adelaide: Government Printer, 1912.

————. "Australian conditions and problems from the standpoint of present anthropological knowledge." *Report of the 14th Meeting AAAS, Melbourne, 1913*, 367–72. Melbourne: Government Printer, 1914.

————. *In Southern Seas: Wanderings of a Naturalist*. London: John Murray, 1924.

————. *Myths and Legends of the Australian Aborigines*. London: Harrap, 1930.

Smyth, R. Brough. "Ozone." *AMJ* 4 (1859): 1–3.

————. *The Aborigines of Victoria, and Other Parts of Australia and Tasmania*, 2 vols. Melbourne: John Currey, O'Neill, 1972 [1876].

Sorokin, P. *Contemporary Sociological Theories Through the First Quarter*. New York: Harper and Row, 1928.

Sowden, William J. *The Northern Territory as It Is: A Narrative of the South Australian Parliamentary Party's Trip*. Adelaide: W. K. Thomas, 1882.

Spencer, W. Baldwin. "Preliminary report on the Aborigines of the Northern Territory." *Commonwealth Parliamentary Papers* 3 (1913).

————. "The Aboriginals of Australia." In *Federal Handbook of the British Association for the Advancement of Science*, ed. G.H. Knibbs, 33–85. Melbourne: Government Printer, 1914.

Spencer, W. Baldwin, and F. J. Gillen. *The Native Tribes of Central Australia*. London: Macmillan, 1899.

————. *Across Australia*, 2 vols. London: Macmillan, 1912.

Springthorpe, J. W. *Unseen Enemies and How to Fight Them* [Australian Health Society Lecture No. 21]. Melbourne: Walker, May, 1891.

————. "Six instances of the use of diphtheria antitoxin." *AMG* 14 (1895): 55–8.

Stephensen, P. R. "The foundations of culture in Australia: An essay towards national self-respect." *Australian Mercury* 1 (1935): 3–42.

————. *The Foundations of Culture in Australia: An Essay Towards National Self-Respect*. Sydney: Angus and Robertson, 1936.

Sterland, W. J. "Hints on the climate of Australia." *Association Medical Journal* 30 (1853): 671–2.

Stirling, E. C. "Anthropology of the central Australian Aborigines." In *Report on the Work of the Horn Scientific Expedition to Central Australia*, ed. W. A. Horn. London: Dulau, 1896.

_____. "Preliminary report on the discovery of native remains at Swanport, River Murray; with an enquiry into the alleged occurrence of a pandemic among the Australian Aboriginals." *Transactions Royal Society of South Australia* 35 (1911): 4–46.

Stirling, J. *Observations on the Climate and Geographical Position of Western Australia, and on Its Adaptation to the Purposes of a Sanatorium for the Indian Army*. London: J. C. Bridgewater, 1859.

Stone, Louis. *Jonah*. London: Methuen, 1911.

Strehlow, T.G.H. *Aranda Traditions*. Melbourne: Melbourne University Press, 1947.

_____. *Dark and White Australians*. Adelaide: South Australian Peace Committee, 1957.

_____. *Songs of Central Australia*. Sydney: Angus and Robertson, 1971.

Sundstroem, E. S. *A Summary of Some Studies in Tropical Acclimatisation* [Department of Health Service Publication No. 6]. Melbourne: Government Printer, n.d. [c. 1924].

_____. *Contribution to Tropical Physiology: With Special Reference to the Adaptation of the White Man to the Climate of North Queensland*. Berkeley: University of California Press, 1926.

Sutton, C. Harvey. "The importance of nationality." *Report of the 13th Meeting AAAS, Sydney, 1911*, 508–10. Sydney: Government Printer, 1912.

_____. "The cure of feeblemindedness." *AMG*, (1913): 556.

_____. "The feebleminded—their classification and importance." *Transactions of the Australasian Medical Congress, 9th Session, Sydney, 1911*, vol. 1, 894–905. Sydney: Government Printer, 1913.

_____. "Modern development of public health—the child as the test of progress" [Presidential Address, Section I, Medical Science and National Health]. *Report of the 20th Meeting AAAS, Brisbane, 1930*, 336–64. Brisbane: Government Printer, 1931.

_____. "Physical education and national fitness." *Australian Rhodes Review* 4 (1939): 56–62.

Syder, C. B. Mingay. *The Voice of Truth in Defence of Nature; and Opinions Antagonistic to Those of Dr Kilgour*. Geelong: Heath and Cordell, 1855.

Tasmanian Parliament. *Military Sanitarium: Report of the Board of Commissioners*. Hobart: Government Printer, 1858.

Taylor, T. Griffith. *The Control of Settlement by Humidity and Temperatures*. Melbourne: Commonwealth Bureau of Meteorology, 1916.

_____. "Geographical factors controlling the settlement of tropical Australia." *Queensland Geographical J.* 32–3 (1918): 1–67.

_____. "The evolution and distribution of race, culture and language." *Geographical Review* 11 (1921): 54–119.

_____. "The distribution of future white settlement: A world survey based on physiographic data." *Geographical Review* 12 (1922): 375–402.

_____. *Environment and Race: A Study of the Evolution, Migration, Settlement and Status of the Races of Man*. London: Oxford University Press, 1927.

_____. *Journeyman Taylor: The Education of a Scientist*. London: Robert Hale, 1958.

Taylor, T. Griffith, and F. Jardine. "Kamilaroi and white: A study of racial mixture in New South Wales." *J. and Proceedings Royal Society of NSW* 58 (1924): 268–92.

Tebbutt, A. H. "Comparative iso-agglutinin index of Australian Aborigines and Australians." *MJA* ii (1923): 346.

_____. "Second report on the comparative iso-agglutinin index of Australian Aborigines and Australians." *Proceedings Pan-Pacific Science Congress*, ed. Gerald Lightfoot, vol. 1, 242–7. Melbourne: Government Printer, 1923.

Tench, Watkin. *Sydney's First Four Years*, ed. L. F. Fitzhardinge. Sydney: Angus and Robertson, 1961 [1789 and 1793].

Thomson, William. *Not Man, but Man-like*. Melbourne: Argus, 1863.

_____. *A Consumptive Voyage to the Medical Society*. Melbourne: Fergusson and Moore, 1870.

_____. *On Phthisis and the Supposed Influence of Climate*. Melbourne: Stillwell and Knight, 1870.

_____. "Notes on the report of the chairman of the Diphtheria Commission." *AMJ* 17 (1872): 244–50.

_____. *Remarks on the Introduction of Diphtheria into Victoria*. Melbourne: Stillwell and Knight, 1872.

_____. *On Typhoid Fever*. Melbourne: George Robertson, 1874.

_____. *Contagion Alone the Cause of Typhoid Fever in Melbourne*. Melbourne: Stillwell, 1880.

_____. *The Germ Theory of Disease Applied to Eradicate Phthisis from Victoria*. Melbourne: Sands and McDougall, 1882.

Tindale, N. B. "Distribution of Aboriginal tribes: A field survey." *Transactions Royal Society of South Australia* 64 (1940): 140–231.

_____. "Survey of the half-caste problem in South Australia." *Proceedings Royal Geographical Society of Australasia, South Australian Branch* 42 (1940–1): 66–161.

_____. *Aboriginal Tribes of Australia: Their Terrain, Environmental Controls, Distribution, Limits and Proper Names*. Canberra: Australian National University Press, 1974.

_____. "A South Australian looks at some beginnings of archaeological research in Australia." *Aboriginal History* 6 (1982): 93–110.

Tindale, Norman B., and Joseph B. Birdsell. "Tasmanoid types in North Queensland." *Records of the South Australian Museum* 7 (1941): 1–9.

Topinard, Paul. "Etudes sur les Tasmaniens." *Mémoires de la Société d'Anthopologie* 3 (1871): 307–31.

_____. *Anthropology*, trans. Robert T. H. Bartley. London: Chapman and Hall, 1878.

Trollope, Anthony. *Australia and New Zealand*, 2 vols. London: Dawson's, 1968 [1873].

Turner, A. Jefferis. "The place of bacteriology in practical medicine." *AMG* 14 (1895): 200–6.

Turner, Duncan. *Is Consumption Contagious?* Melbourne: Melville, Mullen and Slade, 1894.

Turner, W. "Report on the human crania and other bones of the skeletons collected during the voyage of *HMS Challenger*, in the years 1873–76. Part 1: The crania." In *Report of the Scientific Results of the Exploring Voyage of HMS Challenger, 1873–76. Zoology*, vol. 10, 1–130. London: HMSO, 1884.

"Twain, Mark" [Samuel L. Clemens]. *Following the Equator: A Journey around the World*, 2 vols. Hopewell NJ: Ecco Press, 1992 [1879].

Twopeny, Richard. *Town Life in Australia*. London: Elliot Stock, 1883.

Tylor, Edward B. "Preface." In *The Aborigines of Tasmania*, by H. Ling Roth, 2nd edn., i–v. Hobart: Fuller's Bookshop, 1899 [1890].

"Vagabond" [John Stanley James]. *Vagabond Country: Australian Bush and Town Life in the Victorian Age*, ed. Michael Cannon. Melbourne: Hyland House, 1981.

Victorian Central Board of Health. *Typhoid Fever*. Melbourne: Government Printer, 1887.

Vidal de la Blach, P. *Principles of Human Geography*, ed. Emmanuel de Martonne, trans. Millicent T. Bingham. New York: Henry Holt, 1926.

Vries, Hugo de. *Species and Varieties: Their Origin by Mutation,* ed. D. T. MacDougal. Chicago: Open Court Publishers, 1904.

Waite, J. H. "Preliminary report of ankylostomiasis in Papua." *MJA* ii (1917): 221–3.

————. "The Queensland hookworm campaign." *MJA* ii (1918): 505–10.

Waite, J. H., and I. L. Neilson. "A study of the effects of hookworm infection upon the mental development of North Queensland schoolchildren." *MJA* i (1919): 1–8.

Wallace, Alfred R. *Australasia*, 2 vols. London: Edward Stanford, 1893.

Wardlaw, H. S. Halcro. "The energy consumption of Australian students." *MJA* ii (1922): 294.

Wardlaw, H. S. Halcro, and C. H. Horsley. "The basal metabolism of some Australian Aborigines." *Australian J. Experimental Biology and Medical Science* 5 (1928): 263–72.

Wardlaw, H. S. Halcro, H. Whitridge Davies, and M. R. Joseph. "Energy metabolism and insensible perspiration of Australian Aborigines." *Australian J. Experimental Biology and Medical Science* 12 (1934): 63–74.

Wardlaw, H. S. Halcro, H. C. Barry, I. W. McDonald, and A. K. Macintyre. "The haemoglobin and solids of the blood of Australian Aborigines and whites." *Australian J. Experimental Biology and Medical Science* 13 (1935): 1–8.

Watson, J. C. "Our empty north: An unguarded gate." *Lone Hand* (1 August 1907): 420–6.

Weissmann, August. *The Germ Plasm: A Theory of Heredity*, trans. W. Newton Parker and Harriet Rönnfeldt. London: W. Scott, 1893.

Western Australian Parliament. *Dispatches on the Subject of the Establishment of a Sanitarium in Western Australia for British Troops Serving in India.* Perth: Government Printer, 1886.

Westgarth, William. *A Report on the Condition, Capabilities and Prospects of the Australian Aborigines.* Melbourne: William Clarke, 1846.

White, Gilbert. "Some problems of Northern Australia." *Victorian Geographical Journal* 25 (1907): 53–74.

————. *Thirty Years in Tropical Australia.* London: Society for Promoting Christian Knowledge, 1918.

White, J. Aitken. "On the fevers of the Gulf of Carpentaria." *AMJ* 12 (1867): 361–5.

White, John. *Journal of a Voyage to New South Wales,* ed. Alec H. Chisholm. Sydney: Angus and Robertson, 1962 [1790].

Wickens, C. H. "Vitality of white races in low latitudes." *Economic Record* 3 (1927): 117–26.

————. "Dr Huntington and low latitudes." *Economic Record* 6 (1930): 123–7.

Wilkinson, H. L. *The World's Population Problems and a White Australia.* London: P. S. King, 1930.

Wilkinson, W. Camac. "Two cases of diphtheria treated with Behring's antitoxin." *AMG* 14 (1895): 232–3.

Williams, W. Wynne. "Settlement of the tropics." *Economic Record* 11 (1935): 20–34.

————. "The white man in the Australian tropics: History of colonisation." In *Comptes rendus du 15ème Congrès international de Géographie, Amsterdam, 1938,* vol. 2, 337–44. Leiden: E. J. Brill, 1938.

Wilsone, D. H. "Memorandum of a trip to Port Phillip." In *Letters from Victorian Pioneers, being a Series of Papers on the Early Occupation of the Colony,* ed. Thomas Francis Bride. Melbourne: Heinemann, 1969 [1898].

Wood, G. L. "The settlement of northern Australia." *Economic Record* 2 (1926): 1–19.

————. "The immigrant problem in Australia." *Economic Record* 2 (1926): 229–39.

Woodruff, Charles E. *The Effects of Tropical Light on White Men.* New York: Rebman, 1905.

————. "The neurasthenic states caused by excessive light." *Medical Record* 68 (23 December 1905): 1005–9.

Woollard, H., and J. B. Cleland. "Anthropology and blood grouping with special reference to Australian Aborigines." *Man* 29 (1929): 181–8.

Young, W. J. "A note on the black pigment in the skin of an Australian Black." *Biochemical J.* 8 (1914): 460–2.

————. "Fighting tropical diseases in Australia." *Lone Hand* 2 (1 June 1914): 33–6.

————. "Observations upon the body temperature of Europeans living in the tropics." *J. Physiology* 44 (1915): 222–32.

Secondary Sources

Theses and Dissertations

Bolton, Conevery. The "Health of the Country": Body and Environment in the Making of the American West, 1800–60. Ph.D. dissertation, Harvard University, 1998.

Butcher, Barry W. Darwinism and Australia, 1836–1914. Ph.D. thesis, University of Melbourne, 1992.

Harloe, Lori. White Man in Tropical Australia: Anton Breinl and the Australian Institute of Tropical Medicine. B.A. (hons.) thesis, James Cook University of North Queensland, 1987.

Hoare, Michael. Science and Scientific Associations in Eastern Australia; 1820–90. Ph.D. thesis, Australian National University, 1974.

Jones, Ross. "Skeletons in Toorak and Collingwood Cupboards": Eugenics in Educational and Health Policy in Victoria, 1910–39. Ph.D. thesis, Monash University, 2000.

Smith, F. B. Religion and Freethought in Melbourne, 1870 to 1890. M.A. thesis, University of Melbourne, 1960.

Books and Articles

Abbie, A. A. *The University of Adelaide School of Medicine.* Glebe, NSW: Australasian Medical Publishing Co., 1952.

Ackerknecht, Erwin. "Anticontagionism between 1821 and 1867." *Bulletin of the History of Medicine* 22 (1948): 562–93.

————. *History and Geography of the Most Important Diseases.* New York: Hafner Publishing, 1972.

Adams, Mark. "Eugenics in the history of science." In *The Wellborn Science: Eugenics in Germany, France, Brazil and Russia,* eds. Adams et al. New York: Oxford University Press, 1990.

Adas, Michael. *Machines as the Measure of Men: Science, Technology and Ideologies of Western Dominance.* Ithaca: Cornell University Press, 1989.

Allen, Theodore. *The Invention of the White Race, Volume 1: Racial Oppression and Social Control.* London: Verso, 1994.

Alomes, Stephen. *A Nation at Last? The Changing Character of Australian Nationalism, 1880–1988.* Sydney: Angus and Robertson, 1988.

Anderson, Benedict. *Imagined Communities: Reflections on the Origin and Spread of Nationalism.* London: Verso, 1983.

Anderson, Hugh. *The Poet Militant: Bernard O'Dowd.* Melbourne: Hill of Content, 1969.

Anderson, Ian. "Black bit, white bit." *RePublica* 1 (1994): 113–22.

————. "I, the 'hybrid' Aborigine: Film and representation." *Australian Aboriginal Studies* 11 (1997): 4–14.

Anderson, Warwick. "Climates of opinion: Acclimatization in nineteenth-century France and England." *Victorian Studies* 35 (1992): 135–57.

_____. "Excremental colonialism: Public health and the poetics of pollution." *Critical Inquiry* 21 (1995): 640–69.

_____. "'Where every prospect pleases and only man is vile': Laboratory medicine as colonial discourse." In *Discrepant Histories: Translocal Essays on Filipino Cultures*, ed. Vicente Rafael, 83–112. Philadelphia: Temple University Press, 1995.

_____. "Disease, race and empire." *Bulletin of the History of Medicine* 70 (1996): 62–7.

_____. "Immunities of empire: Race, disease and the new tropical medicine." *Bulletin of the History of Medicine* 70 (1996): 94–118.

_____. "Race, geography and nation: Re-mapping 'tropical' Australia, 1890–1920." *Historical Records of Australian Science* 11 (1997): 457–68.

_____. "'The trespass speaks': White masculinity and colonial breakdown." *American Historical Review* 102 (1997): 1433–70.

_____. "Leprosy and citizenship." *Positions: East Asia Cultures Critique* 6 (1998): 707–30.

_____. "Victor G. Heiser." In *American National Biography*, eds. John A. Garraty and Mark C. Carnes, vol. 10, 522–4. New York: Oxford University Press, 1999.

_____. "The natures of culture: Environment and race in the colonial tropics." In *Imagination and Distress in Southern Environmental Projects*, eds. Paul Greenough and Anna L. Tsing. Durham, NC: Duke University Press, forthcoming.

Arnold, David. *Colonizing the Body: State Medicine and Epidemic Disease in Nineteenth-Century India*. Berkeley: University of California Press, 1993.

_____. *The Problem of Nature: Environment, Culture and European Expansion*. Oxford: Blackwell, 1996.

_____, ed. *Imperial Medicine and Indigenous Societies*. Manchester: Manchester University Press, 1988.

_____, ed. *Warm Climates and Western Medicine: The Emergence of Tropical Medicine 1500–1900*. Amsterdam: Rodopi, 1996.

Aronowitz, Robert. *Making Sense of Illness: Science, Society and Disease*. Cambridge: Cambridge University Press, 1998.

Attwood, Bain. *The Making of Aborigines*. Sydney: Allen and Unwin, 1989.

Attwood, Harold, ed. *The History of the Wallaby Club*. Mont Albert, Vic.: Landscape Publications, 1993.

Austin, Tony. "Cecil Cook, scientific thought and 'half-castes.'" *Aboriginal History* 14 (1990): 104–22.

_____. *Simply the Survival of the Fittest: Aboriginal Administration in South Australia's Northern Territory, 1863–1910*. Darwin: Historical Society of the Northern Territory, 1992.

_____. *I Can Picture the Old Home so Clearly: The Commonwealth and "Half-Caste" Youth in the Northern Territory, 1911–39*. Canberra: Aboriginal Studies Press, 1993.

_____. *Never Trust a Government Man: Northern Territory Aboriginal Policy, 1911–39*. Darwin: Northern Territory University Press, 1997.

Bacchi, C. L. "The nature-nurture debate in Australia, 1900–14." *Historical Studies* [Australia] 19 (1980): 199–212.

Baldwin, Peter. *Contagion and the State in Europe, 1830–1930*. Cambridge: Cambridge University Press, 1999.

Barkan, Elazar. *The Retreat of Scientific Racism: Changing Concepts of Race in Britain and the United States Between the World Wars*. Cambridge: Cambridge University Press, 1992.

Bashford, Alison. "Quarantine and the imagining of the Australian nation." *Health* 2 (1998): 387–402.

_____. "Epidemic and governmentality: Smallpox in Sydney, 1881." *Critical Public Health* 9 (1999): 301–16.

Bauman, Zygmunt. *Modernity and Ambivalence*. Cambridge: Polity Press, 1991.

_____. "Gamekeepers turned gardeners." In *The Bauman Reader*, ed. Peter Beilharz, 103–12. Oxford: Blackwell, 2001.

Beckett, Jeremy R., ed. *Past and Present: The Construction of Aboriginality*. Canberra: Aboriginal Studies Press, 1994.

Bell, Peter. *Timber and Iron: Houses in Queensland Mining Settlements, 1861–1920*. St Lucia: University of Queensland Press, 1984.

Birch, Alan. "The implementation of the White Australia Policy in the Queensland sugar industry, 1901–12." *Australian J. Politics and History* 11 (1965): 198–210.

Bird, Carmel. *The Stolen Generation: Their Stories*. Sydney: Random House, 1998.

Blainey, Geoffrey. *A Centenary History of the University of Melbourne*. Melbourne: Melbourne University Press, 1957.

_____. "Climate and Australia's history." *Melbourne Historical J.* 10 (1971): 5–9.

Bolton, G. A. *A Thousand Miles Away: A History of North Queensland to 1920*. Brisbane: Jacaranda Press, 1963.

Borges, Dain. "Puffy, ugly, slothful and inert: Degeneration in Brazilian social thought, 1880–1940." *J. Latin American Studies* 25 (1995): 235–56.

Borrie, W. D. *The Peopling of Australasia: A Demographic History, 1788–1988*. Canberra: Demography Program, Australian National University, 1994.

Bourke, Helen. "Sociology and the social sciences in Australia, 1912–28." *Australian and New Zealand J. of Sociology* 17 (1981): 26–35.

Bowler, Peter J. *The Eclipse of Darwinism: Anti-Darwinian Theories in the Decades around 1900*. Baltimore: The Johns Hopkins University Press, 1983.

_____. *Evolution: The History of an Idea*. Berkeley: University of California Press, 1984.

Branagan, David, and Blaine Lim. "J. W. Gregory, traveller in the Dead Heart." *Historical Records of Australian Science* 6 (1984): 71–84.

Bringing Them Home: Report of the National Inquiry into the Separation of Aboriginal and Torres Strait Islander Children from Their Families. Canberra: Commonwealth of Australia, 1997.

Brown, E. Richard. *Rockefeller Medicine Men: Medicine and Capitalism in America*. Berkeley: University of California Press, 1979.

Brown, Nicholas. "Australian intellectuals and the image of Asia, 1920–60." *Australian Cultural Studies* 9 (1990): 80–92.

Brown-May, Andrew. *Melbourne Street Life: The Itinerary of Our Days*. Melbourne: Australian Scholarly/Arcadia, 1998.

Bryder, Linda. *Below the Magic Mountain: A Social History of Tuberculosis in Twentieth-Century Britain*. Oxford: Oxford University Press, 1988.

Bulloch, William. *The History of Bacteriology*. London: Oxford University Press, 1960.

Burkhardt, Richard W. Jr. *The Spirit of System: Lamarck and Evolutionary Biology*. Cambridge, MA: Harvard University Press, 1977.

Butcher, Barry W. "Darwinism, social Darwinism and the Australian Aborigines: A re-evaluation." In *Darwin's Laboratory: Evolutionary Theory and Natural History in the Pacific*, eds. Roy MacLeod and Philip F. Rehbock, 371–94. Honolulu: University of Hawaii Press, 1994.

————. "Darwin down under: Science, religion and evolution in Australia." In *Disseminating Darwin: The Role of Place, Race, Religion and Gender*, eds. Ronald L. Numbers and John Stenhouse, 39–60. Cambridge: Cambridge University Press, 1999.

Bynum, W. F. "Darwin and the doctors: Evolution, diathesis and germs in nineteenth-century Britain." *Gesnerus* 1–2 (1983): 43–53.

————. *Science and the Practice of Medicine in the Nineteenth Century*. Cambridge: Cambridge University Press, 1994.

Cahn, Audrey. *University Children*. Warrandyte, Vic.: A. Cahn, 1987

Canguilhem, Georges. *The Normal and the Pathological*, trans. Carolyn R. Fawcett. New York: Zone Books, 1989.

Cannon, Michael. *The Land Boomers*. Melbourne: Melbourne University Press, 1966.

Cannon, Susan Faye. "Humboldtian science." In *Science in Culture: The Early Victorian Period*, by Cannon, 73–110. New York: Science History Publications, 1978.

Carter, Paul. *The Road to Botany Bay: An Exploration of Landscape and History*. Chicago: University of Chicago Press, 1987.

Cassedy, James H. "Medical men and the ecology of the Old South." In *Science and Medicine in the Old South*, eds. Ronald L. Numbers and Todd L. Savitt, 166–78. Baton Rouge and London: Louisiana State University Press, 1989.

Castles, Francis. *The Working Class and Welfare: Reflections on the Political Development of the Welfare State in Australia and New Zealand*. Wellington, NZ: Allen and Unwin, 1985.

Cawte, Mary. "Craniometry and eugenics in Australia: R.J.A. Berry and the quest for social efficiency." *Historical Studies* [Australia] 22 (1986): 35–53.

Cell, John. *The Highest Stage of White Supremacy: The Origins of Segregation in South Africa and the American South*. Cambridge: Cambridge University Press, 1982.

Chatterjee, Partha. *The Nation and Its Fragments: Colonial and Postcolonial Histories*. Princeton: Princeton University Press, 1993.

Chernin, Eli. "Patrick Manson (1844–1922) and the transmission of filariasis." *American J. Tropical Medicine and Hygiene* 26 (1977): 1065–70.

Chesterman, John, and Brian Galligan. *Citizens Without Rights: Aborigines and Australian Citizenship*. Cambridge: Cambridge University Press, 1997.

Chinard, Gilbert. "Eighteenth-century theories on America as a human habitat." *Proceedings of the American Philosophical Society* 91 (1947): 27–57.

Christie, Nancy J. "Environment and race: Geography's search for a Darwinian synthesis." In *Darwin's Laboratory: Evolutionary Theory and Natural History in the Pacific*, eds. Roy MacLeod and Philip F. Rehbock, 426–73. Honolulu: University of Hawaii Press, 1994.

Cilento, Raphael. "Medicine in Queensland." *Royal Historical Society of Queensland J.* 6 (1961–2): 866–941.

Clark, C.M.H. *A History of Australia*. Melbourne: Melbourne University Press, 1962.

Cleland, J. B. "Some early references to tuberculosis in Australia." *MJA* i (1938): 256–8.

Clements, F. W. *A History of Human Nutrition in Australia*. Melbourne: Longman Cheshire, 1986.

Cole, Douglas. "'The crimson thread of kinship': Ethnic ideas in Australia, 1870–1914." *Historical Studies* [Australia] 14 (1971): 511–25.

Colley, Linda. *Britons: Forging the Nation, 1707–1837*. New Haven and London: Yale University Press, 1992.

Cooter, Roger. "Anticontagionism and history's medical record." In *The Problem of Medical Knowledge: Examining the Social Construction of Medicine*, eds. Peter Wright and Andrew Treacher, 87–93. Edinburgh: Edinburgh University Press, 1982.

Corris, Peter. "White Australia in action: The repatriation of the Pacific islanders from Queensland." *Historical Studies* [Australia] 15 (1972): 170–5.

————. *Passage, Port and Plantation: A History of the Solomon Islands Labour Migration, 1870–1914*. Melbourne: Melbourne University Press, 1973.

Courtenay, P. P. "The white man and the Australian tropics—a review of some prejudices and opinions of the pre-war years." In *Lectures on North Queensland History*, vol. 2, ed. B.J. Dalton, 57–65. Townsville, Department of History, James Cook University, 1975.

Cowlishaw, Gillian. "Colour, culture and the Aboriginalists." *Man* 22ns (1987): 221–37.

————. *Black, White or Brindle: Race in Rural Australia*. Cambridge: Cambridge University Press, 1988.

Cowlishaw, L. "The first fifty years of medicine in Australia." *Australian and New Zealand J. of Surgery* 6 (1936): 3–17.

Craik, Jennifer. "The cultural politics of the Queensland house." *Continuum* 3 (1990): 188–213.

Crellin, John K. "The dawn of germ theory: Particles, infection and biology." In *Medicine and Science in the 1860s*, ed. F.N.L. Poynter, 57–76. London: Wellcome Institute of the History of Medicine, 1968.

Cronin, Kathryn. *Colonial Casualties: The Chinese in Early Victoria*. Melbourne: Melbourne University Press, 1982.

Crook, David P. *Benjamin Kidd: Portrait of a Social Darwinist*. Cambridge: Cambridge University Press, 1984.

Cumpston, J.H.L. *The Health of the People: A Study in Federalism.* Canberra: Roe-buck, 1978.

_____. *Health and Disease in Australia: A History*, ed. Milton Lewis. Canberra: Australian Government Publishing Service, 1989.

Curson, P. H. *Times of Crisis: Epidemics in Sydney 1788–1900.* Sydney: Sydney University Press, 1985.

Curtin, Philip D. *The Image of Africa: British Ideas in Action, 1780–1950.* Madison: University of Wisconsin Press, 1964.

Davidson, B. R. *The Northern Myth: A Study of the Physical and Economic Limits to Agriculture and Pastoral Development in Tropical Australia.* Melbourne: Melbourne University Press, 1965.

Davis, Vivienne de Wahl. "Sir Harry Allen and the foundation of the Walter and Eliza Hall Institute of Medical Research." *Historical Records of Australian Science* 5 (1983): 31–8.

Davison, Graeme. *The Rise and Fall of Marvellous Melbourne.* Melbourne: Melbourne University Press, 1978.

_____. "Sydney and the bush: An urban context for the Australian legend." *Historical Studies* [Australia] 18 (1978): 191–209.

_____. "The city-bred child and urban reform in Melbourne 1900–40." In *Social Process and the City*, ed. Peter Williams, 143–174. Sydney: George Allen and Unwin, 1983.

Denoon, Donald. "The idea of tropical medicine and its influence in Papua New Guinea." In *Health and Healing in Tropical Australia and New Guinea*, eds. Roy MacLeod and Donald Denoon, 12–22. Townsville: James Cook University, 1991.

Denoon, Donald, with Kathleen Dryan and Leslie Marshall. *Public Health in Papua New Guinea: Medical Possibility and Social Constraint, 1884–1984.* Cambridge: Cambridge University Press, 1989.

Desmond, Adrian. *The Politics of Evolution: Morphology, Medicine and Reform in Radical London.* Chicago: University of Chicago Press, 1989.

_____. *Huxley: From Devil's Disciple to Evolution's High Priest.* London: Penguin, 1998.

Desmond, Adrian, and James Moore. *Darwin.* London: Penguin, 1992.

Dettelbach, Michael. "Humboldtian science." In *Cultures of Natural History*, eds. Nick Jardine, James A. Secord, and Emma Spary, 287–304. Cambridge: Cambridge University Press, 1996.

Dixon, Robert. *Writing the Colonial Adventure: Race, Gender and Nation in Anglo-Australian Popular Fiction, 1875–1914.* Cambridge: Cambridge University Press, 1995.

Docker, John. *The Nervous Nineties: Australian Cultural Life in the 1890s.* Melbourne: Oxford University Press, 1991.

Docker, John, and Gerhard Fischer, eds. *Race, Culture and Identity in Australia and New Zealand.* Sydney: University of New South Wales Press, 2000.

Douglas, Mary. *Purity and Danger: An Analysis of Concepts of Pollution.* London: Routledge, 1966.

Douglas, R. A. "Dr Anton Breinl and the Australian Institute of Tropical Medicine." *MJA* i (1977): 713–6, 748–51, 784–90.

————. "One day in the medical life of Queensland: The opening of the Australian Institute of Tropical Medicine." In *Pioneer Medicine in Australia*, ed. John Pearn, 135–58. Brisbane: Amphion Press, 1988.

Douglass, William A. *From Italy to Ingham: Italians in North Queensland.* St Lucia: University of Queensland Press, 1995.

Dubow, Saul. "Race, civilisation and culture: The elaboration of segregationist discourse in the interwar years." In *The Politics of Race, Class and Nationalism in South Africa*, eds. Shula Marks and Stanley Trapido, 71–94. London: Longman, 1987.

————. *Scientific Racism in Modern South Africa.* Cambridge: Cambridge University Press, 1995.

Duffy, John. *The Sanitarians: A History of American Public Health.* Chicago: University of Illinois Press, 1990.

Duncan, James. "Sites of representation: Place, time and the discourse of the Other." In *Place/Culture/Representation*, eds. James Duncan and David Ley, 39–56. London and New York: Routledge, 1993.

Dunlap, Thomas R. "The acclimatisation movement and Anglo ideas of nature." *J. World History* 8 (1997): 303–19.

Dunstan, David. *Governing the Metropolis: Politics, Technology and Social Change in a Victorian City: Melbourne, 1850–1901.* Melbourne: Melbourne University Press, 1984.

Dyason, Diana. "William Gillbee and erysipelas at the Melbourne Hospital: Medical theory and social actions." *J. Australian Studies* 14 (1984): 3–27.

————. "James Jamieson and the ladies." In *Patients, Practitioners and Techniques: Second National Conference on Medicine and Health in Australia, 1984*, eds. Harold Attwood and R. W. Home, 139–54. Melbourne: Medical History Unit, University of Melbourne, 1985.

————. "The medical profession in colonial Victoria, 1834–1901." In *Disease, Medicine and Empire: Perspectives on Western Medicine and the Experience of European Expansion*, eds. Roy MacLeod and Milton Lewis, 194–216. London: Routledge, 1988.

Dyer, Richard. *White.* London and New York: Routledge, 1997.

Easterby, Harry T. *The Queensland Sugar Industry: An Historical Review.* Brisbane: Government Printer, n.d.

Edwards, Coral, and Peter Read. *The Lost Children.* Sydney: Doubleday, 1989.

Edwards, Graham A. "Sunstroke and insanity in nineteenth-century Australia." In *Reflections on Medical History and Health in Australia*, eds. Harold Attwood and Geoffrey Kenny, 35–42. Melbourne: Medical History Unit, University of Melbourne, 1987.

Elkin A. P., and N.W.G. Macintosh, eds. *Grafton Elliot Smith: The Man and His Work.* Sydney: Sydney University Press, 1974.

Elliott, Brian. "Jindyworobaks and Aborigines." *Australian Literary Studies* 8 (1977): 29–50.

_____. *The Jindyworobaks*. St Lucia: University of Queensland Press, 1979.

Ernst, Waltraud, and Bernard Harris, eds. *Race, Science and Medicine, 1700–1900*. London and New York: Routledge, 1999.

Ettling, John. *The Germ of Laziness: Rockefeller Philanthropy and Public Health in the New South*. Cambridge, MA: Harvard University Press, 1981.

Evans, Raymond, Kay Saunders, and Kathryn Cronin. *Exclusion, Exploitation and Extermination: Race Relations in Colonial Queensland*. Sydney: Australian and New Zealand Book Co., 1975.

Farley, John. *Bilharzia: A History of Imperial Tropical Medicine*. Cambridge: Cambridge University Press, 1991.

Feldberg, Georgina. *Disease and Class: Tuberculosis and the Shaping of Modern North American Society*. New Brunswick: Rutgers University Press, 1995.

Fisher, Fedora Gould. *Raphael Cilento: A Biography*. St Lucia: University of Queensland Press, 1994.

Flannery, Tim. *The Future Eaters: An Ecological History of the Australasian Lands and People*. French's Forest, NSW: Reed New Holland, 1998 [1994].

Ford, Edward. "Medical practice in early Sydney, with special reference to the work and influence of John White, William Redfern and William Bland." *MJA* ii (1955): 41–54.

Foster, Leonie. *High Hopes: The Men and Motives of the Australian Round Table*. Melbourne: Melbourne University Press, 1986.

Foucault, Michel. *Discipline and Punish: The Birth of the Prison*, trans. Alan Sheridan. New York: Pantheon Books, 1967.

_____. *History of Sexuality*, trans. Robert Hurley. New York: Pantheon Books, 1978.

Fredrickson, George W. *The Black Image in the White Mind: The Debate on Afro-American Character and Destiny, 1817–1914*. New York: Harper and Row, 1971.

_____. *A Comparative Study of American and South African History*. New York: Oxford University Press, 1981.

Frost, Alan. "What created, what perceived? Early responses to New South Wales." *Australian Literary Studies* 72 (1975): 185–205.

Gandevia, Bryan. "William Thomson and the history of the contagionist doctrine in Melbourne." *MJA* i (1953): 398–403.

_____. "Land, labour and gold: The medical problems of Australia in the nineteenth century." *MJA* i (1960): 754–62.

_____. "The medico-historical significance of young and developing countries, illustrated by Australian experience." In *Modern Methods in the History of Medicine*, ed. Edwin Clarke, 75–98. London: Athlone Press, 1971.

_____. *Tears Often Shed: Child Health and Welfare in Australia from 1788*. Sydney: Pergamon, 1978.

_____. "The Sir Edward Stirling Memorial Lecture." *Occasional Papers on Medical History Australia*, eds. Harold Attwood, Frank Forster, and Bryan Gandevia, 59–83. Melbourne: Medical History Unit, University of Melbourne, 1984.

Garton, Stephen. "Sir Charles Mackellar: Psychiatry, eugenics and child welfare in New South Wales, 1900–14." *Historical Studies* [Australia] 22 (1986): 21–34.

————. "Sound minds and healthy bodies: Re-considering eugenics in Australia, 1914–40." *Australian Historical Studies* 26 (1994): 163–79.

Geary, Laurence M. "The Scottish-Australian connection, 1850–1900." In *The History of Medical Education in Britain*, eds. Vivian Nutton and Roy Porter, 51–75. Amsterdam: Rodopi, 1995.

Gelder, Ken, and Jane M. Jacobs. *Uncanny Australia: Sacredness and Identity in a Postcolonial Nation*. Melbourne: Melbourne University Press, 1999.

Gellner, Ernest. *Nations and Nationalism*. Oxford: Blackwell, 1983.

Gentilli, J. "A history of meteorological and climatological studies in Australia." *University Studies in History* 5 (1967): 54–79.

Gerstle, Gary. *American Crucible: Race and Nation in the Twentieth Century*. Princeton: Princeton University Press, 2001.

Gibson, Ross. *The Diminishing Paradise: Changing Literary Perceptions of Australia*. Sydney: Sirius Books, 1984.

Gieson, Gerald L. *The Private Science of Louis Pasteur*. Princeton: Princeton University Press, 1995.

Gillbank, Linden. "The Acclimatisation Society of Victoria." *Victorian History J.* 51 (1980): 255–70.

————. "The origins of the Acclimatisation Society of Victoria: Practical science in the wake of the goldrush." *Historical Records of Australian Science* 6 (1986): 359–74.

Gillespie, James. *The Price of Health: Australian Governments and Medical Politics, 1910–60*. Cambridge: Cambridge University Press, 1991.

————. "The Rockefeller Foundation, the hookworm campaign and a national health policy in Australia, 1911–30." In *Health and Healing in Tropical Australia and New Guinea*, eds. Roy MacLeod and Donald Denoon, 64–87. Townsville: James Cook University, 1991.

Glacken, Clarence J. *Traces on the Rhodian Shore: Nature and Culture in Western Thought from Ancient Times to the End of the Eighteenth Century*. Berkeley: University of California Press, 1967.

Glick, Thomas F., ed. *The Comparative Reception of Darwinism*. Chicago: University of Chicago, 1974.

Goldberg, David Theo. *Racist Culture: Philosophy and the Politics of Meaning*. Cambridge: Blackwell, 1993.

Goodman, David. *Gold Seeking: Victoria and California in the 1850s*. Sydney: Allen and Unwin, 1994.

Gordon, Douglas. "Sickness and death at the Moreton Bay convict settlement." *MJA* ii (1963): 473–80.

————. *Mad Dogs and Englishmen Went Out in the Queensland Sun: Health Aspects of the Settlement of Tropical Queensland*. Brisbane: Amphion Press, 1990.

Graham, Richard, ed. *The Idea of Race in Latin America, 1870–1940*. Cambridge: Cambridge University Press, 1990.

Graves, Adrian. "The abolition of the Queensland labour trade: Politics or profits?" In *Essays in the Political Economy of Australian Capitalism*, vol. 4, eds. E. L. Wheelwright and Ken Buckley. Sydney: Australian and New Zealand Book Co., 1980.

————. "Crisis and change in the Queensland sugar industry, 1863–1906." In *Crisis and Change in the International Sugar Economy, 1860–1914*, eds. Bill Albert and Adrian Graves. Edinburgh: Edinburgh University Press, 1984.

Gray, Geoffrey. "From nomadism to citizenship: A. P. Elkin and Aboriginal advancement." In *Citizenship and Indigenous Australians: Changing Conceptions and Possibilities*, eds. Nicolas Peterson and Will Sanders, 55–78. Cambridge: Cambridge University Press, 1998.

Griffiths, Tom. *Hunters and Collectors: The Antiquarian Imagination in Australia*. Cambridge: Cambridge University Press, 1996.

Grmek, Mirko. "Géographie médicale et histoire des civilisations." *Annales: Economies, Sociétés, Civilisations* 18 (1963): 1071–97.

Haebich, Anna. *For Their Own Good: Aborigines and Government in the South West of Western Australia, 1900–40*, 3rd edn. Nedlands, WA: University of Western Australia Press, 1998.

————. *Broken Circles: Fragmenting Indigenous Families 1800–2000*. Fremantle, WA: Fremantle Arts Centre Press, 2000.

Hage, Ghassan. *White Nation: Fantasies of White Supremacy in a Multicultural Society*. Sydney: Pluto Press, 1998.

Hammonds, Evelynn. *Childhood's Deadly Scourge: The Campaign to Control Diphtheria in New York City, 1880–1930*. Baltimore: The Johns Hopkins University Press, 1999.

Hannaway, Caroline. "Environment and miasmata." In *Companion-Encyclopaedia of the History of Medicine*, eds. W. F. Bynum and Roy Porter, vol. 1, 292–308. London: Routledge, 1993.

Haraway, Donna. *Simians, Cyborgs and Women: The Reinvention of Nature*. London: Free Association, 1991.

Hardy, Anne. *The Epidemic Streets: Infectious Disease and the Rise of Preventive Medicine, 1856–1900*. Oxford: Oxford University Press, 1993.

Hardy, Susan. "Ferments, zymes and the west wind: Adapting disease theories and therapies in New South Wales, 1860–80." In *Reflections on Medical History and Health in Australia*, eds. Harold Attwood and Geoffrey Kenny, 43–60. Melbourne: Medical History Unit, University of Melbourne, 1987.

Harloe, Lori. "From north to south: The translocation of the Australian Institute of Tropical Medicine." In *Pioneer Medicine in Australia*, ed. John Pearn, 145–58. Brisbane: Amphion Press, 1988.

————. "Anton Breinl and the Australian Institute of Tropical Medicine." In *Health and Healing in Tropical Australia and New Guinea*, eds. Roy MacLeod and Donald Denoon, 34–46. Townsville: James Cook University, 1991.

Harrison, Mark. *Public Health in British India: Anglo-Indian Preventive Medicine, 1859–1914*. Cambridge: Cambridge University Press, 1994.

_____. "'The tender frame of man': Disease, climate and racial difference in India and the West Indies, 1760–1860." *Bulletin of the History of Medicine* 70 (1996): 68–93.

_____. *Climates and Constitutions: Health, Race, Environment and British Imperialism in India, 1600–1850.* New Delhi: Oxford University Press, 1999.

Hart, Alfred. *History of the Wallaby Club.* Melbourne: Anderson, Gowan, 1944.

Hasluck, Paul. *Shades of Darkness: Aboriginal Affairs, 1925–65.* Melbourne: Melbourne University Press, 1988.

Haynes, Roslynn D. *Seeking the Centre: The Australian Desert in Literature, Art and Film.* Cambridge: Cambridge University Press, 1998.

Henderson, Lyn. "The truth in stereotype? Italians and criminality in north Queensland between the wars." *J. Australian Studies* 45 (1995): 32–40.

Hergenhan, L. T., ed. *A Colonial City: High and Low Life. Selected Journalism of Marcus Clarke.* St Lucia: University of Queensland Press, 1972.

Herle, Anita, and Sandra Rouse, eds. *Cambridge and the Torres Strait: Centenary Essays on the 1898 Anthropological Expedition.* Cambridge: Cambridge University Press, 1998.

Hicks, Neville. *"This Sin and Scandal": Australia's Population Debate, 1891–1911.* Canberra: Australian National University Press, 1978.

Higham, John. "The re-orientation of American culture in the 1890s." In *The Origins of Modern Consciousness,* ed. J. Weiss, 25–48. Detroit: Wayne State University Press, 1965.

Hirst, J. B. "The pioneer legend." *Historical Studies* [Australia] 18 (1978): 316–37.

Hoare, Michael. "Learned societies in Australia: The foundation years in Victoria, 1850–60." *Records of the Australian Academy of Science* 1 (1969): 7–29.

Hobsbawm, E. J. *Nations and Nationalism Since 1780: Programme, Myth, Reality,* 2nd Edition. Cambridge: Cambridge University Press, 1990.

Hofstadter, Richard. *Social Darwinism in American Thought,* rev. edn. New York: George Braziller, 1959 [1945].

hooks, bell. "Representing whiteness: Seeing *Wings of Desire.*" In *Yearnings: Race, Gender and Cultural Politics,* 165–78. London: Turnaround, 1991.

Horrigan, Stephen. *Nature and Culture in Western Discourses.* New York and London: Routledge, 1988.

Howells, W. W. "Memoriam—Earnest Albert Hooton." *American J. Physical Anthropology* 12 (1954): 445–54.

Hunt, Doug. "Exclusivism and unionism: Europeans in the Queensland sugar industry, 1900–10." In *Who Are Our Enemies? Racism and the Australian Working Class,* eds. Ann Curthoys and Andrew Markus, 80–95. Neutral Bay, NSW: Hale and Iremonger, 1978.

Hunter, Ernest. *Aboriginal Health and History: Power and Prejudice in Remote Australia.* Cambridge: Cambridge University Press, 1993.

Hyslop, Anthea. "Insidious immigrant: Spanish influenza and border quarantine in Australia, 1919." In *Migration to Mining: Medicine and Health in Australian History,* ed. Suzanne Parry, 201–15. Darwin: Historical Society of the Northern Territory, 1998.

Immigration Reform Group. *Immigration: Control or Colour Bar? The Background to "White Australia" and a Proposal for Change*, ed. Kenneth Rivett. Melbourne: Melbourne University Press, 1962.

Inglis, K. S. *Hospital and Community: A History of the Royal Melbourne Hospital*. Melbourne: Melbourne University Press, 1958.

————. *C.E.W. Bean, Australian Historian*. St Lucia: University of Queensland Press, 1970.

————. *Anzac Remembered: Selected Writings*, ed. John Lack. Parkville: Department of History, University of Melbourne, 1998.

Jacobs, Patricia. Science and veiled assumptions: Miscegenation in W.A. 1930–37. *Australian Aboriginal Studies* 2 (1986): 15–23.

————. *Mister Neville*. Fremantle, WA: Fremantle Arts Centre Press, 1990.

Jacobson, Mathew Frye. *Whiteness of a Different Color: European Immigrants and the Alchemy of Race*. Cambridge, MA: Harvard University Press, 1998.

Jones, G. Stedman. *Outcast London: A Study of the Relationship between Classes in Victorian Society*. Oxford: Clarendon Press, 1971.

Jones, Greta. *Social Darwinism and English Thought: The Interaction between Biological and Social Theory*. Sussex: Harvester Press, 1980.

Jones, Michael Owen. "Climate and disease: The traveler describes America." *Bulletin of the History of Medicine* 41 (1967): 254–66.

Jones, P. G. "South Australian anthropological history: The Board for Anthropological Research and its early expeditions." *Records of the South Australian Museum* 20 (1987): 71–92.

————. "Obituary for Norman Barnett ('Tinny') Tindale." *Aboriginal History* 18 (1994): 5–8.

Jordanova, L. J. "Earth science and environmental medicine: The synthesis of the late Enlightenment." In *Images of the Earth: Essays in the History of the Environmental Sciences*, ed. L. J. Jordanova and Roy S. Porter, 119–46. Chalfont St. Giles: British Society for the History of Science, 1979.

Joyce, R. B. *Sir William McGregor*. Oxford: Oxford University Press, 1971.

Kennedy, Dane. "The perils of the midday sun: Climatic anxieties in the colonial tropics." In *Imperialism and the Natural World*, ed. John D. Mackenzie, 118–40. Manchester: Manchester University Press, 1990.

Kevles, Daniel. *In the Name of Eugenics: Genetics and the Uses of Human Heredity*. Cambridge MA: Harvard University Press, 1995.

Kidd, Rosalind. *The Way We Civilise: Aboriginal Affairs—The Untold Story*. St Lucia: University of Queensland Press, 1997.

Kirk, David, and Karen Twigg. "Constructing Australian bodies: Social normalisation and school medical inspection, 1909–19." *J. Australian Studies* 40 (1994): 57–74.

Kolakowski, Leszek. *Modernity on Endless Trial*. Chicago: University of Chicago Press, 1990.

Kraut, Alan M. *Silent Travelers: Germs, Genes and the "Immigrant Menace."* New York: Basic Books, 1994.

Kuper, Adam. *The Invention of Primitive Society: Transformations of an Illusion.* London: Routledge, 1988.

Kupperman, Karen Ordahl. "Fears of hot climates in the Anglo-American colonial experience." *William and Mary Quarterly* 41 (1984): 213–40.

Lack, John, and Jacqueline Templeton, eds. *Sources of Australian Immigration History, Volume 1: 1901–45.* Melbourne: History Department, University of Melbourne, 1988.

Lake, Marilyn. "The politics of respectability: Identifying the masculinist context." *Historical Studies* [Australia] 22 (1986): 116–31.

Latour, Bruno. "Give me a laboratory and I will raise the world." In *Science Observed: Perspectives on the Social Study of Science*, eds. Karin Knorr-Cetina and M. Mulkay, 141–70. London: Sage, 1983.

Lawrence, Christopher. *Medicine in the Making of Modern Britain 1700–1920.* London: Routledge, 1994.

Le Souef, J. Cecil. "Acclimatisation in Victoria." *Victorian Historical Magazine* 36 (1965): 8–29.

Leavitt, Judith Walzer. *Typhoid Mary: Captive of the Public's Health.* Boston: Beacon, 1996.

Lendon, A. A. *Jubilee of the Medical School, 1885–1935.* Adelaide: Hassall Press, 1935.

Lesser, Jeffrey. *Negotiating National Identity: Immigrants, Minorities and the Struggle for Ethnicity in Brazil.* Durham: Duke University Press, 1999.

Lewis, Milton. "Editor's Introduction." In *Health and Disease in Australia: A History*, by J.H.L. Cumpston, 1–31. Canberra: Australian Government Publishing Service, 1989.

Lewis, Milton, and Roy MacLeod. "A working man's paradise? Reflections on urban mortality in colonial Australia, 1860–1900." *Medical History* 31 (1987): 387–402.

————. "Medical politics and the professionalisation of medicine in New South Wales, 1850–1901." *J. Australian Studies* 22 (1988): 69–82.

Lewontin, Richard, Steven Rose, and Leon J. Kamin. *Not in Our Genes: Biology, Ideology and Human Nature.* New York: Pantheon Books, 1984.

Link, William. "Privies, progressivism and public schools: Health reform and education in the rural South, 1909–20." *J. Southern History* 54 (1988): 623–42.

Livingstone, David N. "Human acclimatisation: Perspectives in a contested field of inquiry in science, medicine and geography." *History of Science* 25 (1987): 359–94.

————. "Climate's moral economy: Science, race and place in post-Darwinian British and American geography." In *Geography and Empire*, eds. Anne Godlewska and Neil Smith, 132–54. Oxford: Blackwell, 1994.

Love, Harold. *James Edward Neild: Victorian Virtuoso.* Melbourne: Melbourne University Press, 1989.

Macintyre, Stuart. *A Colonial Liberalism: The Lost World of Three Victorian Visionaries.* Oxford: Oxford University Press, 1991.

Mackay, E. Alan. "Medical practice during the goldfields era in Victoria." *MJA* ii (1936): 421–8.

MacKnight, C. C., ed. *The Farthest Coast: A Selection of Writings Related to the History of the Northern Coast of Australia*. Melbourne: Melbourne University Press, 1969.

MacLeod, Roy, and Milton Lewis, eds. *Disease, Medicine and Empire: Perspectives on Western Medicine and the Experience of European Expansion*. London: Routledge, 1988.

Maegraith, B. H. "History of the Liverpool School of Tropical Medicine." *Medical History* 16 (1972): 354–68.

Manderson, Desmond. "'Disease, defilement, depravity': Towards an aesthetic analysis of health. The case of the Chinese in Australia." In *Migrants, Minorities and Health: Historical and Contemporary Studies*, eds. Lara Marks and Michael Worboys, 22–48. London: Routledge, 1997.

Mandle, W. F. "Cricket and Australian nationalism in the nineteenth century." *J. Royal Australian Historical Society* 59 (1973): 225–46.

Manne, Robert. "In denial: The Stolen Generations and the right." *Australian Quarterly Essay* 1 (2001): 1–113.

Manson-Bahr, Philip. *History of the School of Tropical Medicine in London, 1899–1949*. London: H. K. Lewis, 1956.

Markel, Howard. *Quarantine! East European Jewish Immigrants and the New York City Epidemics of 1892*. Baltimore: The Johns Hopkins University Press, 1997.

Markus, Andrew. *Fear and Hatred: Purifying Australia and California, 1850–1901*. Sydney: Hale and Iremonger, 1979.

————. *Governing Savages*. Sydney: Allen and Unwin, 1990.

Marshall, T. H. "Citizenship and social class." In *Citizenship and Social Development*, 1–85. New York: Anchor Books, 1967.

May, Cathy. *Topsawyers: The Chinese in Cairns, 1870–1920* [Studies in North Queensland History No. 6]. Townsville: History Department, James Cook University, 1984.

————. "The Chinese in the Cairns district, 1876–1920." In *Race Relations in North Queensland*, ed. Henry Reynolds, 258–75. Townsville: James Cook University, 1993.

Mayne, A.J.C. *Fever, Squalor and Vice: Sanitation and Social Policy in Victorian Sydney*. St Lucia: Queensland University Press, 1982.

————. "'The dreadful scourge': Responses to smallpox in Sydney and Melbourne, 1881–2." In *Disease, Medicine and Empire: Perspectives on Western Medicine and the Experience of European Expansion*, eds. Roy MacLeod and Milton Lewis, 219–41. London: Routledge, 1988.

McCalman, Janet. *Sex and Suffering: Women's Health and a Women's Hospital: The Royal Women's Hospital, 1856–1996*. Melbourne: Melbourne University Press, 1998.

McCann, D. A., and P. Batterham. "Australian genetics: A brief history." *Genetica* 90 (1993): 81–114.

McGregor, Russell. "The idea of racial degeneration: Baldwin Spencer and the Aborigines of the Northern Territory." In *Health and Healing in Tropical Aus-*

tralia, eds. Roy MacLeod and Donald Denoon, 23–34. Townsville: James Cook University Press, 1991.

_____. "Representations of the half-caste in the Australian scientific literature of the 1930s." *J. Australian Studies* 36 (1993): 51–64.

_____. "The concept of primitivity in the writings of A. P. Elkin." *Aboriginal History* 17 (1993): 95–104.

_____. "Intelligent parasitism: A. P. Elkin and the rhetoric of assimilation." *J. Australian Studies* 50–51 (1996): 188–30.

_____. "An Aboriginal Caucasian: Some uses for racial kinship in early twentieth-century Australia." *Australian Aboriginal Studies* 1 (1996): 11–20.

_____. *Imagined Destinies: Aboriginal Australians and the Doomed Race Theory, 1880–1939*. Melbourne: Melbourne University Press, 1997.

McIntosh, A. M. "Early settlement in northern Australia." *MJA* i (1958): 409–15, 441–9.

McLean, Ian. *White Aborigines: Identity Politics in Australian Art*. Cambridge: Cambridge University Press, 1998.

McQueen, Humphrey. "The Spanish influenza pandemic in Australia, 1918–19." In *Social Policy in Australia: Some Perspectives, 1901–75*, ed. Jill Roe, 131–47. Sydney: Cassell, 1976.

Miller, Genevieve. *"Airs, Waters and Places* in history." *J. History of Medicine* 8 (1962): 129–40.

Mitchell, Ann M. *The Hospital South of the Yarra: A History of the Alfred Hospital, Melbourne, from Its Foundation to the 1940s*. Melbourne: Alfred Hospital, 1977.

Mitchell, Paul. "A short medical history of Townsville." *Health* 3 (1925): 33–42.

Molesworth, B. H. "Kanaka labour in Queensland." *Historical Society of Queensland J.* 3 (1917): 142–54.

Moore, Clive. *Kanaka: A History of Melanesian Mackay*. Port Moresby: Papua-New Guinea University Press, 1985.

Morrison, Toni. *Playing in the Dark: Whiteness and the Literary Imagination*. Cambridge, MA: Harvard University Press, 1992.

Morton, S. R., and D. J. Mulvaney, eds. *Exploring Central Australia: Society, the Environment and the 1894 Horn Expedition*. Chipping Norton, NSW: Surrey Beatty, 1996.

Moyal, Ann. *A Bright and Savage Land: Scientists in Colonial Australia*. Sydney: Collins, 1986.

Mozley, Ann. "Evolution and the climate of opinion in Australia, 1840–76." *Victorian Studies* 10 (1967): 411–30.

Muirden, Bruce. *The Puzzled Patriots: The Story of the Australia First Movement*. Melbourne: Melbourne University Press, 1968.

Mulvaney, D. J. "Australian anthropology: Foundations and funding." *Aboriginal History* 17 (1993): 105–28.

Mulvaney D .J., and J. H. Callaby. *"So Much That Is New." Baldwin Spencer, 1860–1929: A Biography*. Melbourne: Melbourne University Press, 1985.

Mulvaney, D. J., Howard Morphy, and Alison Petch, eds. *"My Dear Spencer": The Letters of F. J. Gillen to Baldwin Spencer*. Melbourne: Hyland House, 1997.

Munro, Craig. "Two boys from Queensland: P. R. Stephensen and Jack Lindsay." In *Culture and History: Essays Presented to Jack Lindsay*, ed. Bernard Smith, 40–71. Sydney: Hale and Iremonger, 1984.

_____. *Wild Man of Letters: The Story of P. R. Stephensen*. Melbourne: Melbourne University Press, 1984.

Nadel, George. *Australia's Colonial Culture: Ideas, Men and Institutions in Mid-Nineteenth-Century Australia*. Melbourne: F. W. Cheshire, 1957.

Nairn, N. B. "A survey of the white Australia policy in the nineteenth century." *Australian Quarterly* 28 (1956): 16–31.

Nichol, W. "The medical profession in New South Wales, 1788–1850." *Australian Economic History Review* 24 (1984): 115–31.

O'Sullivan, D. M. "David J. Thomas: A founder of Victorian medicine." *MJA* i (1956): 1065.

Oldroyd, D. R. *Darwinian Impacts: An Introduction to the Darwinian Revolution*. Kensington, NSW: New South Wales University Press, 1980.

Osborne, Graeme. "A socialist dilemma." In *Who Are Our Enemies? Racism and the Australian Working Class*, eds. Ann Curthoys and Andrew Markus, 112–28. Neutral Bay, NSW: Hale and Iremonger, 1978.

Osborne, Michael A. "A collaborative dimension of the European empires: Australian and French acclimatisation societies and intercolonial scientific cooperation." In *International Science and National Scientific Identity*, eds. R. W. Home and S. G. Kohlstedt, 97–119. Dordrecht: Kluwer Academic, 1991.

_____. "Resurrecting Hippocrates: Hygienic sciences and the French scientific expeditions to Egypt, Morea and Algeria." In *Warm Climates and Western Medicine: The Emergence of Tropical Medicine, 1500–1900*, ed. David Arnold, 80–98. Amsterdam: Clio Medica, 1996.

Osborne, W. A. "George Britton Halford: His life and work." *MJA* i (1929): 64–71.

Packard, Randall M. *White Plague, Black Labor: Tuberculosis and the Political Economy of Health and Disease in South Africa*. Berkeley: University of California Press, 1989.

Palfreeman, A. C. "The White Australia Policy." In *Racism, the Australian Experience: A Study of Race Prejudice in Australia*, ed. F. S. Stevens, vol. 1, 164–72. New York: Taplinger Publications, 1972.

Palmer, Vance. *The Legend of the Nineties*. Melbourne: Melbourne University Press, 1954.

Parker, Andrew. "A 'complete protective machinery'—classification and intervention through the Australian Institute of Tropical Medicine." *Health and History* 1 (1999): 181–200.

Parry, Suzanne. "Tropical medicine and northern identity." In *From Migration to Mining: Medicine and Health in Australian History*, ed. Suzanne Parry, 89–98. Darwin: Historical Society of the Northern Territory, 1998.

Patrick, Ross. *A History of Health and Medicine in Queensland, 1824–1960.* St Lucia: University of Queensland Press, 1987.

Pelling, Margaret. "Contagion/germ theory/specificity." In *Companion Encyclopaedia of the History of Medicine,* eds. W. F. Bynum and Roy Porter, vol. 1, 309–34. New York: Routledge, 1993.

Pensabene, T. S. *The Rise of the Medical Practitioner in Victoria.* Canberra: Australian National University Press, 1980.

Peterson, Nicolas. "'Studying man and man's nature': The history of the institutionalisation of Aboriginal anthropology." *Australian Aboriginal Studies* 2 (1990): 3–19.

Peterson, Nicolas, and Will Sanders, eds. *Citizenship and Indigenous Australians: Changing Conceptions and Possibilities.* Cambridge: Cambridge University Press, 1998.

Pick, Daniel. *Faces of Degeneration: A European Disorder, c.1848—c.1918.* Cambridge: Cambridge University Press, 1989.

Pike, Douglas. *Paradise of Dissent: South Australia, 1829–57.* Melbourne: Melbourne University Press, 1957.

Plomley, N.J.B. *Friendly Mission: The Tasmanian Journals and Papers of George Augustus Robinson, 1829–34.* Kingsgrove, NSW: Halstead Press, 1966.

Porter, Dorothy. *Health, Civilization and the State: A History of Public Health from Ancient to Modern Times.* London and New York: Routledge, 1999.

Powell, Alan. *Far Country: A Short History of the Northern Territory.* Melbourne: Melbourne University Press, 1982.

Powell, J. M. *The Public Lands of Australia Felix: Settlement and Land Appraisal in Victoria, 1834–91.* Melbourne: Oxford University Press, 1970.

————. "Medical promotion and the consumptive immigrant in Australia." *Geographical Review* 63 (1973): 449–76.

————. *Mirrors of the New World: Images and Image-Makers in the Settlement Process.* Canberra: Australian National University Press, 1978.

————. "Taylor, Stefansson and the arid centre: An historical encounter of 'environmentalism' and 'possibilism.'" *J. Royal Australian Historical Society* 66 (1980): 163–83.

————. "National identity and the gifted immigrant: A note on T. Griffith Taylor, 1880–1963." *J. Intercultural Studies* 2 (1981): 43–54.

————. "Protracted reconciliation: Society and the environment." In *The Commonwealth of Science: ANZAAS and the Scientific Enterprise in Australia, 1888–1988,* ed. Roy MacLeod, 249–71. Melbourne: Oxford University Press, 1988.

————. *Griffith Taylor and "Australia Unlimited"* [J. Murtagh Macrossan Lecture 1992]. St Lucia: University of Queensland Press, 1993.

Power, Helen J. *Tropical Medicine in the Twentieth Century: A History of the Liverpool School of Tropical Medicine, 1898–1990.* London: Kegan Paul International, 1999.

Powles, John. "Professional hygienists and the health of the nation." In *The Commonwealth of Science: ANZAAS and the Scientific Enterprise in Australia,*

1888–1988, ed. Roy MacLeod, 292–307. Melbourne: Oxford University Press, 1988.

Pratt, Mary Louise. *Imperial Eyes: Travel Writing and Transculturation*. London and New York: Routledge, 1992.

Prentis, Malcolm D. "From Lemuria to Kow Swamp: The rise and fall of tri-hybrid theories of Aboriginal origins." *J. Australian Studies* 45 (1995): 79–91.

Price, Charles A. *The Great White Walls Are Built: Restrictive Immigration to North America and Australasia, 1836–88*. Canberra: Australian National University Press, 1974.

————. *Southern Europeans in Australia*. Canberra: Oxford University Press and Australian National University Press, 1979.

Proust, A. J. *History of Tuberculosis in Australia, New Zealand and Papua New Guinea*. Canberra: Brolga Press, 1991.

Provine, William B. *The Origins of Theoretical Population Genetics*. Chicago: University of Chicago Press, 1971.

————. "Geneticists and the biology of race crossing." *Science* 182 (1973): 790–6.

Puckrein, Gary. "Climate, health and black labor in the English Americas." *J. American Studies* 13 (1979): 179–93.

Raftery, Judith. "Keeping healthy in nineteenth-century Australia." *Health and History* 1 (1999): 274–97.

Read, Peter. *The Stolen Generations: The Removal of Aboriginal Children in New South Wales, 1833–1969*. Sydney: Government Printer, 1981.

Reekie, Gail, ed. *On the Edge: Women's Experiences of Queensland*. Brisbane: University of Queensland Press, 1994.

Reynolds, Henry. *Frontier: Aborigines, Settler and Land*. Sydney: Allen and Unwin, 1987.

————. "Townspeople and fringe dwellers." In *Race Relations in North Queensland*, ed. Henry Reynolds, 148–57. Townsville: James Cook University, 1993.

Roderick, Colin. *Henry Lawson, A Life*. North Ryde, NSW: Angus and Robertson, 1991.

Rodwell, Grant. "Professor Harvey Sutton: National hygienist as eugenicist and educator." *J. Royal Australian Historical Society* 84 (1998): 164–79.

Roe, Michael. *The Quest for Authority in Eastern Australia*. Melbourne: Melbourne University Press, 1965.

————. "The establishment of the Australian Department of Health." *Historical Studies* [Australia] 17 (1976): 176–92.

————. *Nine Australian Progressives: Vitalism in Bourgeois Social Thought, 1890–1960*. St Lucia: University of Queensland Press, 1984.

————. *Australia, Britain and Migration, 1915–40: A Study of Desperate Hopes*. Cambridge: Cambridge University Press, 1995.

————. *Life over Death: Tasmanians and Tuberculosis*. Hobart: Tasmanian Historical Research Association, 1999.

Roediger, David. *The Wages of Whiteness: Race and the Making of the American Working Class*. London: Verso, 1991.

Rose, Gillian. *Feminism and Geography: The Limits of Geographical Knowledge.* Cambridge: Polity Press, 1993.

Rosen, George. "What is social medicine: A genetic analysis of the concept." *Bulletin of the History of Medicine* 21 (1947): 674–733.

_____. *A History of Public Health*, expanded edn. Baltimore: The Johns Hopkins University Press, 1993.

Rosenberg, Charles E. "The bitter fruit: Heredity, disease and social thought." In *No Other Gods: On Science and American Social Thought*, 25–53. Baltimore: The Johns Hopkins University Press, 1976.

_____. "George M. Beard and American nervousness." In *No Other Gods: On Science and American Social Thought*, 98–108. Baltimore: The Johns Hopkins University Press, 1976.

_____. "The therapeutic revolution: Medicine, meaning and social change in nineteenth-century America." In *The Therapeutic Revolution: Essays in the Social History of American Medicine*, eds. Morris J. Vogel and Charles E. Rosenberg, 3–25. Philadelphia: University of Pennsylvania Press, 1979.

_____. "Charles Benedict Davenport and the irony of American eugenics." *Bulletin of the History of Medicine* 15 (1983): 18–23.

_____. "Pathologies of progress: the idea of civilization as risk." *Bulletin of the History of Medicine* 72 (1998): 714–30.

Rosenberg, Charles E., and Janet Golden, eds. *Framing Disease: Studies in Cultural History.* New Brunswick: Rutgers University Press, 1992.

Rothman, Sheila M. *Living in the Shadow of Death: Tuberculosis and the Social Experience of Illness in American History.* New York: Basic Books, 1994.

Rotundo, E. Anthony. *American Manhood: Transformations in Masculinity from the Revolution to the Modern Era.* New York: Basic Books, 1993.

Rowland, E. C. *The Tropics for Christ: Being a History of the Diocese of North Queensland.* Townsville: Diocese of North Queensland, 1960.

Rowse, Tim. *Australian Liberalism and National Character.* Melbourne: Kibble Books, 1978.

_____. *White Flour, White Power: From Rations to Citizenship in Central Australia.* Cambridge: Cambridge University Press, 1998.

_____. "The collector as outsider—T.G.H. Strehlow as 'public intellectual.'" *Strehlow Research Centre Occasional Papers* 2 (1999): 61–120.

Rupke, Nicolaas. "Humboldtian medicine." *Medical History* 40 (1996): 293–310.

_____, ed. *Medical Geography in Historical Perspective* [*Medical History* Supplement No. 20]. London: Wellcome Trust Centre for the History of Medicine, 2000.

Russell, K. F. "Medicine in Melbourne—the first fifty years." *MJA* ii (1977): 17–21.

_____. *The Melbourne Medical School, 1862–1962.* Melbourne: Melbourne University Press, 1977.

_____. "Richard James Arthur Berry, 1867–1962." In *Festschrift for Kenneth Fitzpatrick Russell*, eds. Harold Attwood and Geoffrey Kenny, 25–44. Melbourne: Queensberry Hill Press, 1978.

Saunders, Kay. "Masters and servants: The Queensland sugar workers' strike, 1911." In *Who Are Our Enemies? Racism and the Australian Working Class*, eds. Ann Curthoys and Andrew Markus, 96–111. Neutral Bay, NSW: Hale and Iremonger, 1978.

————. *Workers in Bondage: The Origins of Unfree Labour in Queensland, 1824–1916.* St Lucia: University of Queensland Press, 1982.

Saunders, Suzanne. "Another dimension: Xavier Herbert in the Northern Territory." *J. Australian Studies* 26 (1990): 52–65.

————. "Isolation: The development of leprosy prophylaxis in Australia." *Aboriginal History* 14 (1990): 168–81.

————. "A duly qualified medical practitioner: Health services in the Northern Territory, 1911–39." In *Peripheral Visions: Essays on Australian Regional and Local History*, ed. B. J. Dalton, 251–67. Townsville: James Cook University, 1991.

Schlomowitz, Ralph. "Epidemiology of the Pacific labour trade." *J. Interdisciplinary History* 19 (1989): 585–610.

Scott, Ernest. *A History of the University of Melbourne.* Melbourne: Melbourne University Press, 1936.

Scott, H. H. *A History of Tropical Medicine,* 2 vols. London: Edward Arnold, 1939.

Scott, James C. *Seeing Like a State: How Certain Schemes to Improve the Human Condition Have Failed.* New Haven: Yale University Press, 1998.

Searle, G. R. *The Quest for National Efficiency: A Study in British Politics and Political Thought, 1899–1914.* Oxford: Blackwell, 1971.

————. *Eugenics and Politics in Britain, 1900–14.* Leyden: Noordhoff International, 1976.

Semmler, Clement. *The Banjo of the Bush: The Life and Times of A. B. Paterson.* St Lucia: University of Queensland Press, 1974.

Serle, Geoffrey. *The Golden Age: A History of the Colony of Victoria, 1851–61.* Melbourne: Melbourne University Press, 1963.

————. *The Rush to Be Rich: A History of the Colony of Victoria, 1883–9.* Melbourne: Melbourne University Press, 1971.

Sherrington, George. *Australia's Immigrants, 1788–1978.* Sydney: George Allen and Unwin, 1980.

Sicherman, Barbara. "The uses of a diagnosis: Doctors, patients and neurasthenia." *J. History of Medicine* 32 (1977): 33–54.

Skidmore, Thomas E. *Black into White: Race and Nationality in Brazilian Thought.* New York: Oxford University Press, 1974.

Smith, Bernard. *European Vision and the South Pacific, 1768–1850.* London: Oxford University Press, 1969.

Smith, F. B. *The People's Health, 1830–1910.* London: Croom Helm, 1979.

————. *The Retreat of Tuberculosis, 1850–1950.* New York: Croom Helm, 1988.

————. "Australian public health during the depression of the 1930s." *Australian Cultural History* 16 (1997–8): 96–106.

————. "Comprehending diphtheria." *Health and History* 1 (1999): 139–61.

Spencer, Margaret. *John Howard Lidgett Cumpston, 1880–1954: A Biography*. Tenterfield: n.p., 1987.

Spillett, Peter G. *Forsaken Settlement: An Illustrated History of the Settlement of Victoria, Port Essington, North Australia, 1838–49*. Melbourne: Lansdowne, 1972.

Stanner, W.E.H. "The history of indifference thus begins." *Aboriginal History* 1 (1977): 3–26.

Stepan, Nancy. *The Idea of Race in Science: Great Britain, 1800–1960*. Hamden CT: Archon Books, 1982.

_____. "Biology and degeneration: Races and proper places." In *Degeneration: The Dark Side of Progress*, eds. J. Edward Chamberlin and Sander L. Gilman, 97–120. New York: Columbia University Press, 1985.

_____. *"The Hour of Eugenics": Race, Gender and Nation in Latin America*. Ithaca: Cornell University Press, 1991.

Stern, Alexandra Minna. "Secrets under the skin: New historical perspectives on disease, deviation and citizenship." *Comparative Studies in Society and History* 41 (1999): 589–96.

Stewart, Ken, ed. *The 1890s: Australian Literature and Literary Culture*. St Lucia: University of Queensland Press, 1996.

Stewart, Mart A. "'Let us begin with the weather?': Climate, race, and cultural distinctiveness in the American South." In *Nature and Society in Historical Context*, eds. Mikulas Teich, Roy Porter and Bo Gustafsson, 240–56. Cambridge: Cambridge University Press, 1997.

Stocking, George W. Jr. *Race, Culture and Evolution: Essays in the History of Evolution*. London: Collier-Macmillan, 1968.

_____. *After Tylor: British Social Anthropology, 1888–1951*. Madison: University of Wisconsin Press, 1995.

Stoler, Ann Laura. *Race and the Education of Desire: Foucault's History of Sexuality and the Colonial Order of Things*. Durham and London: Duke University Press, 1995.

Stoler, Ann Laura, and Frederick Cooper, "Between metropole and colony: Rethinking a research agenda." In *Tensions of Empire: Colonial Cultures in a Bourgeois World*, eds. Frederick Cooper and Ann Laura Stoler, 1–56. Berkeley: University of California Press, 1997.

Stratton, Jon. "Deconstructing the Territory." *Cultural Studies* 3 (1989): 38–57.

_____. "The colour of Jews: Jews, race and the white Australia policy." *J. Australian Studies* 50–51 (1996): 51–65.

_____. *Race Daze: Australia in Identity Crisis*. Sydney: Pluto Press, 1998.

Temkin, Owsei. "An historical analysis of the concept of infection." In *The Double Face of Janus*, 456–71. Baltimore: The Johns Hopkins University Press, 1977.

Thomas, B., and B. Gandevia. "Dr Francis Workman, emigrant, and the history of taking the cure for consumption in the Australian colonies." *MJA* ii (1959): 1–10.

Tomes, Nancy. *The Gospel of Germs: Men, Women and the Microbe in American Life*. Cambridge, MA: Harvard University Press, 1998.

Torgovnick, Marianna. *Gone Primitive: Savage Intellects, Modern Lives.* Chicago: University of Chicago Press, 1990.

Tovell, Ann, and Bryan Gandevia. "Early Australian medical associations." *MJA* i (1962): 756–9.

Trautmann, Thomas R. *Lewis Henry Morgan and the Invention of Kinship.* Berkeley: University of California Press, 1987.

Tregenza, J. M. *Professor of Democracy.* Melbourne: Melbourne University Press, 1968.

Tunchon, Gregory. "Germ theory: Practical implications for medicine in Victoria." In *Patients, Practitioners and Techniques: Second National Conference on Medicine and Health in Australia, 1984* , eds. Harold Attwood and R. W. Home, 139–54. Melbourne: Medical History Unit, University of Melbourne, 1985.

Turnbull, Paul. "Ramsay's regime: The Australian Museum and the procurement of Aboriginal bodies, c. 1874–1900." *Aboriginal History* 15 (1991): 108–21.

_____. *Science, National Identity and Aboriginal Body Snatching in Nineteenth Century Australia* [Working Paper in Australian Studies No. 65]. London: Institute of Commonwealth Studies, 1991.

Turner, Bryan. "Contemporary problems in the theory of citizenship." In *Citizenship and Social Theory*, ed. Bryan S. Turner. London: Sage, 1993.

Valencius, Conevery Bolton. "Histories of medical geography." In *Medical Geography in Historical Perspective* [*Medical History* Supplement No. 20], ed. Nicolaas Rupke, 3–28. London: Wellcome Trust Centre for the History of Medicine, 2000.

_____. "The geography of health and the making of the American West: Arkansas and Missouri 1800–60." In *Medical Geography in Historical Perspective* [*Medical History* Supplement No. 20], ed. Nicolaas Rupke, 121–45. London: Wellcome Trust Centre for the History of Medicine, 2000.

Verso, Murray. "Airs, waters and places." *Victorian Historical J.* 48 (1977): 6–22.

Walker, David. *Dream and Disillusion: A Search for Australian Cultural Identity.* Canberra: Australian National University Press, 1976.

_____. "The getting of manhood." In *Australian Popular Culture*, eds. Peter Spearritt and David Walker, 121–44. Sydney: Allen and Unwin, 1979.

_____. "Modern nerves, nervous moderns: Notes on male neurasthenia." *Australian Cultural History* 6 (1987): 49–63.

_____. "Climate, civilization and character in Australia, 1880–1940." *Australian Cultural History* 16 (1997–8): 77–95.

_____. *Anxious Nation: Australia and the Rise of Asia, 1850–1939.* St Lucia: University of Queensland Press, 1999.

Walker, M. H. *"Come Wind, Come Weather": A Biography of Alfred Howitt.* Melbourne: Melbourne University Press, 1971.

Wallace, V. H. "The Eugenics Society of Victoria (1936–61)." *Eugenics Review* 53 (1962): 215–18.

Ward, Russel. *The Australian Legend.* Melbourne: Oxford University Press, 1958.

Warner, John Harley. *The Therapeutic Perspective: Medical Practice, Knowledge and Identity in America, 1820–85*. Cambridge, MA: Harvard University Press, 1986.

————. "The idea of Southern medical distinctiveness: Medical knowledge and practice in the Old South." In *Science and Medicine in the Old South*, eds. Ronald L. Numbers and Todd L. Savitt, 179–205. Baton Rouge and London: Louisiana State University Press, 1989.

Watts, Rob. "Beyond nature and nurture: Eugenics in twentieth-century Australian history." *Australian J. Politics and History* 40 (1994): 318–34.

Weickhardt, Len. *Masson of Melbourne*. Melbourne: Royal Australian Chemical Institute, 1989.

Wersky, Gary. *The Visible College*. London: Allen Lane, 1978.

White, K. N. "Negotiating science and liberalism: Medicine in nineteenth-century Australia." *Medical History* 43 (1999): 173–91.

White, Richard. *Inventing Australia: Images and Identity, 1688–1980*. Sydney: George Allen and Unwin, 1981.

Whitelock, Derek. *Adelaide, 1836–1976: A History of Difference*. St Lucia: University of Queensland Press, 1977.

Whyte, Malcom. *A Global Scientist: Douglas H. K. Lee*. Gundaroo: Brolga Press, 1995.

Wiebe, Robert H. *The Search for Order, 1877–1920*. New York: Hill and Wang, 1967.

Wilburd, C. R. "Notes on the history of maritime quarantine in Queensland, 19th century." *Historical Society of Queensland J.* 3 (1945): 369–83.

Willard, Myra. *History of the White Australia Policy to 1920*. Melbourne: Melbourne University Press, 1923.

Williams, Raymond. "Ideas of nature." In *Problems in Materialism and Culture*. London: Verso, 1981.

Willis, Evan. *Medical Dominance: The Division of Labour in Australian Health Care*. Sydney: Allen and Unwin, 1983.

Winslow, C.-E. A. *The Conquest of Epidemic Disease*. Princeton: Princeton University Press, 1943.

Wise, Tigger. *The Self-Made Anthropologist: A Life of A. P. Elkin*. Sydney: Allen and Unwin, 1985.

Wolfe, Patrick. *Settler Colonialism and the Transformation of Anthropology: The Politics and Poetics of an Ethnographic Event*. London: Cassell, 1999.

Woolcock, Helen. "'Our salubrious climate': Attitudes to health in colonial Queensland." In *Disease, Medicine and Empire: Perspectives on Western Medicine and the Experience of European Expansion*, eds. Roy MacLeod and Milton Lewis, 176–93. London: Routledge, 1988.

Worboys, Michael. "The emergence of tropical medicine: A study in the establishment of a scientific specialty." In *Perspectives in the Emergence of Scientific Disciplines*, eds. G. Lemaine et al., 75–98. The Hague: Mouton, 1976.

————. "Manson, Ross and colonial medical policy: Tropical medicine in London and Liverpool, 1899–1914." In *Disease, Medicine and Empire: Perspec-*

tives on Western Medicine and the Experience of European Expansion, eds. Roy MacLeod and Milton Lewis, 21–37. London: Routledge, 1988.

Yarwood, A. T. "Sir Raphael Cilento and *The White Man in the Tropics*." In *Health and Healing in Tropical Australia and New Guinea*, eds. Roy MacLeod and Donald Denoon, 47–63. Townsville: James Cook University, 1991.

Yarwood, A. T., and M. J. Knowling. *Race Relations in Australia: A History*. North Ryde, NSW: Methuen Australia, 1982.

Young, J. A., A. J. Sefton, and Nina Webb. *Centenary Book of the University of Sydney Faculty of Medicine*. Sydney: Sydney University Press, 1984.

Young, Robert J. C. *Colonial Desire: Hybridity in Theory, Culture and Race*. London and New York: Routledge, 1995.

INDEX